Molecular Biology of Diabetes

I. Autoimmunity and Genetics; Insulin Synthesis and Secretion

Molecular Biology of Diabetes

I. Autoimmunity and Genetics; Insulin Synthesis and Secretion

Edited by

Boris Draznin, MD, PhD
University of Colorado Health Sciences Center, Denver, CO

Derek LeRoith, MD, PhD
National Institute of Diabetes and Digestive and Kidney Disease, National Institutes of Health, Bethesda, MD

Humana Press **Totowa, New Jersey**

999 Riverview Drive, Suite 208
Totowa, New Jersey 07512

This publication is printed on acid-free paper. ∞
ANSI Z39.48-1984 (American National Standards Institute) Permanence of Paper for Printed Library Materials.

Printed in the United States of America. 10 9 8 7 6 5 4 3 2 1

Library of Congress Cataloging in Publication Data

Molecular biology of diabetes / edited by Boris Draznin, Derek LeRoith.
p. cm.
Includes index.
Contents: [v. 1.] Autoimmunity and genetics; insulin synthesis and secretion.
ISBN 0-89603-286-8 (alk. paper)
1. Diabetes—Molecular aspects. I. Draznin, Boris. II. LeRoith, Derek, 1945– .
[DNLM: 1. Diabetes Mellitus—immunology. 2. Diabetes Mellitus—genetics. 3. Insulin—physiology. WK 810 M7182 1994]
RC660.M5614 1994
616.4'62—dc20
DNLM/DLC
for Library of Congress 94-27263
CIP

Preface

In a rapidly evolving and extremely important area of medical science, it is often difficult for the student, teacher, and researcher to keep abreast of all the important advances. The purpose of *Molecular Biology of Diabetes, Parts I and II* is to bring to these individuals the latest knowledge of diabetes-related research in a comprehensive, yet concise manner. To this end, we have assembled chapters, written by most of the world's experts in the field, that we believe comprehensively survey and synthesize a coherent understanding of the subject.

Studies of the etiology of type I and type II diabetes are extremely exciting and essential, since we hope to one day prevent the disease using gene therapy. These aspects are covered in *Molecular Biology of Diabetes: I. Autoimmunity and Genetics; Insulin Synthesis and Secretion*. In type II diabetes, an abnormality in pancreatic secretion exists concomitantly with peripheral insulin resistance. This abnormality of insulin secretion is believed to be related to a defect(s) in glucose sensing. Uncoupling of glucose sensing from insulin secretion may be the crucial step in the pathogenesis of noninsulin-dependent diabetes. In this volume, we have invited authors to describe their studies on all known factors affecting β-cell function, including autoimmunity and genetics of diabetes, as well as molecular mechanisms of insulin synthesis and secretion.

In the last few years, the most rapidly advancing area of research in diabetes has been, in fact, related to insulin action. The isolation and characterization of endogenous substrates of the insulin receptor, including IRS-1 and various tyrosine and serine kinases, as well as specific phosphatases, has given us new insights into insulin action and also afforded us with potential target sites for new therapeutic agents. At the same time, discoveries in the cascade of insulin signaling made an unprecedented impact on our understanding of the mechanism of action of other growth factors such as IGF-1 and EGF. Molecular and cellular aspects of insulin action are discussed in

Molecular Biology of Diabetes: II. Insulin Action, Effects on Gene Expression and Regulation, and Glucose Transport.

Finally, new advances have been recently made in the understanding of the mechanism of the insulin-stimulated glucose uptake. Molecular mechanisms of insulin action on translocation and activation of GLUT-4 in the insulin target tissues are thoroughly discussed in the second volume.

We believe that *Molecular Biology of Diabetes, Parts I and II* constitute a comprehensive modern text that will be of great help to those who wish to increase their knowledge in the molecular biology of diabetes and insulin action, as well as all those who simply wish to keep up-to-date with this extremely rapidly advancing field.

Boris Draznin
Derek LeRoith

Contents

Contents

Molecular Biology of Diabetes II: Insulin Action, Effects on Gene Expression and Regulation, and Glucose Transport

Contributors

ILLANI ATWATER • *National Institute of Diabetes and Digestive and Kidney Disease, National Institutes of Health, Bethesda, MD*

DEBORAH L. BENNETT • *Department of Clinical Biochemistry, University of Cambridge, UK*

DONNA BERNER • *Diabetes Research Center, University of Pennsylvania, Philadelphia, PA*

AUBREY E. BOYD III • *Division of Endocrinology, New England Medical Center Hospitals, Boston, MA*

PETER C. BUTLER • *Endocrine Research Unit, Mayo Clinic, Rochester, MN*

FILIPPO CALCINARO • *Barbara Davis Center for Childhood Diabetes, University of Colorado Health Sciences Center, Denver, CO*

JOSEPH S. DILLON • *Division of Endocrinology, New England Medical Center Hospitals, Boston, MA*

NORMAN L. EBERHARDT • *Endocrine Research Unit, Mayo Clinic, Rochester, MN*

GEORGE S. EISENBARTH • *Barbara Davis Center for Childhood Diabetes, University of Colorado Health Sciences Center, Denver, CO*

SARAH FERBER • *Departments of Chemistry and Internal Medicine, Gifford Labs for Diabetes Research, University of Texas, Dallas, TX*

MICHAEL S. GERMAN • *Hormone Research Institute, University of California, San Francisco, CA*

RONALD G. GILL • *Barbara Davis Center for Childhood Diabetes, University of Colorado Health Sciences Center, Denver, CO*

DANLING GU • *Department of Neuropharmacology, Scripps Research Institute, La Jolla, CA*

STEVEN D. HUGHES • *Departments of Chemistry and Internal Medicine, Gifford Labs for Diabetes Research, University of Texas, Dallas, TX*

JOHN C. HUTTON • *Department of Clinical Biochemistry, University of Cambridge, UK*

JOHN H. JOHNSON • *Departments of Chemistry and Internal Medicine, Gifford Labs for Diabetes Research, University of Texas, Dallas, TX*

PRABAKARAN KESAVAN • *Diabetes Research Center, University of Pennsylvania, Philadelphia, PA*
ANJANEYULU KOWLURU • *Clinical Sciences Center, University of Wisconsin, Madison, WI*
MANUEL KUKULJAN • *University of Valparaíso, Chile*
KEVIN J. LAFFERTY • *Barbara Davis Center for Childhood Diabetes, University of Colorado Health Sciences Center, Denver, CO*
GUIZHU LI • *Diabetes Research Center, University of Pennsylvania, Philadelphia, PA*
YIN LIANG • *Diabetes Research Center, University of Pennsylvania, Philadelphia, PA*
MING LU • *Department of Cell Biology, Baylor University, Houston, TX*
MARK A. MAGNUSON • *Department of Molecular Physiology and Biophysics, Vanderbilt University, Nashville, TN*
FRANZ M. MATSCHINSKY • *Diabetes Research Center, University of Pennsylvania, Philadelphia, PA*
PAOLO MEDA • *Department of Morphology, Institute of Histology and Embryology Center Medical University, Geneva, Switzerland*
STEWART A. METZ • *Clinical Sciences Center, University of Wisconsin, Madison, WI*
HABIBA NAJAFI • *Diabetes Research Center, University of Pennsylvania, Philadelphia, PA*
CHRISTOPHER B. NEWGARD • *Departments of Chemistry and Internal Medicine, Gifford Labs for Diabetes Research, University of Texas, Dallas, TX*
KEVIN D. NISWENDER • *Department of Molecular Physiology and Biophysics, Vanderbilt University, Nashville, TN*
TIMOTHY D. O'BRIEN • *Endocrine Research Unit, Mayo Clinic, Rochester, MN*
L. KARL OLSON • *Department of Medicine, University of Minnesota, Minneapolis, MN*
ELIA MARTHA PÉREZ-ARMENDARIZ • *Department of Neuroscience, Albert Einstein College of Medicine, Bronx, NY*
CATHLEEN C. PETTEPHER • *Department of Molecular Physiology and Biophysics, Vanderbilt University, Nashville, TN*
MASSIMO PIETROPAOLO • *Barbara Davis Center for Childhood Diabetes, University of Colorado Health Sciences Center, Denver, CO*
CHRISTIAN QUAADE • *Departments of Chemistry and Internal Medicine, Gifford Labs for Diabetes Research, University of Texas, Dallas, TX*
J. BRUCE REDMON • *Department of Medicine, University of Minnesota, Minneapolis, MN*

R. PAUL ROBERTSON • *Department of Medicine, University of Minnesota, Minneapolis, MN*
PETER RONNER • *Diabetes Research Center, University of Pennsylvania, Philadelphia, PA*
NORA SARVETNICK • *Department of Neuropharmacology, Scripps Research Institute, La Jolla, CA*
BERNARD THORENS • *Institute of Pharmacology and Toxicology, Lausanne, Switzerland*
HOWARD C. TOWLE • *Department of Medicine, University of Minnesota, Minneapolis, MN*
LIJUN WANG • *Diabetes Research Center, University of Pennsylvania, Philadelphia, PA*
DALE R. WEGMANN • *Barbara Davis Center for Childhood Diabetes, University of Colorado Health Sciences Center, Denver, CO*
MICHAEL B. WHEELER • *Division of Endocrinology, New England Medical Center Hospitals, Boston, MA*
HUI-JIAN ZHANG • *Department of Medicine, University of Minnesota, Minneapolis, MN*

Molecular Mechanisms of Autoimmunity and Genetics of Diabetes

Chapter 1

Molecular Targets of the Autoimmunity of Type I Diabetes

Massimo Pietropaolo and George S. Eisenbarth

Introduction

One feature of many autoimmune diseases is a humoral autoimmune response against multiple antigens of a given tissue. Although the pathogenic significance of autoantibodies in type I diabetes is unclear, they serve both as essential markers that an autoimmune response has been initiated and as probes to identify their target autoantigens *(1–5)*.

In type I diabetes or insulin-dependent diabetes mellitus (IDDM), the immunological events leading to pancreatic β-cell destruction appear to be predominantly dependent on the activity of T-cells. A large body of data indicates that type I diabetes develops in genetically susceptible individuals, and that the immune process results in selective lymphocyte-mediated autoimmune β-cell damage. Over time, a large number of β-cells are destroyed until essentially all insulin secretion is lost. Prior to the clinical onset of IDDM, the loss of β-cells is reflected by loss of insulin secretion after an intravenous glucose challenge test.

From: *Molecular Biology of Diabetes, Part I*
Edited by: B. Draznin and D. LeRoith

The disease process is associated with the development of islet-cell antibodies (ICA) in the sera of individuals often years before the clinical onset of the disease. Although the nature of the ICA antigen(s) has not been completely clarified, there is compelling evidence that subcellular organelles such as the secretory granules, as well as islet synaptic-like microvesicles, are both prominent targets of IDDM autoantibodies. Lately, a large effort in diabetes research has been made to identify the target molecules responsible for driving an islet-specific immune response, and a growing list of novel antigens, some of known identity, have been discovered (Table 1). One of the purposes of the identification of autoantigens is to use these molecules as sources for developing biochemical autoantibody assays. Thus far, ICA remains the "gold standard" immune marker of IDDM, but with the optimization of combinatorial biochemical assays we believe that in the near future it will be possible to improve the ability to predict type I diabetes in asymptomatic individuals. Such prediction is a fundamental prerequisite for antigen-specific approaches to prevent IDDM, an effort that is also dependent on the characterization of islet autoantigens.

Target Molecules

Molecularly Characterized Autoantigens

Insulin

Palmer first reported in 1983 *(6)* that insulin autoantibodies were detectable in newly diagnosed diabetic patients before any insulin treatment. These autoantibodies are also detectable years before the development of IDDM, and their presence in ICA-positive first degree relatives, particularly having an impaired first phase insulin response (FPIR), is highly associated with an increased risk for developing the clinical onset of IDDM. Insulin autoantibodies are more commonly elevated in children developing diabetes than in adults, and elevated levels tend to correlate with younger age and with a faster progression of IDDM in preclinical relatives of IDDM patients *(7)*.

Insulin autoantibodies in first degree relatives of diabetic patients share common target epitope(s), namely amino acid residues B1–B3 and A8–A13 *(8)*, which suggests that a common pathogenic mechanism for production of such antibodies may exist (Fig. 1).

Table 1
Major Islet Cell Autoantigens Related to Type I Diabetes Mellitus

Autoantigen	Localization	Significance
Insulin	Secretory granules of pancreatic β-cells	Insulin autoantibodies in ~100% of young children (<age 5) before the clinical onset of IDDM. Correlation with younger age and with faster progression of IDDM in preclinical relatives of IDDM patients. Prophylactic sc injection of insulin may prevent IDDM. T-cells from islets of NOD mice react with insulin.
64 kDa/GAD	Small vesicles of islet cells (GAD also in neurons, testis, ovary, adrenal, pituitary, thyroid)	Autoantibodies to 64 kDa/GAD in ~70% of subjects with preclinical IDDM or with new onset type I diabetes. Only a subset of anti-64 kDa antibodies recognizes GAD. Inverse correlation between GAD autoantibodies and T-cell proliferation to GAD.
ICA69	Rat pancreatic β-cells (ICA69 transcripts present also in brain, heart, kidney, liver)	Autoantibodies to ICA69 in ~50% of preclinical relatives of IDDM patients, and in ~50% of newly diagnosed IDDM patients detectable by Western blotting. Similarities with bovine serum albumin, hypothesized to be environmental trigger factor.
Ganglioside GM2-1	Pancreatic islet cells	Autoantibodies to GM2-1 in ~80% of preclinical IDDM relatives.
37/40 kDa tryptic fragment of 64 kDa/not GAD	Pancreatic islet cells	Precursors of 37/40 kDa tryptic fragment are proteins (not GAD) of M_r 64,000. ~70% of identical twins developing IDDM express anti-37/40 kDa antibodies.
38 kDa	Secretory granules of rat insulinoma tissue (brain?)	Reactivity with T-cell lines of peripheral blood from 8 of 10 new onset IDDM patients.
Carboxypeptidase H	Neuroendocrine secretory cell granules (pancreatic β-cells, adrenal, pituitary)	Autoantibodies to carboxypeptidase H in ~20% of preclinical IDDM relatives.

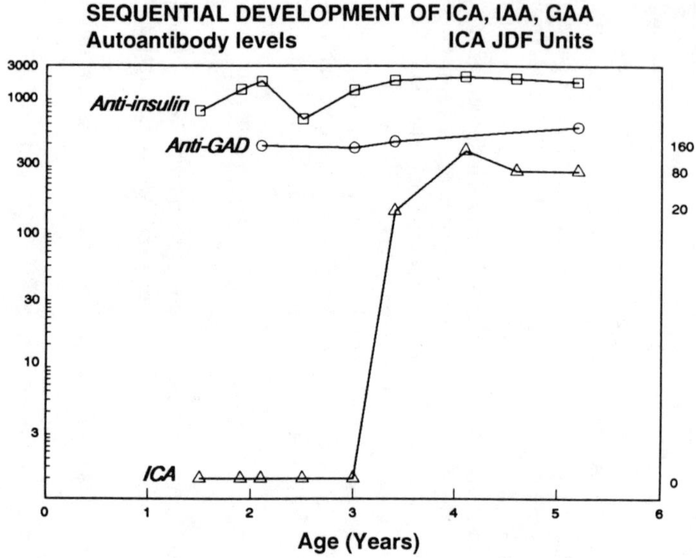

Fig. 1. ICA, anti-insulin, and anti-GAD autoantibodies can precede by years the development of other anti-islet autoantibodies.

To date, insulin is the only known β-cell specific autoantigen associated with type I diabetes. Wegmann and coworkers have found that a major subset of T-cells infiltrating islets of the NOD mouse respond to insulin *(8a)*. Oral feeding of insulin prevents the clinical onset of diabetes in the nonobese diabetic (NOD) mouse, but does not completely prevent insulitis *(9)*. This oral "tolerization" may provide a potential therapy for an autoimmune disease such as IDDM, similar to what is observed in the experimental autoimmune encephalomyelitis (EAE) model in which Lewis rats fed with myelin basic protein (MBP) were resistant to the subsequent induction of experimental autoimmune encephalitis following immunization with MBP. This form of oral tolerance may result from an activation of TGF-β producing regulatory cells *(10)*.

It is noteworthy that polymorphisms of the insulin gene are associated with genetic risk of type I diabetes. These polymorphisms of the 3' region of the insulin gene, and proximal to the insulin-like growth factor II (IGF2) region on chromosome 11 (INS locus) suggest that regulation of insulin expression gene is a major determinant of disease *(11)*.

Glutamic Acid Decarboxylase (GAD) GAD_{65}, GAD_{67}

The 64 kDa autoantigen associated with type I diabetes has recently been identified as GAD by Baekkeskov et al. *(12)*. Pancreatic β-cells and the γ-aminobutyric acid (GABA)-secreting neurons both express comparable levels of GAD. In addition, α-cells of human but not rat islets express GAD. This enzyme catalyzes the conversion of glutamic acid into GABA and is found in β-cells, brain, kidney, thyroid, adrenal, pituitary, testes, ovary, and liver *(13,14)*. GAD autoantibodies were first described in subjects with stiff man syndrome (SMS), a rare neurological disease probably caused by an impairment of GABA-ergic pathways, which is associated with polyendocrine autoimmunity, including IDDM *(15)*. GAD autoantibodies can be detected prior to and at the onset of IDDM, whereas very high titers of GAD antibodies in first degree relatives of patients with type I diabetes paradoxically seem to correlate with the lack of progression to overt disease *(16,17)*.

Two genetically distinct GAD molecules have been described, namely GAD_{65} and GAD_{67}, which are the product of two different genes differing predominantly at their N-terminal domains. GAD_{65} is synthesized as a hydrophilic molecule, which is then palmitoylated, becoming membrane anchored *(13)*. In pancreatic β-cells, GAD_{65} is localized to the membrane of small vesicles that are identical in size to the small synaptic-like microvesicles of neurons. The larger protein termed GAD_{67} is expressed in low levels in rat islets and, unlike GAD_{67}, is always hydrophilic. The role of GAD in the β-cells remains elusive; however, since GABA receptors are found in glucagon-producing α-cells, it has been postulated that GABA may play a role on the glucose-induced inhibition of the glucagon secretion in the α-cells *(18)*. GAD_{65} serves as the main immunogenic isoform of GAD in IDDM, in view of the fact that in human islets only a single isoform, GAD_{65}, is expressed *(19)*. It has been reported that sera from 38 patients with IDDM mostly reacted with the recombinant GAD_{65}, and that the reactivity of 8 of the 38 sera with recombinant GAD_{67} may be a result of crossreactivity of certain epitopes common to both isoforms *(20)*. One possible explanation of the different antigenicity of GAD_{65} and GAD_{67} seems to be owing to the biochemical difference between the two isoforms. The different NH_2-terminal domain of GAD_{65} confers hydrophobic modifications, palmitoylation, and consequent membrane anchoring, whereas GAD_{67} is a soluble molecule. This selective localization of GAD_{65} in the microvesicle membrane compartment (a cytoplasmic, not cell surface compartment) may account for the involvement in autoimmunity of GAD_{65} rather than GAD_{67} *(13)*. It is of interest that palmitoylated influenza peptides, unlike nonpalmitoylated peptides, are potent inducers of a T-cell proliferation in vivo *(21)*.

It is noteworthy that humoral and cellular response to GAD appear to be inversely related *(16)*. High levels of circulating GAD autoantibodies that react with native GAD are associated with low proliferation of peripheral blood T-cells to recombinant GAD, whereas low levels of autoantibodies to GAD are associated with high proliferation of T-cells from IDDM patients to GAD (Fig. 2). This dichotomy of the immune response to GAD led Harrison to speculate that autoimmunity to GAD in IDDM might either be deviated predominantly to a cellular response, without a remarkable antibody production, but with the involvement of CD4 positive T_H1 cells that produce γ-interferon (IFN γ), and interleukin 2 (IL-2) to mediate delayed-type hypersensitivity reactions, or might be deviated to high titer antibody production, with the involvement of CD4 positive T_H2 cells that produce IL-4, IL-5, and IL-10. One hypothesis of the pathogenic role in autoimmunity of GAD is that subjects prone to IDDM that have a peripheral T-cell response to GAD could have a predominant T_H1-like response, whereas in low risk individuals, such as polyendocrine or SMS patients whose titer of GAD autoantibodies is particularly high, the T-cell response may be deviated to T_H2-like response, which is leading to high titer antibody production.

Prognostically significant heterogeneity of ICA in relatives of patients with type I diabetes has been reported *(17)*. In particular, a proportion of first degree relatives of IDDM patients with high titers of ICA do not progress to overt type I diabetes or lose first phase insulin secretion on prospective followup. This particular ICA pattern (that gives β-cell specific staining of rat pancreas frozen sections and that fails to react with mouse islets) was termed "restricted" ICA. There is evidence that the autoantigen of ICA is glutamic acid decarboxylase *(22)*.

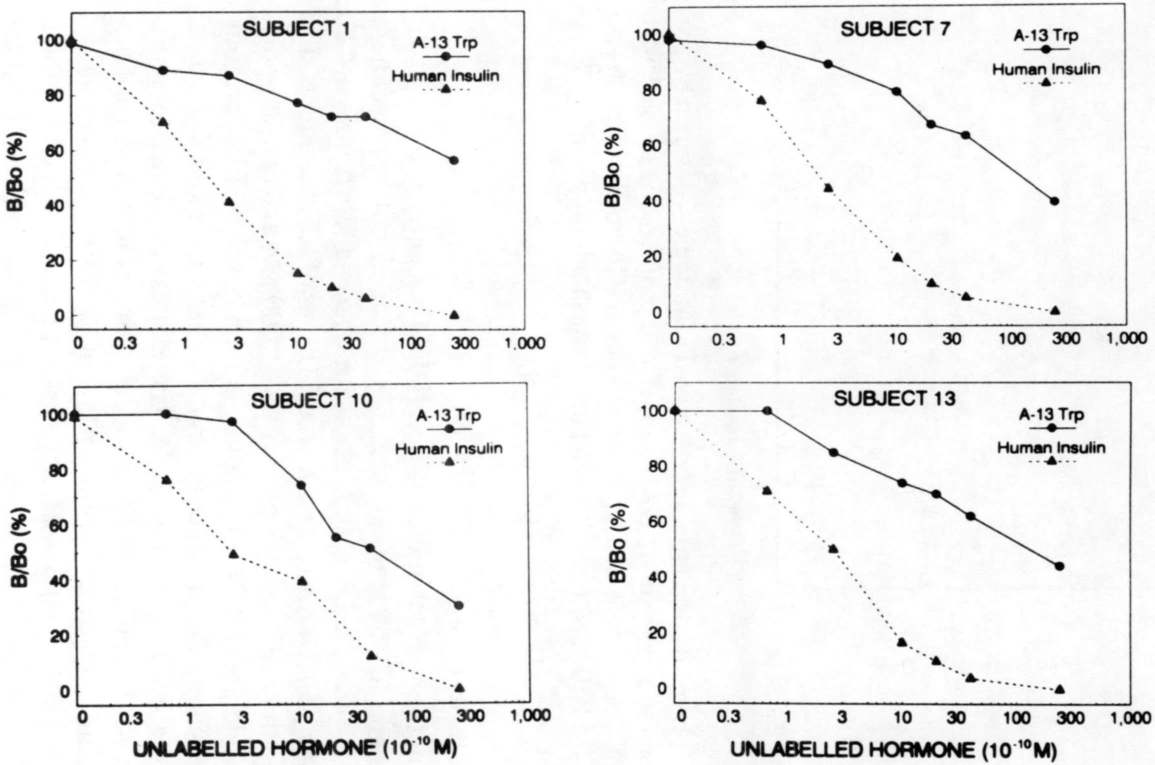

Fig. 2. Inhibition of ^{125}I-human insulin binding by human unlabeled insulin and an A-13 (Trp) insulin analog with concentration ranging from 10^{-11} to $10^{-7}M$ in several first degree relatives of IDDM patients. Binding is expressed as B/Bo (B-NSB)/(Bo-NSB). From Castaño et al. *(8)*.

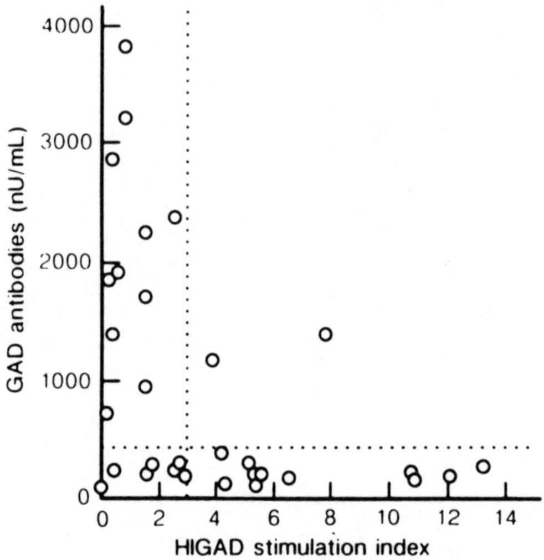

Fig. 3. Inverse correlation between GAD antibodies (detected by precipitation of fetal pig brain GAD), and T-cell proliferation to the central region of recombinant GAD_{67} fusion protein in ICA positive first degree relatives of IDDM patients. Broken lines = thresholds for positivity. From Harrison et al. *(16)*.

Islet Cell Autoantigen 69 (ICA69)

Another target molecule of IDDM recently cloned is the autoantigen ICA69 (Fig. 3) *(23)*. ICA69 was identified screening a human islet λgt11 cDNA expression library using sera from Islet Cell Antibody (ICA) positive first degree relatives of IDDM patients. The deduced molecular mass of ICA69 is 54,600 *Mr*, and on SDS-polyacrylamide gel (PAGE) the molecule migrates at 69 kDa, presumably because of the presence of strongly charged regions throughout the whole lengh of the molecule. The expression of ICA69 on rat islets is β-cell specific. The β-cell localization of ICA69 and its function remain unknown. Approximately 50% of first degree relatives of IDDM patients followed to the onset of the disease carry antibodies to ICA69, and 50% of newly diagnosed diabetic patients are positive for ICA69. It is of interest that ICA69 shares two short regions of identity of 5 and 4 amino acid residues with bovine serum albumin (BSA) (Fig. 4), and is basically identical in sequence to clones of the cows' milk-related p69 studied by Dosch and coworkers *(24)*. It has been reported that new onset diabetic patients carry antibodies to BSA, mostly in a particular region, the "ABBOS" peptide *(24)* (Fig. 5). ICA69 and the ABBOS peptide share minimal similarity in the region of BSA corresponding to the 8 amino acid residues EFKADEKK of ABBOS (Fig. 5).

It has been reported *(25)* that the octapeptide of ABBOS specifically drives T-cell proliferation in lymphocytes from new onset diabetic patients. The region of ICA69 homologous to ABBOS is identical in only 4 amino acid residues. Such similarities of peptides are enough to induce a T-cell response in experimental immune disorders *(26)*. These shared antigenic determinants between ICA69 and BSA may play a role in the induction of an autoimmune response that targets islets following neonatal exposure to cows' milk, or may possibly be a cause of crossreactivity between anti-ICA69 antibodies or anti-BSA/ABBOS antibodies.

Ganglioside GM2-1

Gangliosides are sialic acid containing glycolipids that are components of the plasma membrane and cytoplasm, which may be involved in cell contact and interaction with hormones, toxins, viruses, and antibodies. Gangliosides are formed by a hydrophilic portion (the oligosaccharide chain), and a hydrophobic tail (the ceramide), with at least one sialic acid residue. IgM antibodies to gangliosides are found to be elevated in patients with motor neuron diseases and other neuropathies, and it has been postulated that they might induce a T-cell independent B-lymphocyte response in these patients *(27)*.

Autoantibodies to the GM2-1 autoantigen, a novel pancreatic monosialoganglioside structure (*N*-acetyl-neuraminic acid-galactose-galactosamine-galactosamine-glucose-ceramide) that migrates between GM2 and GM1 standards (GM2-1), are detectable in the sera of ICA positive first degree relatives of IDDM patients before the overt disease *(28,29)*. The fact that ICA positive relatives with markedly increased diabetes risk carry GM2-1 autoantibodies suggests that this may represent an additional marker for the identification of individuals at risk to develop type I diabetes.

Carboxypeptidase H

Carboxypeptidase H is distributed in multiple tissues of neuroendocrine origin, including the secretory granules of the pancreatic β-cells, in which it is one of the most abundant proteins after proinsulin/insulin. Carboxypeptidase H seems to be involved in the

```
A
      CGGGCGGGGATACCCCAGGAGATGGGGTCGAGGAGAGACCCCGGGAGTAGAGAGAGAGAAACTCACTCCCCGAGTCCCCGACCCTCCCCAAG -178
CAAGGTTATAATATAACTTATCCTCTCATGCTTTTTCCTGCCCCTTCTCCCCAAATCATCAACAATAGAAGAAGAAGAAAAC ATG TCA GGA CAC   12
                                                                                   Met Ser Gly His    4

AAA TGC AGT TAT CCC TGG GAC TTA CAG GAT CGA TAT GCT CAA GAT AAG TCA GTT GTA AAT AAG ATG CAA CAG AGA   87
Lys Cys Ser Tyr Pro Trp Asp Leu Gln Asp Arg Tyr Ala Gln Asp Lys Ser Val Val Asn Lys Met Gln Gln Arg   29
                                            AMD                                         CK2
TAT TGG GAG ACG AAG CAG GCC TTT ATT AAA GCC ACA GGG AAG AAG GAA GAT GAA CAT GTT GTT GCC TCT GAC GCG  162
Tyr Trp Glu Thr Lys Gln Ala Phe Ile Lys Ala Thr Gly Lys Lys Glu Asp Glu His Val Val Ala Ser Asp Ala   54

GAC CTG GAT GCC AAG CTA GAG CTG TTT CAT TCA ATT CAG AGA ACC TGT CTG GAC TTA TCG AAA GCA ATT GTA CTC  237
Asp Leu Asp Ala Lys Leu Glu Leu Phe His Ser Ile Gln Arg Thr Cys Leu Asp Leu Ser Lys Ala Ile Val Leu   79
                                CK2
TAT CAA AAG AGG ATA TGT TTC TTG TCT CAA GAA GAA AAC GAA CTG GGA AAA TTT CTT CGA TCC CAA GGT TTC CAA  312
Tyr Gln Lys Arg Ile Cys Phe Leu Ser Gln Glu Glu Asn Glu Leu Gly Lys Phe Leu Arg Ser Gln Gly Phe Gln  104
                                            PKC
GAT AAA ACC AGA GCA GGA AAG ATG ATG CAA GCG ACA GGA AAG GCC CTC TGC TTT TCT TCC CAG CAA AGG TTG GCC  387
Asp Lys Thr Arg Ala Gly Lys Met Met Gln Ala Thr Gly Lys Ala Leu Cys Phe Ser Ser Gln Gln Arg Leu Ala  129
                                                    PKC
TTA CGA AAT CCT TTG TGT CGA TTT CAC CAA GAA GTG GAG ACT TTT CGG CAT CGG GCC ATC TCA GAT ACT TGG CTG  462
Leu Arg Asn Pro Leu Cys Arg Phe His Gln Glu Val Glu Thr Phe Arg His Arg Al.. Ile Ser Asp Thr Trp Leu  154

ACG GTG AAC CGC ATG GAA CAG TGC AGG ACG GAA TAT AGA GGA GCA CTA TTA TGG ATG AAG GAC GTG TCT CAG GAG  537
Thr Val Asn Arg Met Glu Gln Cys Arg Thr Glu Tyr Arg Gly Ala Leu Leu Trp Met Lys Asp Val Ser Gln Glu  179

CTT GAT CCA GAC CTC TAC AAG CAA ATG GAG AAG TTC AGG AAG GTG CAA ACA CAA GTG CGC CTT GCA AAA AAA AAC  612
Leu Asp Pro Asp Leu Tyr Lys Gln Met Glu Lys Phe Arg Lys Val Gln Thr Gln Val Arg Leu Ala Lys Lys Asn  204

[TTT GAC AAA TTG AAG ATG GAT GTG TGT] CAA AAA GTG GAT CTT CTT GGA GCG AGC AGA TGC AAT CTC TTG TCT CAC  687
[Phe Asp Lys Leu Lys Met Asp Val Cys] Gln Lys Val Asp Leu Leu Gly Ala Ser Arg Cys Asn Leu Leu Ser His  229

ATG CTA GCA ACA TAC CAG ACC ACT CTG CTT CAT TTT TGG GAG AAA ACT TCT CAC ACT ATG GCA GCC ATC CAT GAG  762
Met Leu Ala Thr Tyr Gln Thr Thr Leu Leu His Phe Trp Glu Lys Thr Ser His Thr Met Ala Ala Ile His Glu  254
PKC                                         PKC         CK2
AGT TTC AAA GGT TAT CAA CCA TAT GAA TTT ACT ACT TTA AAG AGC TTA CAA GAC CCT ATG AAA AAA TTA GTT GAG  837
Ser Phe Lys Gly Tyr Gln Pro Tyr Glu Phe Thr Thr Leu Lys Ser Leu Gln Asp Pro Met Lys Lys Leu Val Glu  279
                                                                                            CK2
AAA GAA GAG AAG AAG AAA ATC AAC CAG CAG GAA AGT ACA GAT GCA GCC GTG CAG GAG CCG AGC CAA TTA ATT TCA  912
Lys Glu Glu Lys Lys Lys Ile Asn Gln Gln Glu Ser Thr Asp Ala Ala Val Gln Glu Pro Ser Gln Leu Ile Ser  304
                                    AMP     PKC                                         CK2
TTA GAG GAA GAA AAC CAG CGC AAG GAA TCC TCT AGT TTT AAG ACT GAA GAT GGA AAA AGT ATT TTA TCT GCC TTA  987
Leu Glu Glu Glu Asn Gln Arg Lys Glu Ser Ser Ser Phe Lys Thr Glu Asp Gly Lys Ser Ile Leu Ser Ala Leu  329
```

```
GAC AAA GGC TCT ACA CAT ACT GCA TGC TCA GGA CCC ATA GAT GAA CTA TTA GAC ATG AAA TCT GAG GAA GGT GCT 1062
Asp Lys Gly Ser Thr His Thr Ala Cys Ser Gly Pro Ile Asp Glu Leu Leu Asp Met Lys Ser Glu Glu Gly Ala  354

TGC CTG GGA CCA GTG GCA GGG ACC CCG GAA CCT GAA GGT GCT GAC AAA GAT GAC CTG CTG CTG TTG AGT GAG ATC 1137
Cys Leu Gly Pro Val Ala Gly Thr Pro Glu Pro Glu Gly Ala Asp Lys Asp Asp Leu Leu Leu Leu Ser Glu Ile  379
     *          CK2
TTC AAT GCT TCC TCC TTG GAA GAG GGC GAG TTC AGC AAA GAG TGG GCC GCT GTG TTT GGA GAC GGC CAA GTG AAG 1212
Phe Asn Ala Ser Ser Leu Glu Glu Gly Glu Phe Ser Lys Glu Trp Ala Ala Val Phe Gly Asp Gly Gln Val Lys  404

GAG CCA GTG CCC ACT ATG GCC CTG GGA GAG CCA GAC CCC AAG GCC CAG ACA GGC TCA GGT TTC CTT CCT TCG CAG 1287
Glu Pro Val Pro Thr Met Ala Leu Gly Glu Pro Asp Pro Lys Ala Gln Thr Gly Ser Gly Phe Leu Pro Ser Gln  429
                                            CK2
CTT TTA GAC CAA AAT ATG AAA GAC TTA CAG GCC TCG CTA CAA GAA CCT GCT AAG GCT GCC TCA GAC CTG ACT GCC 1362
Leu Leu Asp Gln Asn Met Lys Asp Leu Gln Ala Ser Leu Gln Glu Pro Ala Lys Ala Ala Ser Asp Leu Thr Ala  454
                                            CK2                     PKC
TGG TTC AGC CTC TTC GCT GAC CTC GAC CCA CTC TCA AAT CCT GAT GCT GTT GGG AAA ACC GAT AAA GAA CAC GAA 1437
Trp Phe Ser Leu Phe Ala Asp Leu Asp Pro Leu Ser Asn Pro Asp Ala Val Gly Lys Thr Asp Lys Glu His Glu  479

TTG CTC AAT GCA TGA ATCTGTACCCTTCGGAGGGCACTCACATGCCGCCCCAGCAGCTCCCCTGGGGGCTAGCAGAAGTATAAAGTGATCAGT 1531
Leu Leu Asn Ala END                                                                                    483

ATGCTGTTTTAATAATTATGTGCCATTTTAATAAAATGAAAGGGTCAACGGCCCTGTTAAAAAAAAAAAAAAAAAA                    1607
```

B

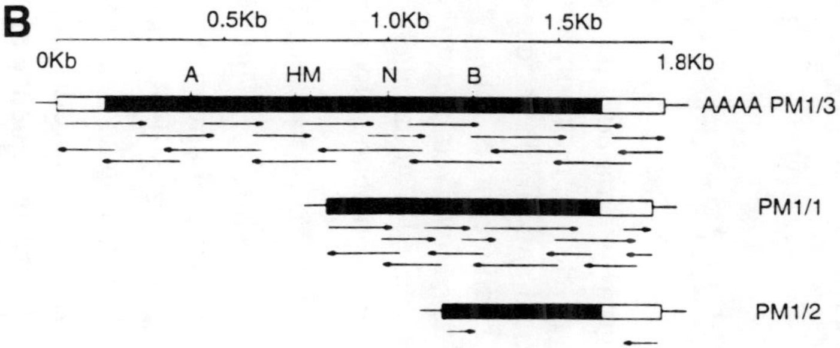

Fig. 4. Complete nucleotide and deduced amino acid sequence of the ICA69 molecule (**A**), and schematic representation for sequencing cDNA encoding for ICA69 (**B**). Underlined are the first upstream in frame stop codon *(TAA)* at nucleotide -75 and the polyadenylation signal 29 bp upstream of the poly (A) tail. Homologous subunits with BSA are in boxes. A potential N-linked glycosylation site is indicated by an asterisk. Potential phosphorylation sites are as follows: PKC (protein kinase C), CK2 (casein kinase II), and AMP (cAMP/cGMP-dependent kinase). A potential amidation site is indicated as AMD. From Pietropaolo et al. *(23)*.

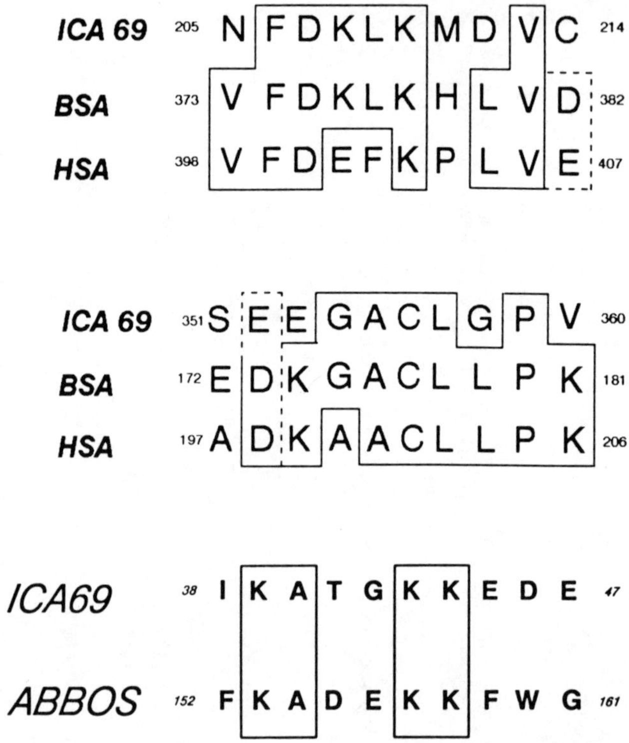

Fig. 5. Regions of similarity between ICA69 molecule, BSA, human serum albumin (HSA) precursor, and the ABBOS peptide. Solid lines enclose identical amino acid residues. Dashed lines enclose amino acid residues with similar charge. Similarity between the BSA peptide ABBOS hypothesized to be involved in cows' milk-induced autoimmunity in type I diabetes, and the islet autoantigen ICA69. Numbers correspond to the amino acid residue numbers. Modified from Pietropaolo et al. *(23)*.

cleavage of proinsulin *(30)*. This enzyme has been termed carboxypeptidase E and enkephalin convertase, and is found in other neuroendocrine secretory cells. This potential IDDM-related antigen was identified screening a rat islet λgt11 expression library *(31)*, and subsequently the plaque-producing antigen (corresponding to approx 1/3 of the whole linear sequence of carboxypeptidase H) reacted with 5 of the 20 sera from other first degree relatives of IDDM patients, and with 0 of the 14 control sera. The percentage of positives among relatives of IDDM patients should increase if the whole length of the molecule is used to be detected by other assay formats, like radioassay (RIA), or ELISA. The molecular mass of the glycosylated membrane-bound form of carboxypeptidase H is 52 kDa *(32)*.

Uncharacterized Autoantigens

64 kDa Antigens (not GAD)

Christie recently reported detection of pancreatic islet 64 kDa autoantigens in type I diabetes distinct from glutamic acid decarboxylase *(33)*. Trypsin digestion of islet protein immunoprecipitated by antibodies of IDDM patients generates three major proteolytic fragments of M_r 37,000, 40,000, and 50,000. There is evidence that the 50,000 M_r component derives from GAD, whereas the precursors of the 37/40 kDa tryptic fragments seem to be proteins of M_r 64,000. Moreover, 37,000/40,000 M_r fragments are detectable after trypsin treatment of immunoprecipitates from insulinoma cells that lack expression of GAD isoforms. Detailed analysis on two-dimensional electrophoresis gel of the 64 kDa immune complexes revealed at least three different proteins (designated α, β, displaying charge heterogeneity, and γ, negatively charged). The 64 kDa (not GAD) autoantigens do not appear related to heat shock proteins. Antibodies to 37/40 kDa tryptic fragments are detectable in approx 70% of identical twins followed to the clinical onset of diabetes *(34)*. Further characterization of the 64 kDa islet precursors of the 37/40 kDa antigen tryptic fragments is required.

38 kDa Antigen(s)

Several investigators have reported reactivity of sera from IDDM patients to potentially different 38 kDa molecules. One such antigen, an undefined 38 kDa component of the insulin secretory granule membranes of rat insulinoma tissue, was suggested as a possible target antigen associated with IDDM. T-cell lines of peripheral blood from 8 of 10 new onset IDDM patients, and one ICA-positive nondiabetic subject, showed proliferation to a preparation of the 38 kDa protein isolated from the insulin secretory granule membranes, as compared to none of the 10 controls. Honeyman et al. recently reported that the 38 kDa antigen is the factor jun-B *(35)*. This molecule has been identified by screening human islet and placenta λgt11 expression libraries using high titer anti-38,000 M_r serum from recent-onset IDDM patients. A recombinant fragment of jun-B (amino acids 1–180) specifically exhibits proliferation in peripheral blood T-cells in new onset IDDM subjects. Jun-B is a ubiquitous nuclear transcription protein, but the relevance of autoantibodies to this molecule is unclear.

Pak et al. identified a human islet protein whose M_r is 38,000, blotting with a monoclonal antibody generated by immunizing Balb/c mice with human cytomegalovirus (CMV) *(36)*. This raises the possibility that the pathogenesis of type I diabetes is related to CMV molecular mimicry. It is of interest that jun-B shares similarities with human CMV in a region close to the NH_2 terminal domain.

52 kDa Antigen

Carboxypeptidase, whose molecular mass is 52 kDa, is one of the potential 52 kDa autoantigens. It is of interest that antibodies reacting with a 52 kDa (p52) rat insulinoma (RIN) protein have been found in sera from both NOD mice and humans with IDDM, and appear to be related with Rubella virus because antirubella capsid antibodies crossreact with this protein *(37)*. Interestingly, antibodies raised to a synthetic peptide sequence corresponding to the N-terminal domain of p52 react with the insulin secretory granules in RIN cells. The potential predictive value of antibodies to p52, and its role in T-cell activation is unknown.

128 kDa Antigen

McEvoy and coworkers reported displacement of radiolabeled mouse antirat insulinoma cell (RIN5F) monoclonal antibody from RIN5F cells by serum from newly diagnosed IDDM patients, but not by sera from control children *(38)*. The antigen is present in rat islets as two bands on Western blots, and in human islets as a single band of approx 128 kDa *(39)*. This assay may detect pancreatic β-cell surface antigens not reactive using the conventional immunofluorescence assay on sections of human pancreas.

Additional Potential Autoantigens

A series of additional islet autoantigens may play a role in the pathogenesis of IDDM. Sulfatides appear to be expressed in the secretory granules of both α- and β-cells, detected by a specific antisulfatide monoclonal antibody, and have been suggested as a possible autoantigen *(40)*.

Johnson et al. reported that immunoglobulins G from patients with new-onset IDDM significantly reduced high K_m glucose transport of rat islet cells *(41)*. This inhibitory activity could be specifically abolished by incubation of immunoglobulins from diabetic patients with either cells or cell membranes, such as hepatocytes or β-cells, which express the GLUT-2 glucose transporter, but not with cells or membranes that do not express GLUT-2 (erythrocytes or kidney brush border cells). These observations taken together suggest, but do not demonstrate, that immunoglobulins G from new onset IDDM patients react with the GLUT-2 glucose transporter or with a β-cell protein functionally related to GLUT-2.

Recently, indirect evidence for the involvement of a *superantigen* in the pathogenesis of IDDM has be postulated after studying the pancreas of an infant who died of ketoacidosis *(42)*. The nucleotide sequence of the majority of the T-cell islet infiltrate revealed identity with Vβ7 T-cell receptors. This has led to speculation that *superantigens* may play a role in the pathogenesis of IDDM.

Heat shock proteins (HSPs), or stress proteins, whose synthesis is induced when a cell undergoes a sudden increase in temperature, are possible candidates in the generation of autoimmunity in IDDM *(43–45)*. HSPs can be divided into four major groups, namely 90, 70, 60, and 10–30 kDa. Most of the interest has focused on the 60 and 70 kDa group members. Evidence that HSPs may have a role in autoimmunity in different autoimmune diseases has been presented *(45)*. In particular, humoral autoimmunity has been reported to HSP65 in rheumatoid arthritis, to HSP70, and to HSP90 in systemic lupus erythematosus, but the role of HSPs as an autoantigen in IDDM is not generally accepted. Two well documented papers identified the 64,000 *Mr* autoantigens as glutamic acid decarboxylase *(12)*, and as 64 kDa precursors of the 37/40 kDa tryptic fragments *(33)*, rather than HSP65 *(44)*.

Boitard et al. reported that NOD mice carry circulating autoantibodies to peripherin, a neuronal protein whose molecular mass is 58 kDa, detected by Western blotting of RIN5F cell extracts *(46)*. A monoclonal antibody against peripherin was used to characterize its expression in cell lines of different origins, and none of the cell lines tested (including thymic, fibroblastic, and pituitary cell lines) expressed peripherin.

Use of Humoral Markers to Characterize Autoantigens in Type I Diabetes Prediction

The identification of the molecular structure of autoantigens in type I diabetes and the optimization of biochemical assays to detect specific autoantibodies to molecularly characterized autoantigens can form the basis for improving the prediction of IDDM. Several biochemical assays have been developed using single islet molecules as antigens, namely insulin, GAD, ICA69 *(47)*, and the 37,000- and 40,000-*Mr* islet-antigen tryptic fragment *(33)*. In particular, if we combine three biochemical assays for three autoantibodies (autoantibodies to insulin, GAD, and ICA69) in first degree relatives of diabetic patients and in newly diagnosed diabetic patients, we can detect positivity for at least one of these three autoantibodies in 100% of relatives followed to the onset of IDDM, as well as in 100% of new-onset diabetic patients. Approximately 18% of ICA negative relatives who have not developed diabetes (commonly considered at low risk to develop IDDM) and 3% of the control population are positive for at least one of the three autoantibodies. If we consider positivity for two or three autoantibodies to insulin, GAD, or ICA69, the percentage of positivity is approx 90% either in preclinical diabetic patients or new-onset diabetics, and, importantly, is only 4% in ICA negative relatives who have not developed IDDM, and 0% in a control population. Therefore, using three biochemically characterized assays in combination, one can obtain high sensitivity and specificity. Combinatorial assays should enhance specificity as well as sensitivity in the assessment of diabetes risk *(47,48)*. There are other interesting islet autoantigens, such as the ganglioside GM2-1 *(29)*, which may improve the predictive value of humoral markers in type I diabetes particularly in combination with other molecularly characterized islet autoantigens. Combined analyses of specific anti-islet humoral markers may be a prerequisite for the development of simple predictive screening for IDDM *(49)*.

Pathogenic Significance

Basic Questions

The identification of a series of islet autoantigens leads to the obvious question as to which antigens are central to the pathogenesis of IDDM. Subsidiary questions include: Which antigens are involved in the initiation and perpetuation of autoimmunity? Which share epitopes with environmental factors potentially initiating disease (e.g., bovine albumin, viruses)? Which humoral response to antigen(s) is important as a predictive marker of IDDM? None of these questions, except for the use of islet autoantigens in prediction, can be answered to date.

How can this plethora of autoantigens related to type I diabetes be rationalized? Comprehensive analysis of the repertoire of autoantibodies in systemic autoimmune diseases has revealed that most autoimmune diseases are associated with a spectrum of autoantibodies against specific subcellular antigens. This diversity of autoantibody species among different autoimmune diseases was difficult to rationalize until the molecular structure and subcellular localization of the autoantigens was discovered. For instance, in scleroderma subcellular particles (34 kDa protein, 40 kDa protein) localized in the nucleolus organizer region have been identified, and this subcellular organelle seems to be an important structure involved in the induction of the scleroderma-related autoimmune responses *(50)*.

In systemic lupus erythematosus, antibodies to Sm antigen, originally defined by immunodiffusion analysis, turned out to be a complex of several autoantibodies reactive with the core proteins of small ribonucleoprotein particles involved in pre-mRNA splicing *(5)*. In IDDM the humoral autoimmune response may well be the result of a complex of several autoantibodies reactive against several components of islet subcellular particles. In IDDM the pancreatic β-cell secretory granules (containing insulin and carboxypeptidase H), or the synaptic-like microvesicles (containing GAD) are considered prominent target organelles involved in the induction of a specific autoimmune response. The diversity of autoantibodies in autoimmune diseases could be explained by the type of antigen-driven autoimmune response that could be related in each disease to the particular type of subcellular particle targeted.

These observations suggest that a complex of single autoantigens driving an immune response are likely to be aggregates of molecules forming subcellular particles. Therefore autoimmunity could be induced by several components of these particles.

We favor the hypothesis that insulin is a central molecule for the pathogenesis of type I diabetes (Fig. 1). The sequential timing of the

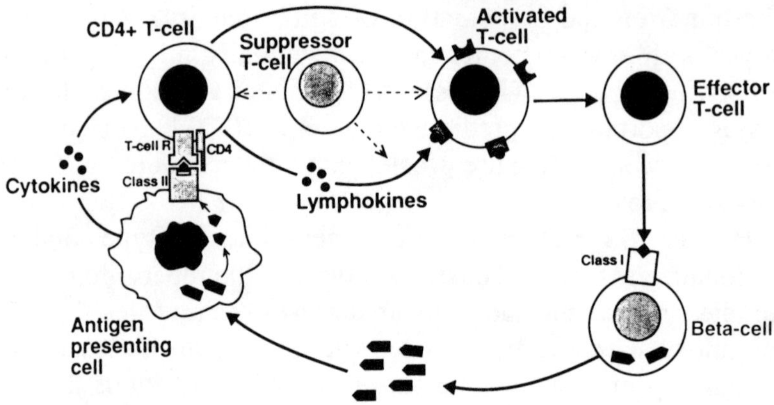

Fig. 6. The T-cell regulatory cascade. Defining the primary activation step of the anti-β-cell autoimmune reaction is a prerequisite of any logical strategy to induce tolerance. From Boitard *(51)*.

appearance of autoantibodies is not yet fully defined, but insulin autoantibodies frequently precede other autoantibodies. Polymorphisms of the insulin gene contribute to diabetes risk. Levels of insulin autoantibodies correlate with the age at which type I diabetes develops. Anti-insulin reactive T-cells are prominent within islets of NOD mice.

Molecular Testing of Pathogenic Role of Autoantigens

Understanding the primary activation step of the anti-islet cell autoimmune reaction cascade *(51)* has been one of the major interests in diabetes research (Fig. 6). Extensive research has focused on the characterization of which peptide(s) within the class II molecule cleft on antigen-presenting cells is able to drive a specific anti-islet immune response.

The general approach developed to address the role of autoantigens in T-cell activation in IDDM has essentially been the establishment of T-cell lines and clones that proliferate in response to specific islet autoantigens.

To date for IDDM, insulin is the only β-cell specific autoantigen. A peculiar feature of IDDM is that insulitis occurs only if β-cells remain within islets. Thus, if an antigen (e.g., GAD) is expressed in non-β-cells of human islets it cannot be sufficient to mediate T-cell infiltration. One animal model of IDDM that is similar to human type I diabetes is the NOD mouse. These mice develop spontaneous insulin-dependent diabetes mainly because of a T-cell involvement in the islet autoimmune process. Wegmann has recently reported *(8a)* that T-cell lines derived from CD4 T-cell islet lesions generated in the NOD mouse with islet stimulation do not transfer the disease when injected intraperitoneally into the NOD-severe-combined immunodeficient (SCID) mouse. A high proportion of T-cells within these lines proliferate to insulin. CD4 T-cell clones, particularly those of Haskins and coworkers, derived from splenocytes that do not respond to insulin, are able to transfer diabetes in nondiabetic mice *(52)*. In humans, Roep and coworkers have reported T-cell responses to a 38 kDa secretory granule protein from rat insulinoma *(53)*, which has not yet been characterized, whereas responses to GAD *(54,55)*, or HSP65 *(43)* have been described.

An extensive characterization of T-cell reactivity to autoantigens related to IDDM, including epitope mapping, is now required. This is an easier task in animal models of IDDM than in human IDDM. One important approach that may overcome this obstacle to the study of human islet specific cell-mediated immunity (CMI) utilizes immunodeficient mice. It has been reported that the peritoneal injection of mononuclear blood cells (MBCs) from newly diagnosed type I diabetic patients into CD-1 *nu/nu* mice recipients is able to induce significant mononuclear cell infiltrate around the mouse islets *(56)*. When islet specific T-cell lines and clones are established from these infiltrates, we will have an important tool to evaluate the human T-cell proliferation to molecularly characterized islet autoantigens, and therefore to better define their pathogenic role in the human disease process.

Genetics of Autoimmunity in IDDM, Transgenic Studies

Genes with the closest correlation with diabetes susceptibility are HLA class II genes, or immune response genes, which in humans correspond to DP, DQ, and DR. It is noteworthy that the same HLA allele may protect from one disorder, for instance, HLA DR2, DQA1*0102, DQB1*0602 is rare in patients with IDDM, whereas it is associated with multiple sclerosis *(57,58)*. Therefore it seems that susceptibility linked by alleles within the HLA region may influence the likelihood to develop specific disorders rather than induce autoimmunity in general. This implies that if HLA alleles play a role in the disease susceptibility by their function as immune response genes, selective targeting is likely.

An alternative way by which HLA alleles may determine susceptibility for autoimmune disease is by altering the development of the T-cell repertoire. Recent observations in a transgenic mouse model provide evidence that the predilection for MHC is due to the way the T-cell receptor repertoire is derived. In the thymus thymocytes during their development express a multitude of T-cell receptors and only thymocytes that express a receptor weakly reactive with self MHC antigens presented in the thymus mature further. This process (termed positive selection) can potentially enhance selection of autoreactive T-cells. Expression of specific HLA molecules also leads to intrathymic clonal deletion of certain T-cell receptor families that might otherwise contribute to the anti-islet autoimmune response. Those developing thymocytes with high affinity for self MHC transduce a signal that leads to programmed cell death (apoptosis).

The NOD mouse is an important model in which hypotheses on how autoimmunity in IDDM develops can be tested. It has been postulated that NOD mice transgenic for MHC class II I-E molecule do not develop insulitis or diabetes because of the intrathymic clonal deletion of certain TCR V_β families that might otherwise contribute to the pathogenesis of insulitis *(59,60)*. Further experiments, however, demonstrate that markedly skewing the T-cell receptor repertoire does not diminish autoimmunity in NOD mice *(61)*, providing evidence that the protective effect of the I-E gene in NOD mice may not be mediated by the clonal deletion of particular V_β families, but rather by other mechanisms. Therefore, an intact TCR repertoire appears to not be essential in the pathogenesis of insulitis in the NOD mouse, although T-cells are certainly required for the development of insulitis.

The observation that less than 100% of monozygotic twins are concordant for the development of type I diabetes led to speculation that environmental factors can influence disease susceptibility. In addition to environmental factors, monozygotic twins are not identical after the maturation of their immune system because they differ in T-cell and immunoglobulin gene rearrangements *(62)*. In addition, lymphoid somatic mutations may contribute to clones of cells escaping tolerance induction.

Effector Mechanisms of β-Cell Destruction

Humoral and cell-mediated immunity are the two fundamental effector arms of the immune system. For many autoimmune disorders one or the other of these effector mechanisms predominates in the disease-related pathogenic mechanism. There are many different mechanisms by which human autoantibodies can induce pathology, including inhibiting the functional activity of the antigen (e.g., blocking the functional activity of insulin receptor associated with insulin autoantibodies) or stimulation of the functional activity of the antigen (e.g., Graves' disease with stimulatory anti-TSH autoantibodies). To date, in type I diabetes there is no compelling evidence that autoantibodies influence the function of important domains of autoantigens, but T-cell-mediated immunity seems to play a key role in the pathogenesis of the disease process.

Transfer of Disease

Transfer models have been developed to study cell mediated effector mechanisms of β-cell destruction. Transfer of diabetes occurs following injection of spleen cells from diabetic NOD donors into both 8-wk-old male NOD recipients *(63)*, and naive neonates *(64)*. In recipient neonates the first event was the expression of class II MHC antigens on endothelial cells. Insulitis was characterized by the presence of CD4 positive T-cells followed by recruitment of CD8 positive cells. Both CD4 and CD8 positive cells are required to transfer diabetes to neonate and NOD recipients, as confirmed by the prevention of transfer by treatment of preirradiated adult recipients with anti-CD4, anti-CD8 *(65,66)*, or anti-CD3 monoclonal antibodies. The involvement of B-lymphocytes is not required in the transfer of diabetes in NOD mice *(67)*, because the treatment of recipients with a monoclonal antibody against the μ chain of IgM prior to and after the birth did not reduce the transfer efficiency of purified T-cells from diabetic NOD mice, despite the presence of a β-cell damage. CD4 positive anti-islet T-cell clones are sufficient to transfer diabetes *(68)*.

Beside the involvement of T-cells, potential inflammatory mediators, such as lymphokines and nitric oxide *(69)*, may play a role in the pathogenesis of IDDM.

Autoimmune diabetes can be induced in transgenic mice in which the pancreatic β-cells express interferon-α (IFN-α) and the insulitis as well as the clinical features of diabetes in these mice are prevented by a neutralizing antibody to IFN-α. It is important to highlight that because this model has similarities with the IFN-α expression described in islet cells in human diabetes *(70)*, expression of IFN-α may be a causal factor in the development of this disease in humans. Thus, once the inflammatory process initiates in the islet microenvironment by the production of IFN-α, a powerful inflammatory reaction involving T- and B-cells as well as NK cells may occur.

The involvement of IFN-γ in the genesis of insulitis is supported by the presence of IFN-γ in human pancreatic islet lesions *(71)*, and from the fact that IFN-γ in β-cells of transgenic mice leads to hypoinsulinemic diabetes *(72)*.

It is of interest that treatment with Complete Freund's adjuvant (CFA) in NOD mice inhibits the development of diabetes, but not insulitis *(73)*. CFA treatment may lead to a "deviation" of the autoimmune response toward TH_2 activation because it negatively regulates IFN-γ production that is required from T-cell mediated islet damage *(74)*. The low frequency of IFN-γ-producing cells in the islet cell infiltrate is associated with nondestructive islet lesions as well as with high frequency of IL4-producing cells.

Although in vitro studies have shown that interleukin 1 (IL-1) selectively damages ß-cells in vitro, and inhibits insulin secretion of isolated perfused pancreata *(75,76)*, studies in vivo demonstrated that exposure to cytokines of syngeneic islets in contact with allogeneic islets grafted under the kidney capsule does not lead to their destruction *(77)*. Moreover tumor necrosis factor α or IL-1 treatment is able to prevent diabetes in NOD mice *(78,79)*.

Tolerance Induction

A number of immunomodulatory therapies have been investigated as potential treatment for type I diabetes. Administration of oral autoantigens is one potential approach to induce antigen-driven peripheral immune tolerance. Autoimmune diseases, such as EAE,

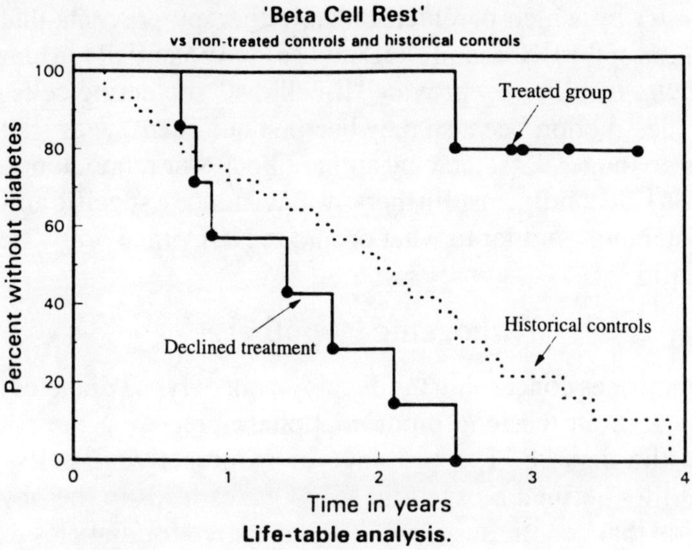

Fig. 7. Life table results of a pilot trial of prevention of type I diabetes with low dose insulin therapy of high risk (anti-islet autoantibodies plus loss of first phase insulin secretion) relatives of patients with type I diabetes. From Keller et al. *(85)*. The *y*-axis plots the percentage of relatives remaining nondiabetic and the *x*-axis, years of followup.

multiple sclerosis *(10,80,81)*, experimental autoimmune uveoretinitis *(82)*, and adjuvant- and collagen-induced arthritis *(83)* are important examples of induction of systematic immunologic hyporesponsiveness antigen- and peptide-dependent. It has been found that oral administration of porcine insulin in NOD mice over 1 yr dramatically delays the clinical onset of IDDM *(9)*. Furthermore, splenic T-cells from animals orally treated with insulin inhibited adoptive transfer of the disease, indicating that oral insulin generates active cellular mechanisms that suppress the disease. Oral tolerance is particularly attractive because of lack of known toxicity and specificity of its immunologic effect.

Following studies in BB rats *(84)*, in humans an insulin prophylactic pilot study in individuals at high risk of type I diabetes has started, and the findings show that low-dose subcutaneous insulin injection in the treated group may have been effective in preventing diabetes during a followup ranging from 2.3 to 3.3 yr *(85)* (Fig. 7).

The manner by which parenteral insulin therapy prevents diabetes and insulitis of the BB rat and NOD mouse, and potentially in humans, is unknown. Insulin may provide "β-cell rest" protecting cells from immune destruction because they become quiescent, with islet-cell antigens no longer detectable by autoantibodies or monoclonal antibodies *(86)*. Secondly, insulin therapy may induce a specific antigen-driven tolerance, similar to what occurs in NOD mice orally treated with insulin.

Pathogenic Hypotheses

Hypotheses concerning the development of type I diabetes must take into account the long prodromal phase preceding the clinical onset of the disease. The presence of autoreactive T-cells with susceptibility defined by specific MHC genes leads to the obvious conclusion that genetic susceptibility is required for diabetes development in humans and in animal models. The presence of autoreactive T-cells may result from defective selection of the T-cell repertoire (e.g., abnormal positive selection). The role of T-cell selection in determining the peripheral T-cell repertoire and autoimmune susceptibility has been reported in a collagen arthritis model *(87)*, but remains hypothetical in human IDDM.

Evidence for a triggering role of environmental factors such as bovine albumin of milk or viral infection has also been postulated. Viral infection may initiate *(88)* or prevent *(89)* activation of autoimmunity from experiments in animals, but several studies in humans also suggest that persistent viral infection (e.g., rubella virus, coxsackie B4, cytomegalovirus, Epstein-Barr, and so on) may be involved in some cases of IDDM. The role of viruses in the pathogenesis of IDDM is also supported by direct isolation of virus from the pancreas of an infant who died of diabetic ketoacidosis *(90)*. Horn et al. reported that a sequence of E1 protein of the rubella virus shares five amino acid residues identical (GPPAA) to a segment encoded by the IDDM associated DQw8 allele *(91)*, suggesting that this shared peptide may serve as an autoantigenic target for crossreactive response to the pathogen. The lack of a rationale as to why crossreactivity with a ubiquitous MHC molecule should specifically induce diabetes, however, detracts from this hypothesis. On the other hand, suppression of islet autoimmunity in experimental diabetes by Epstein-Barr viral infection could be explained with the fact that Epstein-Barr virus shares homology with interleukin 10, a cytokine with potent suppressive effect on the immune system *(92)*.

The hypothesis that cows' milk is a possible trigger associated with type I diabetes *(24,93,94)* (supported by epidemiological findings indicating that early exposure to cows' milk proteins in childhood may be associated with increased risk of IDDM *[95]*) requires further study. With the cloning of the islet related molecule (ICA69), such studies should be facilitated *(23)*.

The fact that multiple antigens related to IDDM have been identified should be not a surprise, in view of observations in other endocrine autoimmune disorders *(5)*. Their association with clinical subtypes of a given autoimmune disease implies that islet-specific T-cells or antibodies may correlate with different rates of progression to IDDM. Thus, heterogeneity of type I diabetes may be explained by a heterogeneity of anti-islet antigen autoimmune responses.

Ongoing studies in first degree relatives of diabetic patients suggest that autoantibodies against biochemically characterized autoantigens (insulin, GAD_{65}, and ICA69) appear independently *(47)* and the pattern of autoantibody expressed may influence the progression to overt disease. Therefore, it appears that breaking tolerance in type I diabetes is not simply an all-or-none phenomenon, but is both quantitative and antigen selective. With the detection of autoantibodies and T-cell responses to multiple autoantigens, criteria need to be developed to define "pathogenic" autoantigens, namely antigens sufficient to generate an autoimmune response or sufficient to maintain autoimmunity once initiated. Table 2 lists several criteria to distinguish between antigens sufficient to maintain or generate an autoimmune disorder. It is likely that there are also many antigens for which an autoimmune response is secondary to tissue destruction but does not contribute to disease.

How can autoantigens participate in an autoimmune process? In conditions in which a humoral or cellular response is directed against membrane-bound or cell surface antigens, such as pemphigus vulgaris, it is reasonable to consider that they could be involved in the pathogenesis of the disease. In many autoimmune diseases, such as

Table 2
Criteria to Distinguish Between Autoantigens Sufficient (but not Necessary) to Maintain or Generate an Autoimmune Response

	Maintain	Generate
Autoantibodies–autoreactive T-cells are found	X	X
Autoantibody or T-cells responses appear first		X
Autoantigen is specific for cell targeted	X	X
Autoantibodies or T-cells target tissue in vitro	X	X
Autoantibodies or T-cells transfer disease to immunodeficient mice	X	
Ectopic transgenic induced production of autoantigen targets ectopic tissue	X	
Induction of tolerance to antigen blocks disease		X

IDDM, some antigens are intracellular (e.g., GAD), and are in "privileged" sites that are normally inaccessible either to T-cells or circulating autoantibodies. Insulin is expressed both on the surface and intracytoplasmically. It is not completely clear how these antigens become involved in pathogenesis. However, certain intracellular molecules that escape autolytic degradation are released into the extracellular milieu. In this case epitopes of these molecules are capable of reacting either with T-cells or circulating autoantibodies thus generating and maintaining an inflammatory process.

Table 3 summarizes our current view of the pathogenesis of type I diabetes. The disease develops in the setting of genetic susceptibility determined by alleles both within and outside of the major histocompatibility complex. The disease is the result of progressive plaque-like destruction of beta cells within individual islets (insulitis) and overt hypoglycemia develops only after extensive beta cell destruction. During the process of beta cell destruction, a family of autoantigens (present in insulin secretory granules and synaptic-like microvesicles are targeted). Any pathogenic scheme at present is only an outline of the disease process. In particular, the genes creating diabetes susceptibility outside of the major histocompatibility complex are unknown. It is likely that within this decade, this lack of knowledge will be overcome. Hopefully, safe prevention of the disorder will come with a better understanding of the molecular pathology of type I diabetes.

Table 3
Pathogenesis of Type I Diabetes

Event	Potential determinants
Altered T-cell/B-cell development ↓	Non-MHC genes (e.g., Insulin gene polymorphisms, ? genes influencing apoptosis?) Somatic mutations
Altered T-cell regulation ↓	T_H2 vs T_H1 responses (e.g., Adjuvant-like exposure)
Antigen presentation by B-lymphocytes and monocytes to B- and T-cells ↓	Class II MHC genes
Expansion anti-islet CD4 T-lymphocytes ↓	Islet damage/β-cell secretion
Perpetuation/regulation autoimmunity ↓	Immunoglobulin gene mutations DR4 haplotypes: high response to insulin and other autoantigens Local lymphokine production Enhanced vascular permeability Enhanced Class I, Class II expression
β-cell toxicity ↓	Lymphokines Free radicals CD4/CD8 T-cells NK cells Macrophages
Progressive plaque-like β-cell destruction ↓	
Type I diabetes	

References

1. Eisenbarth GS: Type I diabetes mellitus: a chronic autoimmune disease. *N Engl J Med* 314:1360–1368, 1986.
2. Bottazzo GF, Genovese S, Bosi E, Dean BM, Christie MR, Bonifacio E: Novel considerations on the antibody/autoantigen system in type I (insulin-dependent) diabetes mellitus. *Ann Med* 23:453–461, 1991.
3. Harrison LC: Islet cell antigens in insulin-dependent diabetes: Pandora's box revisited. *Immunol Today* 13:348–352, 1992.
4. Maclaren N, Lafferty K: Perspectives in diabetes: The 12th international immunology and diabetes workshop. *Diabetes* 42:1099–1104, 1993.
5. Tan EM: Autoantibodies in pathology and cell biology. *Cell* 67:841–842, 1991.
6. Palmer JP, Asplin CM, Clemons P, et al.: Insulin antibodies in insulin-dependent diabetics before insulin treatment. *Science* 222:1337–1339, 1983.
7. Ziegler AG, Ziegler R, Vardi P, Jackson RA, Soeldner JS, Eisenbarth GS: Life table analysis of progression to diabetes of anti-insulin autoantibody-positive relatives of individuals with type I diabetes. *Diabetes* 38:1320–1325, 1989.

8a. Wegmann D, Norbury-Glaser M, and Daniel D: Insulin specific T cells are a predominant component of islet-specific T cells isolated from islet infiltrates of pre-diabetic NOD mice. *Eur J Immunol,* in press.

8. Castaño L, Ziegler A, Ziegler R, Shoelson S, Eisenbarth GS: Characterization of insulin autoantibodies in relatives of patients with insulin-dependent diabetes mellitus. *Diabetes* 42:1202–1209, 1993.
9. Zhang JZ, Davidson L, Eisenbarth GS, Weiner HL: Suppression of diabetes in non-obese diabetic mice by oral administration of porcine insulin. *Proc Natl Acad Sci USA* 88:10252–10256, 1991.
10. Miller A, Lider O, Roberts AB, Sporn MB, Weiner HL: Suppressor T cells generated by oral tolerization to myelin basic protein suppress both in vitro and in vivo immune responses by the release of transforming growth factor B after antigen-specific triggering. *Proc Natl Acad Sci USA* 421:425, 1992.
11. Todd JA, Mijovic C, Fletcher J, Jenkins D, Bradwell AR, Barnett AH: Identification of susceptibility loci for insulin-dependent diabetes mellitus by trans-racial gene mapping. *Nature* 338:587–589, 1989.
12. Baekkeskov S, Aanstoot H, Christgau S, et al.: Identification of the 64K autoantigen in insulin dependent diabetes as the GABA-synthesizing enzyme glutamic acid decarboxylase. *Nature* 347:151-156, 1990.
13. Christgau S, Aanstoot HJ, Schierbeck H, et al.: Membrane anchoring of the autoantigen GAD65 to microvesicles in pancreatic beta-cells by palmitoylation in the NH2-terminal domain. *J Cell Biol* 118(2):309–320, 1992.
14. Karlsen AE, Hagopian WA, Grubin CE, et al.: Cloning and primary structure of a human isoform of glutamic acid decarboxylase from chromosome 10. *Proc Natl Acad Sci USA* 88:8337–8341, 1991.
15. Solimena M, Folli F, Denis-Donini S, et al.: Autoantibodies to glutamic acid decarboxylase in a patient with stiffman syndrome, epilepsy, and type I diabetes mellitus. *N Engl J Med* 318:1012–1020, 1988.

16. Harrison LC, Honeyman MC, DeAizpurua HJ, et al.: Inverse relation between humoral and cellular immunity to glutamic acid decarboxylase in subjects at risk of insulin-dependent diabetes. *Lancet* 341:1365–1369, 1993.
17. Gianani R, Pugliese A, Bonner-Weir S, et al.: Prognostically significant heterogeneity of cytoplasmic islet cell antibodies in relatives of patients with type I diabetes. *Diabetes* 41:347–353, 1992.
18. Rorsman P, Berggren PO, Bokvist K, et al.: Glucose-inhibition of glucagon secretion involves activation of GABA-receptor chloride channels. *Nature* 341:233,234, 1989.
19. Petersen JS, Russel S, Marshall MO, et al.: Differential expression of glutamic acid decarboxylase in rat and human islets. *Diabetes* 42:484–495, 1993.
20. Velloso LA, Kampe O, Hallberg A, Christmanson L, Betsholtz C, Karlsson FA: Demonstration of GAD-65 as the main immunogenic isoform of glutamate decarboxylase in type I diabetes and determination of autoantibodies using a radiogland produced by eukaryotic expression. *J Clin Invest* 91:2084–2090, 1993.
21. Deres K, Schild H, Wiesmuller KH, Jung G, Rammensee HG: In vivo priming of virus-specific cytotoxic T lymphocytes with lipopeptide vaccine. *Nature* 342:561–564, 1989.
22. Gianani R, Jackson R, Eisenbarth GS: Evidence that the autoantigen of restricted ICA is GAD. *Diabetes Res Clin Prac* 14(suppl 1):S13 (abstract), 1991.
23. Pietropaolo M, Castaño L, Babu S, et al. Islet cell autoantigen 69 kD (ICA69): Molecular cloning and characterization of a novel diabetes associated autoantigen. *J Clin Invest* 1993; 92:359–371.
24. Karjalainen J, Martin JM, Knip M, et al.: A bovine albumin peptide as a possible trigger of insulin-dependent diabetes mellitus. *N Engl J Med* 327:302–307, 1992.
25. Karjalainen J, Cheung R, Vandermeulen J, Martin JM, Knip M: T cell proliferation response against bovine albumin (BSA) follows the natural course and is restricted to the linear ABBOS sequence in insulin-dependent diabetes mellitus (IDDM). *Autoimmunity* (suppl):62 (abstract), 1993.
26. Luo A-M, Garza KM, Hunt D, Tung KSK: Antigen mimicry in autoimmune disease. Sharing of amino acid residues critical for pathogenic T cell activation. *J Clin Invest* 92:2117–2123, 1993.
27. Freimer ML, McInstosh K, Adams RA, Alving CR, Drachman DB: Gangliosides elicit a T-cell independent antibody response. *J Autoimmun* 6:281–289, 1993.
28. Dotta F, Colman PG, Nayak RC, et al.: Ganglioside expression in human pancreatic islets. *Diabetes* 38:1478–1483, 1989.
29. Dotta F, Gianani R, Dionisi S, Tiberti C, Eisenbarth GS, DiMario U: Expression of anti-GM2-1 islet ganglioside antibodies in ICA+ relatives of type I diabetics. *Autoimmunity* (suppl):70 (abstract), 1993.
30. Davidson HW, Rhodes CJ, Hutton JC: Intraorganellar calcium and pH control proinsulin cleavage in the pancreatic A cell via two distinct site-specific endopeptidases. *Nature* 333:93–96, 1988.
31. Castaño L, Russo E, Zhou L, Lipes MA, Eisenbarth GS: Identification and cloning of a granule autoantigen (carboxypeptidase H) associated with type I diabetes. *J Clin Endocrinol Metab* 73:1197–1201, 1991.

32. Davidson HW, Hutton JC: The insulin-secretory-granule carboxypeptidase H. *Biochem J* 245:575–582, 1993.
33. Christie MR, Hollands JA, Brown TJ, Michelsen BK, Delovitch TL: Detection of pancreatic islet 64,000 M_r autoantigens in insulin-dependent diabetes distinct from glutamate decarboxylase. *J Clin Invest* 92:240–248, 1993.
34. Christie MR, Richard YM, Tun RYM, et al.: Antibodies to GAD and tryptic fragments of islet 64K antigen as distinct markers for development of IDDM: Studies with identical twins. *Diabetes* 41:782–787, 1992.
35. Honeyman MC, Cram DS, Harrison LC: Transcription factor jun-B is target of autoreactive T-cells in IDDM. *Diabetes* 1993 (in press).
36. Pak CY, Cha CY, Rajotte RV, McArthur RG, Yoon YW: Human pancreatic islet cell specific 38 kilodalton autoantigen identified by cytomegalovirus-induced monoclonal islet cell autoantibody. *Diabetologia* 33:569–572, 1990.
37. Karounos DG, Simmerman L, Hickman SL, Jacob RJ: Identification of the p52-Rubella related autoantigen as an insulin secretory granule protein. *Diabetes* 42 (Suppl 1):221A (abstract), 1993.
38. Thomas NM, Ginsberg-Fellner F, McEvoy RC: Strong association between diabetes and displacement of mouse anti-rat insulinoma cell monoclonal antibody by human serum in vitro. *Diabetes* 39:1203–1211, 1990.
39. Pan Y-X, Thomas NM, McEvoy RC: Purification and partial characterization of 160 kD and 155 kD B cell membrane antigens detected by MAb 1A2. *Autoimmunity* (suppl):77 (abstract), 1993.
40. Buschard K, Josefsen K, Horn T, Larsen S, Fredman P: Sulphatide and anti-sulphatide antibodies in type I diabetes mellitus. *Diabetes* 42 (Suppl 1):5A (abstract), 1993.
41. Johnson JH, Crider BP, McCorkle K, Alford M, Unger RH: Inhibition of glucose transport into rat islet cells by immunoglobulins from patients with new-onset insulin-dependent diabetes mellitus. *N Engl J Med* 322:653–659, 1990.
42. Trucco M, Ricordi C, Weidman E, Rodriquez-Rilo H, Trucco G, Finegold D: Involvement of superantigens in the etiology of IDDM. *Diabetes* 42(Suppl 1):4A, 1993.
43. Elias D, Reshef T, Birk OS, Zee R, Walker MD, Cohen IR: Vaccination against autoimmune mouse diabetes with a T-cell epitope of the human 65-kD heat shock protein. *Proc Natl Acad Sci USA* 88:3088–3091, 1991.
44. Jones DB, Hunter NR, Duff GW: Heat-shock protein 65 as a B cell antigen of insulin-dependent diabetes. *Lancet* 336:583–585, 1990.
45. Kaufman SHE: Heat shock proteins and the immune response. *Immunol Today* 11:129–136, 1990.
46. Boitard C, Villa MC, Becourt C, et al.: Peripherin: An islet antigen that is cross-reactive with non-obese diabetic mouse class II gene products. *Proc Natl Acad Sci USA* 89:172–176, 1992.
47. Pietropaolo M, Buelow R, Gianani R, Yu L, Eisenbarth GS: Independent assortment of biochemically defined autoantibodies in prediabetic relatives. *J Immunol* 150:166A (abstract), 1993.

48. Bingley PJ, Christie MR, Bonfanti R, et al.: Combined analysis of autoantibodies enhances prediction of IDDM in islet cell antibody (ICA) positive relatives. *Autoimmunity* (suppl):67 (abstract), 1993.
49. Eisenbarth GS, Verge CF, Allen H, Rewers MJ: Perspectives in diabetes: The design of trials for the prevention of IDDM. *Diabetes* 42:941–947, 1993.
50. Maul GG, French BT, van Venrooij WJ, Jimenez SA: Topoisomerase I identified by scleroderma 70 antisera: enrichment of topoisomerase I at the centromere in mouse mitotic cells before anaphase. *Proc Natl Acad Sci USA* 83:5245–5149, 1986.
51. Boitard C: The differentiation of the immune system towards anti-islet autoimmunity. Clinical aspects. *Diabetologia* 35:1101–1112, 1992.
52. Haskins K, McDuffie M: Acceleration of diabetes in young NOD mice with a CD4+ islet-specific T cell clone. *Science* 249:1433–1436, 1990.
53. Roep BO, Kallan AA, Hazenbos WLW, et al.: T-cell reactivity to 38 kD insulin-secretory-granule protein in patients with recent-onset type 1 diabetes. *Lancet* 337:1439–1441, 1991.
54. Atkinson MA, Kaufman DL, Campbell L, et al.: Response of peripheral-blood mononuclear cells to glutamate decarboxylase in insulin-dependent diabetes. *Lancet* 339:458,459, 1992.
55. Latchman D: No diabetes link to hsp65? *Nature* 356:114, 1992.
56. Calcinaro F, Hao L, Chase HP, Klingensmith G, Lafferty KJ: Detection of cell-mediated immunity in type I diabetes mellitus. *J Autoimmun* 5:137–147, 1992.
57. Erlich HA, Griffith RL, Bugawan TL, Ziegler R, Alper C, Eisenbarth GS: Implication of specific DQB1 alleles in genetic susceptibility and resistance by identification of IDDM siblings with novel HLA-DQB1 allele and unusual DR2 and DR1 haplotypes. *Diabetes* 40:478–481, 1991.
58. Atkinson MA, Maclaren NK: What causes diabetes? *Sci Am* 263:62–71, 1990.
59. Nishimoto H, Kikutani H, Yamamura K, Kishimoto T: Prevention of autoimmune insulitis by expression of I-E molecules in NOD mice. *Nature* 328:432–434, 1987.
60. Reich EP, Janeway C, Rath S, Sherwin RS: Islet specific T cell clones from diabetes NOD mice can cause histological insulitis. *Diabetes* 38(Suppl 2):13A, 1989.
61. Lipes MA, Rosenzweig A, Tan K, et al.: Progression to diabetes in non-obese diabetic (NOD) mice with transgenic T cell receptors. *Science* 259:1165–1169, 1993.
62. Strominger JL: Biology of the human histocompatibility leukocyte antigen (HLA) system and a hypothesis regarding the generation of autoimmune disease. *J Clin Invest* 77:1411–1415, 1986.
63. Wicker LS, Miller BJ, Mullen Y: Transfer of autoimmune diabetes mellitus with splenocytes from non-obese diabetic (NOD) mice. *Diabetes* 35(8): 855–860, 1986.

64. Bendelac A, Carnaud C, Boitard C, Bach JF: Syngeneic transfer of autoimmune diabetes from diabetic NOD mice to healthy neonates. Requirement for both L3T4+ and Lyt-2+ T-cells. *J Exp Med* 166:823–832, 1987.
65. Miller BJ, Appel MC, O'Neil JJ, Wicker LS: Both the LYT-2+ and L3T4+ T cell subsets are required for the transfer of diabetes in non-obese diabetic mice. *J Immunol* 140:52–58, 1992.
66. Hutchings P, Simpson E, O'Reilly LA, Lund T, Waldmann H, Cooke A: The involvment of Lyt2+ T cells in beta cell destruction. *J Autoimmun* 3:101–109, 1990.
67. Bendelac A, Boitard C, Bedossa P, Bazin H, Bach JF, Carnaud C: Adoptive T cell transfer does not require recruitment of host B lymphocytes. *J Immunol* 141:2625–2628, 1988.
68. Candeias S, Katz J, Benoist C, Mathis D, Haskins K: Islet-specific T cell clones from non-obese diabetic mice express heterogenous T cell receptors. *Proc Natl Acad Sci USA* 88:6167, 1991.
69. Nomikos IN, Wang Y, Lafferty KJ: Involvement of O_2 radicals in "autoimmune" diabetes. *Immun Cell Biol* 67:85–87, 1989.
70. Stewart TA, Hultgren B, Huang X, Pitts-Meek S, Hully J, Maclachlan NJ: Induction of type I diabetes by interferon-a in transgenic mice. *Science* 260:1942–1946, 1993.
71. Debray-Sachs M, Carnaud C, Boitard C, et al.: Prevention of diabetes in NOD mice treated with antibody to murine IFN-g. *J Autoimmun* 4:237–248, 1991.
72. Sarvetnick N, Liggitt D, Pitts SL, Hansen SE, Stewart TA: Insulin-dependent diabetes mellitus induced in transgenic mice by ectopic expression of class II MHC and interferon-g. *Cell* 52:773–782, 1988.
73. Shehadeh NN, LaRosa F, Lafferty KJ: Altered cytokine activity in adjuvant inhibition of autoimmune diabetes. *J Autoimmun* 6:291–300, 1993.
74. Foulis AK, McGill M, Farquharson MA: Insulitis in type I (insulin-dependent) diabetes mellitus in man-macrophages, and interferon-g containing cells. *J Pathol* 165:97–103, 1991.
75. Bendtzen K, Mandrup-Poulsen T, Nerup J, Nielsen JH, Dinarello CA, Svenson M: Cytotoxicity of human p17 interleukin-1 for pancreatic islets of Langerhans. *Science* 232:1545–1547, 1986.
76. Mandrup-Poulsen T, Bendtzen K, Nerup J, Dinarello CA, Svenson M, Nielsen JH: Affinity-purified human interleukin-1 is cytotoxic to isolated islets of Langerhans. *Diabetologia* 29:63–67, 1986.
77. Sutton R, Gray DWR, McShane P, Dallman P, Morris PJ: The specificity of rejection and the absence of susceptibility of pancreatic islet beta cells to nonspecific immune destruction in mixed strain islets grafted beneath the renal capsule in the rat. *J Exp Med* 170:751–762, 1989.
78. Campbell IL, Oxbrow L, Harrison LC: Reduction in insulitis following administration of IFN-g and TNF-alpha in the NOD mouse. *J Autoimmun* 4:249–262, 1991.
79. Jacob CO, Also S, Michie S, McDevitt HO, Acha-Orbea H: Prevention of diabetes in non-obese diabetic mice by tumor necrosis factor (TNF):

similarities between TNF-alpha interleukin 1. *Proc Natl Acad Sci USA* 87:968–972, 1990.
80. Weiner HL, Mackin GA, Matsui M, et al.: Double-blind pilot trial of oral tolerization with myelin antigens in multiple sclerosis. *Science* 1321: 1324, 1993.
81. Gaur A, Wiers B, Liu A, Rothbard J, Fathman CG: Amelioration of autoimmune encephalitis by myelin basic protein synthetic peptide-induced anergy. *Science* 258:1491–1494, 1992.
82. Nussenblatt RB, Caspi R, Mahdi R, et al.: Inhibition of S-antigen induced experimental autoimmune uveoretinitis by oral induction of tolerance with S-antigen. *J Immunol* 144:1689–1695. 1990.
83. Zhang JZ, Lee CS, Lider O, Weiner HL: Suppression of adjuvant arthritis in Lewis rats by oral administration of type II collagen. *J Immunol* 145:2489–2493, 1990.
84. Gottsfredsen CF, Buschard K, Frandsen EK: Reduction of diabetes incidence of BB Wistar rats by early prophylactic insulin treatment of diabetes-prone animals. *Diabetologia* 28:933–935, 1985.
85. Keller RJ, Eisenbarth GS, Jackson RA: Insulin prophylaxis in individuals at high risk of type I diabetes. *Lancet* 341:927–928, 1993.
86. Appel MC, Dotta F, O'Neill J, Eisenbarth GS: Beta cell activity regulates the expression of islet antigen determinant. *Diabetologia* 32:461A (abstract), 1989.
87. Anderson GD, Banerjee S, Luthra HS, David CS: Role of Mls-1 locus and clonal deletion of T cells in susceptibility to collagen-induced arthritis in mice. *J Immunol* 147:1189–1193, 1991.
88. Guberski DL, Thomas VA, Shek WR, et al.: Induction of type 1 diabetes by Kilham's rat virus in diabetes-resistant BB/Wor rats. *Science* 254:1010–1013, 1991.
89. Oldstone C: Prevention of type I diabetes in non-obese diabetic mice by virus infection. *Science* 239:500–502, 1987.
90. Horn GT, Bugawan TL, Long CM, Erlich HA: Allelic sequence variation of the HLA-DQ loci: Relationship to serology and to insulin-dependent diabetes mellitus susceptibility. *Proc Natl Acad Sci USA* 85:6012–6016, 1988.
91. Yoon JW, Austin M, Onodera T, Notkins AL: Isolation of a virus from the pancreas of a child with diabetic ketoacidosis. *N Engl J Med* 300(21): 1173–1179, 1979.
92. Howard M, O'Garra A: Biological properties of interleukin 10. *Immunol Today* 13:198–200, 1992.
93. Elliott RB, Martin JM: Dietary protein: a trigger of insulin dependent diabetes in the BB rat. *Diabetologia* 26:297–299, 1984.
94. Martin JM, Trink B, Daneman D, Dosch H, Robinson B: Milk proteins in the etiology of insulin-dependent diabetes mellitus (IDDM). *Ann Med* 23:447–452, 1991.
95. Kostraba JN, Cruickshanks KJ, Lawler-Heavner J, et al.: Early exposure to cow's milk and solid foods in infancy, genetic predisposition and risk of IDDM. *Diabetes* 42:288–295, 1993.

Chapter 2

Murine Transgenic Models of IDDM

Danling Gu and Nora Sarvetnick

Introduction

Insulin-dependent diabetes mellitus (IDDM) is an autoimmune disease. To study the immune responses leading to the breakdown of tolerance to islet β-cells, genes of putative causative agents and of major histocompatibility complex (MHC) are linked to insulin promoter and incorporated into the germ line of a mouse. The expression of transgenes are tissue specific (β-cell-specific) and their actions are analyzed during the life span of the "host" animals. These transgenic mice not only serve as models of IDDM but also provide new powerful tools for studying the many aspects of peripheral tolerance.

The technology that allows the incorporation of a selected foreign gene into a germ line of an animal and the consequences of the expression of this alien gene (transgene) being investigated in the whole organism has opened up an exciting frontier in biomedical research. For the study of diabetes, especially IDDM (type I diabetes), the gene transfer technique has gained new insights into the etiology of IDDM. Recent advances in our understanding of IDDM have made IDDM a ripe subject to be exploited by means of transgenic animals. For example, the structure of insulin gene and the mechanisms regulating its expression have been known for some

From: *Molecular Biology of Diabetes, Part I*
Edited by: B. Draznin and D. LeRoith © 1994 Humana Press Inc., Totowa, NJ

time, making it possible for the study of cell-type (β-cell) specific transgene expression *(1–3)*. Additionally, the autoimmune nature of IDDM has been established and the hypothesis for the mechanisms leading to IDDM has been formulated, providing a theoretical ground for generating transgenic mouse models *(4)*. Furthermore, genetic mutant animal models for human IDDM, nonobese diabetic (NOD) mouse, and Biological Breeding (BB) rats have afforded the investigators to use transgenes in defining the regions and the mutations that constitute the genetic makeup of susceptibility and resistance to diabetes (*see* ref. *5* for BB; *see* ref. *6* for NOD). And finally, the complex interplay of multiple genes and environmental factors such as the one seen in the development of IDDM are best analyzed in vivo with respect to the function of a particular gene in question *(7)*. In this regard, the usefulness of transgenic animals has also been amply illustrated in the studies of other human diseases plagued by complex etiology of genetic nature: hepatitis B virus induced heptocarcinoma *(8)*, rheumatoid arthritis *(9)*, systemic lupus erythematosus *(10)*. Indeed, the transgenic animals serve not only as models for human disease but also provide a powerful tool for looking into the intricate inner workings of various biological processes, such as autoimmunity, differentiation, cell lineage, tumorigenesis, and many others *(7,11)*.

The immense interest shown in diabetic transgenic mice following the first attempt using such mice as models for autoimmune responses related to IDDM in 1987 has resulted in voluminous reports and a number of reviews *(12)*. Additional materials related to this topic are referred to in the following reviews: generation of transgenic mice *(13,14)*; previous reviews of transgenic mouse models for autoimmune diseases and diabetes *(11,15–18)*; transgenic NOD mouse models *(19–21)*; and the possible applications of gene therapy in diabetes *(22)*.

Human IDDM is a result of selective destruction of pancreatic islet β-cells. The development of disease has environmental and genetic components *(23,24)*. We shall limit the scope of this chapter to the recent developments concerning three major facets of IDDM:

1. Environmental factors—viral transgenes and IDDM;
2. Autoimmunity—transgenes of autoimmune responses in relation to IDDM; and

3. Genetic predisposition—analyses of genetic background of IDDM-prone NOD mice by transgenic technology.

Viral Transgenes and IDDM

Viral infection is considered one of the major environmental factors in the initiation of autoimmune responses leading to IDDM *(4)*. The effects of viral infection in β-cells can be mimicked by a transgene linking a viral gene to the promoter segment of insulin gene. The fusion of a transgene to the insulin promoter results in tissue specific (β-cell) transgene expression *(3,25,26)*. Hanahan and his colleagues generated transgenic mice to large T-antigen (Tag) of simian virus 40 (SV 40) for the studies of tumorigenesis, cell lineage analysis, and autoimmunity *(3,12)*. They showed that Tag was produced exclusively in β-cells and its presence caused islet hyperplasia and β-cell tumors. Since the Tag gene is integrated into the mouse germ line and is heritable, its protein product would be regarded as "self" and granted tolerance by the immune system. However, three out of four Tag transgenic mouse lines developed autoimmune responses characterized by the presence of circulating antibody specific to Tag protein and lymphocytic infiltration (insulitis) causing islet damage. The islet destruction did not lead to diabetes, probably because the islet loss was balanced and eventually overtaken by the islet hyperplasia. The loss of tolerance was related to the timing of the Tag expression. The tolerant mice expressed the Tag gene before birth or during neonatal life. In contrast, the nontolerant mice expressed the Tag gene much later in life. However, not all of the late-expression mice had autoimmune responses, suggesting that some other factors are involved contributing to the susceptibility of a portion of the population. The results of this study were interpreted to show the importance of the timing of an autoantigen appearance in the induction of tolerance during ontogeny of susceptible mice. It is not clear how tolerance is established or lost in Tag transgenic mice. These issues are addressed and clarified to some extent in other transgenic mouse models.

Roman and her colleagues produced transgenic mice that expressed influenza virus hemagglutinin (HA) in β-cells *(27)*. All three lines, ranging from 13 to 27%, developed diabetes at mature age. The development of hyperglycemia in HA transgenic mice displayed all the features that characterize human IDDM. The diabetes in all cases were insulin dependent and responded to insulin regimen. The hyperglycemia was accompanied by polydipsia/polyuria, and in severely diabetic mice showed a high incidence (70%) of ketonuria. Damage to β-cells was associated with insulitis and was preceded by the presence of antibodies to HA, β-cell surface, and cytoplasmic antigens. The results suggested that hyperglycemia in HA transgenic mice is a consequence of autoimmune destruction of β-cells. The HA transgenic mice, as in the case of Tag transgenic mice, showed only a fraction of population, with loss of tolerance to transgene product. This fact again suggested that additional factors contribute to the susceptibility of certain individuals. One such factor could be the segregation of genes of the MHC. One of three HA transgenic lines with a homozygous H-2d locus of class I MHC had a much earlier onset and a higher incidence of diabetes. The MHC I molecules encoded by H-2d locus have been shown to be extremely efficient in their ability to serve as restriction elements in the recognition of HA by cytotoxic T-lymphocytes (CTL) *(28)*. The subject of susceptibility will be discussed further later. It should be noted that HA transgenic mice expressed HA gene in fetus at the time of pancreas diverticulum formation. In contrast to Tag transgenic mice, early transgene expression did not result in tolerance.

In other viral transgenic mice efforts to duplicate the major processes of human IDDM were attempted by using genes coding either lymphocytic chlorimeningitis virus (LCMV) glycoprotein (GP) or LCMV nucleoprotein (NP) as transgenes *(29)*. LCMV transgenic mice (both GP and NP) expressed extremely low levels of GP or NP and did not develop tolerance or autoimmunity. Among mature mice, only 6% were diabetic and 2% had a low titer antibody against LCMV. When normoglycemic mice were injected with LCMV, 88% developed autoimmune diabetes evidenced by high-titered antibody to "self antigen" LCMV, hyperglycemia, insulitis, and β-cell destruction. The lymphocyte infiltrates were $CD8^+$ and $CD4^-$ of Thy1,2 lineage. Several cultured $CD8^+$ lymphocyte lines showed CTL activity that was LCMV specific and MHC restricted. Their findings were substantiated by another study of LCMV-GP transgenic mice *(30)*. Taken together, these results indicate that the apparent "peripheral tolerance" of lymphocytes to the "transgenic self" can break down after the challenge of the immunogenic form of virus. The latter group examined the mechanism of T-cell mediated tolerance further by crossing GP transgenic mice with other transgenic mice expressing T-cell receptor (TCP) specific for GP. The self reactive T-cells in the double transgenic mice were not removed by either clonal deletion or aborted by clonal anergy (functional paralysis), but instead, existed in a state of "functional unresponsiveness" owing to the absence of appropriate activation. Their view, in essence, advocates that peripheral tolerance has never been established, and does not exist. Infection of LCMV in both GP and GP-TCR transgenic mice readily abolishes the peripheral unresponsiveness resulting in $CD8^+$CTL mediated diabetes. The induction of self tolerance or lack of it plays a critical role in manifestation of autoimmune diseases such as IDDM. The transgenic mouse models of tissue specific antigen expression provide an in vivo system to elucidate the mechanisms of peripheral tolerance *(18,31,32)*.

Transgenic Models of IDDM in Relation to MHC

One avenue by which the immune system responds to antigens is by the presentation of antigens on MHC class I (H-2) and class II (I-A and I-E) molecules to T-cells ($CD8^+$, CTL for class I; $CD4^+$ cells, T-helper cells for class II) that express T-cell receptors (TCR) specific for these antigens. MHC class I molecules are expressed at a low level in all tissues including β-cells, whereas MHC class II genes are not expressed by β-cells but only on the cells of thymic origin such as B-lymphocytes and the cells of macrophage-dendritic lineage that usually function as antigen-presenting cells (APC) in immune responses.

There is strong evidence to suggest that MHC molecules play a central role in the β-cell destruction and the progression to overt IDDM *(4)*. There have been many different theories put forth to explain how the peripheral tolerance is maintained and broken down *(18,19,33)*. One of the most vigorously tested hypotheses is that the immune system maintains tolerance to peripheral autoantigens simply by lack of efficient presentation of autoantigens to the autoreactive T-cells. To explain how IDDM develops, it was hypothesized that the viral injury to β-cells and the subsequent local cytokine production by inflammatory cells causes aberrant expression of MHC II molecules by β-cells. The β-cells then function as APC presenting autoantigens and stimulate antigen-specific T-cells leading to autoimmune destruction of β-cells *(4)*. If the hypothesis is correct, the induced expression of MHC class II molecules on β-cells would result in autoimmunity to β-cells and IDDM. This hypothesis is in agreement with the findings that β-cells from newly diagnosed IDDM patients exhibited strong MHC expression *(34,35)*. In Bottazzo's hypothesis, MHC II molecules expressed on β-cells play an obligatory role in the development of IDDM. On the other hand, hyperexpression of class I molecules on β-cells may also involve in the initiation of autoimmune responses leading to the activation of $CD8^+$ CTL resulting in IDDM *(33,36)*.

Several groups independently generated transgenic mice to express class II molecules *(37–39)*, or to augment the expression of class I molecules in β-cells *(33,40)*. All four transgenic mice expressed high levels of MHC molecules and all developed severe diabetes characterized by hyperglycemia and hyperinsulinemia. However, to everyone's surprise, there was no evidence of any immune reactions involved. There was no mononuclear lymphocyte infiltration in islets of any of these transgenic mice. It was learned later that high levels of MHC molecule production in β-cells by itself is detrimental to β-cells by reduction of insulin mRNA synthesis *(41)* and by impairing insulin secretion *(15,40–42)*. Indeed, when MHC II molecules were expressed at the normal physiological level as expressed in resting splenic B-lymphocytes, there was no β-cell destruction and no immune involvement *(39)*. The results of MHC transgenic mouse models clearly showed that the induction of MHC molecules alone would not transform β-cells into antigen presenting cells. These findings considerably weakened Bottazzo's hypothesis. However, the transgenic expression of MHC molecules on β-cells is not exactly the same as the induction of MHC expression in IDDM. For one thing, in the development of IDDM, macrophages and lymphocytes appear in association with environmental factors such as viral infection. Both macrophages and lymphocytes, when activated, are a rich source of cytokines. These cytokines, in addition to the presumed function to upregulate MHC gene expression on β-cells, may act alone or in concert to activate T-cells, so the presentation of autoantigens by

MHC-expressed β-cells can proceed *(43,44)*. The role of cytokines in the context of MHC function in the development of IDDM is discussed later.

One of the best examples applying the transgenic approach to study cytokine participation in IDDM is the insulin linked interferon-γ (IFN-γ) transgenic mice *(14,38)*. Two of three IFN-γ mouse lines developed diabetes accompanied by polyurea, polyposia, and weight loss. The onset of hyperglycemia began between 10–20 wk of age in one line and approx 5 mo of ages in the other line. The islets from the mice with early onset of diabetes showed infiltrating lymphocytes at around 4 wk of age, well before the onset of hyperglycemia. The infiltrating lymphocytes are composed of macrophages and natural killer cells (5%), helper T-cells (70%), and cytotoxic T-cells (25%). In old mice, lymphocytes were also scattered in the acinar tissue and the islets were obliterated or difficult to locate in the midst of massive lymphocyte accumulation and the presence of interstitial tissue and the numerous pancreatic ducts. The transgenic mice rejected MHC-matched islet grafts indicating that the destruction of islets is immune mediated specifically sensitized to islet cells. The effects of transgenic IFN-γ and the mechanisms of islet destruction are not clear. Several possibilities have been proposed:

1. IFN-γ may exert direct toxicity to β-cells;
2. IFN-γ may facilitate the lymphocyte recruitment by inducing high endothelial cells;
3. IFN-γ may upregulate MHC genes;
4. IFN-γ may activate already existing autoreactive T-cells which otherwise remain unresponsive; and
5. IFN-γ may induce the expression of costimulatory molecules *(14,45)*.

In a series of studies conducted by Allison and her colleagues, three transgenic mouse strains were generated, each carried MHC class I, interleukin-2 (IL-2), and MHC class I-specific TCR transgenes, respectively. Double and triple transgenic mice were then produced by mating among them *(36,46–48)*. The results of these studies demonstrated that:

1. MHC transgenic mice developed nonimmune mediated diabetes as mentioned earlier *(36)*;

2. IL-2 mice developed massive lymphocyte infiltration but not diabetes or autoimmunity *(47)*;
3. IL-2 × MHC double transgenic mice accepted skin grafts bearing MHC molecules *(46)*.
4. MHC × MHC-specific TCR transgenic mice rejected skin grafts bearing high density of MHC molecules but ignored low density MHC molecules on the β-cells in islets *(47)*; and
5. Triple transgenic mice developed severe diabetes as early as one week after birth, whereas IL-2 mice or IL-2 × TCR double transgenic mice did not develop diabetes.

Based on the results of these studies, the authors proposed that the immunocompetent autoreactive T-cells to MHC class I molecules were not completely deleted in thymus but existed in the periphery neither tolerated nor immunized by MHC molecules, and local production of IL-2 can stimulate an antigen-specific autoimmune response *(48)*.

Another cytokine transgenic mice harboring tumor necrosis factor (TNF-α) gene linked to insulin gene also showed massive lymphocyte infiltration *(49)*. The TNF-α transgenic mice did not develop diabetes. The infusion of TNF-α mice with IFN-γ or introduction of LCMV by mating with LCMV transgenic mice *(30)* failed to illicit diabetes. These results led authors to conclude that insulitis may be necessary but not sufficient to cause diabetes.

Transgenic NOD Mice: Studies of Susceptibility and Resistance to IDDM

The NOD mouse is the animal model of human IDDM *(19,20)*. Both humans and NOD mice have genetically inherited predisposition to IDDM. In humans, the HLA (the major histocompatibility complex of human) class II genes DR3 and DR4 (DR is the human counterpart of murine I-E) are associated with susceptibility to IDDM, whereas DR2 genes are associated with resistance. In addition, DQβ chain (murine I-Aβ chains) with aspartic acid (Asp) at 57 position are prevalent to IDDM. A substitution of Asp57 with such noncharged amino acids as serine or valine have been observed in IDDM patients. In NOD mice, three loci are identified as contributing to diabetes susceptibility. One of the three loci is closely linked to class II MHC region on chromosome 17. The haplotype of MHC class II identified with susceptibility has two unusual features distinguished by no expression of I-E molecules because of a deletion in the promoter region of the Eα gene, whereas Eβ gene functions normally but its product cannot express on the cell surface without Eα; and the I-A molecule has two amino acid changes at position 56 and 57 from pro-Asp to His-Ser, which are unique to NOD mice. The lack of I-E gene expression in NOD mice was an obvious "defect" to be considered for diabetes susceptibility. To determine if the introduction of the I-Eα gene to NOD mice would result in the prevention of diabetes, NOD mice were mated with transgenic mice for I-Eα^d or I-Eα^κ. The F1 progeny were then backcrossed to NOD mice. Among the F2 offspring it was found that NOD mice with intact I-E molecules did not development insulitis *(50,51)*. The protective effect of I-E has also been confirmed in Eα transgenic NOD by direct incorporation of Eα gene into NOD germ line *(52,53)*.

A similar approach using transgenic mice was also employed to assess the diabetogenic effect of NOD I-A molecules. NOD transgenic mice with the "nonsusceptible" I-A gene (I-A$^\kappa$) expressing both Aα^κ and Aβ^κ showed significant reduction in the incidence of insulitis *(53,54)*. The similar reduction of insulitis was observed when NOD transgenic mice expressed I-A$^\kappa$ carrying muted I-Aα^κ leaving serine residue at position 57 *(54)*. The same protective effect was also obtained when NOD transgenic mice carried muted Aβ^{nod} resulting in substituting histidine with proline *(53)*. These results suggest that histidine at position 56 may play a role in determination of Aβ^{nod} conformation responsible for diabetogenesis.

Conclusion

The transgenic mouse studies have been extremely useful in the understanding of how immune tolerance is established or broken down, which is the fundamental question underlying the pathogenic processes of IDDM. The advances in our knowledge of human IDDM through transgenic models not only help us understand the basic principle of immune tolerance but also lay out a blueprint for studies of other autoimmune diseases. We are hopeful that from the results of the research via transgenic mice briefly described above and the continuing efforts along these lines, a complete composite picture of IDDM may emerge in the near future, and that genetic manipulation technology can be applied directly to the prevention and the treatment of human IDDM.

References

1. Bell G, Santerre RF, Rutter RJ, Cordell B, Tisscher E, Goodman HM: Sequence of the human insulin gene. *Nature* 284:26–32, 1980.
2. Edlund T, Walker MD, Barr PJ, Rutter WJ: Cell-specific expression of the rat insulin gene: evidence for role of two distinct 5' flanking elements. *Science* 230:912–916, 1985.
3. Hanahan D: Heritable formation of pancreatic β-cell tumours in transgenic mice expressing recombinant insulin/simian virus 40 oncogenes. *Nature* 315:115–122, 1985.
4. Bottazzo GF, Pujol-Borrell, R, Hanafusa T, Feldmann M: Role of aberrant HLA-DR expression and antigen presentation in induction of endocrine autoimmunity. *Lancet* 2:1115–1119, 1983.
5. Nakhooda AF, Like AA, Chappel CI, Wei CN, Marliss EB: The spontaneously diabetic Wister rat (the "BB" rat). *Diabetologia* 14:199–207, 1978.
6. Makino S, Kunimoto K, Muraoka Y, Mizushima Y, Kattagiri K, Tochino Y: Breeding of a nonobese diabetic strain of mice. *Exp Anim* 29:1–13, 1980.
7. Hanahan D: Transgenic mice as probes into complex systems. *Science* 246:1265–1275, 1989.
8. Chisari FV, Klopchin K, Moriyama T, et al.: Molecular pathogenesis of hepatocellular carcinoma in hepatitis B virus transgenic mice. *Cell* 59:1145–1156, 1989.
9. Iwakura Y, Tosu M, Yoshida E, Takiguchi M, Sato K, Kitajima I, et al.: Induction of inflamatory arthropathy resembling rheumatoid arthritis in mice transgenic for HTLV-1. *Science* 253: 1026–1028, 1991.
10. Strasser A, Whittingham S, Vaux DL, Bath ML, Adams JD, Cory S, Harris AW: Enforced BCL2 expression in β-lymphoid cells prolongs antibody responses and elicits autoimmune disease. *Proc Natl Acad Sci USA* 88: 8661–8665, 1991.
11. Lee M-S, Sarvetnick N: Transgenes in autoimmunity. *Curr Opin Immunol* 4: 723–727, 1992.
12. Adams TE, Susan A, Hanahan D: Non-tolerance and autoantibodies to a transgenic self antigen expressed in pancreatic β-cells. *Nature* 325:223–228, 1987.
13. Palmiter RD, Brinster RL: Germ line transformation of mice. *Annu Rev Genet* 20:465–499, 1986.
14. Sarvetnick N, Shizuru J, Liggitt D, Martin L, McIntyre B, Gregory A, Parslow T, Stewart T: Loss of pancreatic islet tolerance induced by β-cell expression of interferon-γ. *Nature* 346:844–847, 1990.
15. Parham P: Intolerable secretion in tolerant transgenic mice. *Nature* 333: 500–503, 1988.
16. Pujol-Borrell R, Bottazzo GF: Puzzling diabetic transgenic mice: a lesson for human type I diabetes? *Immunol Today* 9:303–306, 1988.
17. Lipes MA, Eisenbarth GS: Transgenic mouse models of Type I diabetes. *Diabetes* 39:879–884, 1990.

18. Lo D: Immune responses to tissue-restricted self antigens: studies on T cell tolerance and autoimmunity to pancreatic beta cells. *Curr Topics Microb Immun* 164:71–90, 1990.
19. Slattery R: Transgenic approaches to understanding the role of MHC genes in insulin dependent diabetes mellitus. II. The nonobese diabetic (NOD) mouse. *Bailliere's Clin Endocrinol Metabol* 50:449–454, 1991.
20. Kikutani H, Makino S: The murine autoimmune diabetes model: NOD and related strains. *Adv Immunol* 51:285–322, 1992.
21. Yamamura K-L, Miyazaki T, Uno M, Miyazaki J-I: Transgenic mouse as a tool for the study of autoimmune disease: insulin-dependent diabetes mellitus. *Int J Immunopharmacology* 14:451–455, 1992.
22. Newgard CB: Cellular engineering for the treatment of metabolic disorders: prospects for therapy in diabetes. *Biotechnol* 10:1112–1120, 1992.
23. Eisenbarth GS: Type I diabetes mellitus. A chronic autoimmune disease. *N Engl J Med* 314:1360–136, 1986.
24. Baekkeskov S, Hansen B: Human diabetes. *Curr Topics Microbiol Immunol* 164:1–193, 1990.
25. Bucchini D, Ripoche M-A, Stinnakre MG, Desbois P, Lore D, Montehioux E, Absil J, Lepesant J-A, Pictet R, Jami J: Pancreatic expression of human insulin gene in transgenic mice. *Proc Natl Acad Sci USA* 83:2511–2515, 1986.
26. Seldon RF, Skoskiewicz MJ, Howie KB, Russel PS, Goodman HM: Regulation of human insulin gene expression in transgenic mice. *Nature* 321:525–528, 1986.
27. Roman LM, Simons LF, Hammer RE, Sambrook JF, Gething M-JH: The expression of influenza virus hemagglutinin in the pancreatic β-cells of transgenic mice results in autoimmune diabetes. *Cell* 61:383–396, 1990.
28. Braciale TL, Sweetser MT, Morrison LA, Kittesen DJ, Braciale VL: Class I major histocompatibility complex-restricted cytotoxic T-lymphhocytes recognize a limited number of sites on the influenza hemagglutinin. *Proc Natl Acad Sci USA* 86:277–281, 1989.
29. Oldstone MBA, Nerenberg M, Southern P, Price J, Lewicke H: Virus infection triggers insulin-dependent diabetes mellitus in a transgenic model: role of anti-self (virus) in immune response. *Cell* 65:319–331, 1991.
30. Ohashi PS, Oehen S, Buerki K, Pircher H, Ohashi CT, Odematt B, Malissen B, Zinkernagel RM, Hengartner H: Ablation of tolerance and induction of diabetes by viral infection in viral antigen transgenic mice. *Cell* 65:305–317, 1991.
31. Schonrich G, Kallinke U, Momburg F, Malissen M, Schmitt-Verhuist A-M, Malissen B, Hammerling GJ, Arnold B: Down-regulation of T cell receptors on self-reactive T cells as a novel mechanism for extrathymic tolerance induction. *Cell* 65:293–304, 1991.
32. Lo D, Freedman J, Hesse S, Palmiter RD, Brinster RL, Sherman LA: Peripheral tolerance to an islet cell-specific hemagglutinin transgene affects both CD4+ and CD8+ T cell. *Eur J Immunol* 22:1013–1022, 1992.

33. Harrison LC: Transgenic approaches to understanding the role of MHC genes in insulin dependent diabetes mellitus. Immune and nonimmune mechanisms of B cell destruction. *Bailliere's Clin Endocrinol Metabol* 5: 439–448, 1991.
34. Bottazzo GF, Dean BM, McNally JM, MacKay EH, Switt PGF, Gamble DR: In situ characterization of autoimmune phenomenon and expression of HLA molecules in the pancreas of diabetic insulitis. *N Engl J Med* 313:353–360, 1985.
35. Foulis AK, Farguharson MA, Hardman R: Abberant expression of class II major histocompatibility complex molecules by B cells and hyperexpression of class I major histocompatibility complex molecules by insulin containing islets in type 1 (insulin dependent) diabetes mellitus. *Diabetologia* 30:333–343, 1987.
36. Allison J, Campbell IL, Morahan G, Mandel TE, Harrison LC, Miller JFAP: Diabetes in transgenic mice resulting from over-expression of class I histocompatibility molecules in pancreatic B cells. *Nature* 333:529–533, 1988.
37. Lo D, Burkly LC, Widera G, Cowing C, Flavell RA, Palmiter RD, Brinster RL: Diabetes and tolerance in transgenic mice expressing class II MHC molecules in pancreatic B cells. *Cell* 53:159–168, 1988.
38. Sarvetnick N, Liggitt D, Pitts SL, Hansen SE, Stewart TA: Insulin-dependent diabetes mellitus induced in transgenic mice by expression of class II MHC and interferon-γ. *Cell* 52:773–782, 1988.
39. Bohme J, Haskins K, Stecha P, van Ewijk W, LeMeur M, Gerlinger P, Benoist C, Mathis D: Transgenic with I-A on islet cells are normoglycemic but immunologically intolerant. *Science* 244:1179–1183, 1989.
40. Miller JFAP, Allison J, Morahan G: Tolerance and diabetes in transgenic mice over-expressing class I histocompatibility molecules in pancreatic β cells. *J Autoimm* 3(suppl):87–90, 1990.
41. Gortz J, Eibel H, Kohler G: Non-tolerance and differential susceptibility to diabetes in transgenic mice expressing major histocompatibility class II genes on pancreatic B cells. *Eur J Immunol* 20:1677–1683, 1990.
42. Allison J, Malcolm L, Culvenor J, Bartholomeusz RK, Holmberg K, Miller JFAP: Overexpression of B2-microglobulin in transgenic mouse islet β-cell results in defective insulin secretion. *Proc Natl Acad Sci USA* 88:2070–2074, 1991.
43. Campbell IL, Harrison LC: Molecular pathology of type I diabetes. *Mol Biol Med* 7:299–309, 1990.
44. Harrison LC, Campbell IL, Colman PG, Chosich N, Kay TWH, Tait BD, et al.: Type 1 diabetes: Immune mechanisms and immune therapies. *Adv Endocrinol Metabol* 1:35–94, 1990.
45. Sarvetnick N, Shizuru J, Liggitt D, Stewart T: Inflammatory destruction of pancreatic β cells in γ-interferon transgenic mice. *Cold Spring Harbor Symp Quant Biol* 54:837–842, 1989.
46. Morahan G, Allison J, Miller JFAP: Tolerance of class I histocompatibility antigen expressed extrathymically. *Nature* 339:622–624, 1989.

47. Allison J, Malcolm L, Chosich N, Miller JFAP: Inflammation but not autoimmunity occurs in transgenic mice expressing constitutive levels of interleukin-2 in islet β cells. *Eur J Immunol* 22:1115–1121, 1992.
48. Heath WR, Allison J, Hoffman MW, Schoenrich G, Haemmering G, Arnold B, Miller JFAP: Autoimmune diabetes as a consequence of locally produced interleukin-2. *Nature* 359:547–549, 1992.
49. Higuchi Y, Herrera P, Muniesa P, Huarte J, Belin D, Ohashi P, Aichele P, Orci L, Vassalli J-D, Vassalli P: Expression of a tumor necrosis factor a transgene in murine pancreatic β cells results in severe and permanent insulitis without evolution towards diabetes. *J Exp Med* 176:1719–1731, 1992.
50. Nishimoto H, Kikutani H, Yamamura K, Kishimoto T: Prevention of autoimmune insulitis by expression of I-E molecules in NOD mice. *Nature* 328:432-434, 1987.
51. Bohme J, Schuhbaur B, Kanagawa O, Benoist C, Mathis D: MHC-linked protection from diabetes dissociated from clonal deletion of T-cells. *Science* 249:293–295,1990.
52. Uehira M, Uno M, Kurner T et al.: Development of autoimmune insulitis is prevented in $E\alpha^d$ but not $A_\beta{}^\kappa$ NOD transgenic mice. *Int Immunol* 1:209–213, 1989.
53. Lund T, O'Reilly L, Hutchings P, Kanagawa O, Simpson E, Gravely R, et al.: Prevention of insulin dependent diabetes mellitus in nonobese diabetic mice by transgenes encoding modified I-A beta chain or I-E alpha chain. *Nature* 345:727–729,1990.
54. Miyazaki T, Uno M, Uehira M, Kikutani H, Kishimoto T, Kimoto M, Nishimoto H, Miyazaki J, Yamamura K: Direct evidence of the contribution of the unique $I\text{-}A^{nod}$ to the development of insulitis in nonobese diabetic mice. *Nature* 345:722–724,1990.

Chapter 3

Pancreatic Islet Transplantation

Ronald G. Gill

Introduction

Type I diabetes represents a unique problem for the field of transplantation. The rationale for pancreatic islet grafting is to prevent the debilitating complications associated with the disease process. Indeed, islet transplantation has been shown to prevent or arrest diabetic complications *(1–3)*. However, unlike other conditions of end-stage organ failure where transplantation is necessary, diabetes is not immediately life-threatening with the advent of exogenous insulin therapy. Thus, for type I diabetes, the risks associated with current regimens of immunosuppression used in transplantation, such as nephrotoxicity, opportunistic infections, and neoplasia, may rival the consequences of disease-associated complications. Therefore, the criteria for islet transplantation in diabetic recipients prior to the manifestations of disease complications must be more stringent than those for patients with other forms of organ failure. This problem is reflected by the current status of clinical islet transplantation where islet grafts are usually performed in diabetic patients receiving simultaneous solid organ grafts (usually kidney) with concomitant immunosuppression *(4)*. The future goal of islet transplantation, however, must be the grafting of islets in the diabetic recipient prior to the onset of disease complications using minimal host immunosuppression.

From: *Molecular Biology of Diabetes, Part I*
Edited by: B. Draznin and D. LeRoith

Technical advances in pancreatic islet isolation and purification are making islet transplantation an increasingly feasible treatment for type I diabetes *(4)*. However, three important obstacles hamper the routine use of islet grafting in diabetes. Two of these barriers result from immune-mediated damage to the graft: *transplantation immunity*, resulting in graft rejection, and *disease recurrence*, the reenactment of the underlying autoimmune pathogenesis that can destroy islet grafts both in humans *(5)* and in animal models of autoimmune diabetes, the NOD mouse *(6)*, and the BB rat *(7)*. The nature of disease pathogenesis in islet transplants is a focus of another contribution of this edition *(8)*, and so will not be primarily addressed here. A third, more logistical problem in islet transplantation results from the shortage of available clinical tissue for transplantation. This problem requires the consideration of tissue from other species (xenografts) as a potential source of donor material. This discussion will center on the nature of the immune response, which results in the rejection of islet allografts and xenografts. Understanding of the processes resulting in islet damage will be crucial for developing future strategies to circumvent these responses.

The Role of MHC Antigens in Allograft Immunity: The Transplantation Paradox

The Two-Signal Hypothesis for T-Cell Activation

According to the classic view of allograft immunity, major histocompatibility complex (MHC) antigens are inherently strong immunogens, and binding of these antigens drives T-cell activation *(9)*. Although allograft rejection clearly represents a response to transplantation antigen, especially MHC antigen, there has been a persistent problem with this classic view. Early attempts to isolate and characterize transplantation antigens found them to be quite weak immunogens *(10)*. Later studies by Batchelor et al. *(11)* demonstrated that MHC antigens, either class I or class II, isolated from the cell surface were poor immunogens. These observations lead us to a *transplantation paradox*: Allograft immunity represents a violent response to antigens that are inherently weak immunogens.

The solution to this paradox was provided by the proposition of Lafferty and Cunningham that two signals were required for T-cell activation *(12)*, a concept derived from the original two-signal model

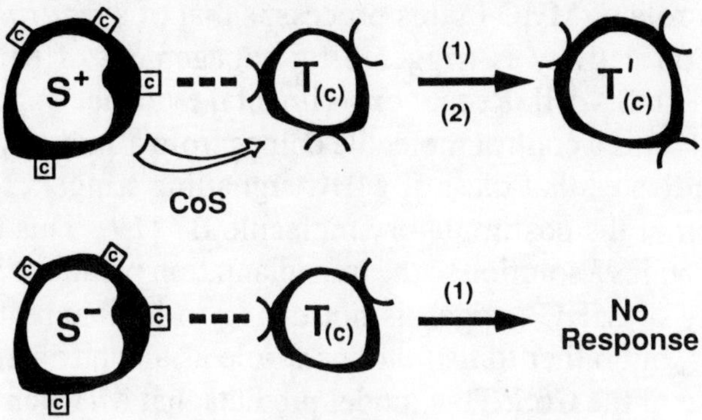

Fig. 1. The stimulator cell model. Alloantigens presented by an S+ cell will provide a source of both signals (antigen and costimulator) required for T-cell activation (T-cell specificity indicated by the parentheses). Alloantigen presented on the surface of an S– cell will not be directly immunogenic because these cells cannot provide a source of the second signal. According to this model, costimulator activity is triggered by engagement of a control structure ("C") on the surface of the S+ cell.

for self-nonself discrimination developed by the Bretscher/Cohn model *(13)*. According to the Lafferty/Cunningham model, signal one (antigen) was provided by binding of the T-cell receptor and signal two was provided by an inductive molecule, or *costimulator* (CoS), produced by a metabolically active antigen-presenting cell (APC), or *stimulator* cell (Fig. 1). Whereas previous studies showed that cytokines can demonstrate CoS activity in vitro *(14)*, recent work has brought attention to the role of the accessory molecule interactions between T-cells and APC involved in providing costimulatory signals required for T-cell activation. Key cell-surface molecules involved in this process are CD28 *(15)* and CTLA-4 *(16)*, which are expressed by T-cells interacting with the B7/BB1 molecule, which are in turn expressed by APCs and activated B-cells *(17)*. Other accessory molecules expressed by APCs, such as ICAM-1 and LFA-3 *(18)*, may also have important costimulatory functions. Regardless of the exact nature of costimulatory signals, cells capable of exhibiting CoS activity will have a stimulatory (S+) phenotype, whereas other cells, such as tissue parenchymal cells, which express the same antigens but do not produce CoS activity, will have a nonstimulatory phenotype (S-).

The role of MHC in this process is that of a *control* structure; that is, CoS activity is triggered by engagement of MHC on the surface of an S+ cell. Recent experimental evidence supporting the role of MHC as a control molecule comes from a study by Nabavi et al. that indicates that class II MHC signalling triggers the surface expression of the costimulatory molecule B7 *(19)*. This two-signal model provides a solution to the transplantation paradox. The immunogenicity of MHC antigen is not owing to its inherent antigenic properties, but rather to its *functional* role as a control structure for the release of the CoS. This model predicts that MHC antigens will only be immunogenic while on the surface of metabolically active S+ cells; isolated MHC antigens or MHC antigens on the surface of S– cells will not be immunogenic. The significant contribution of this two-signal hypothesis to transplantation biology is the concept that alloantigen alone is not the barrier to allografting. Rather, tissue immunogenicity will be a function of S+ cells, or "passenger leukocytes," resident within the graft *(20)*.

Alteration of Tissue Immunogenicity

The notion that alloantigen presentation between S+ and S– cells within the graft represents qualitatively different forms of antigen presentation led back to an early concept that graft immunogenicity can be reduced by appropriate tissue pretreatment *(10)*. That is, selective depletion of S+ cells within the graft should lead to prolonged graft acceptance. Tissue pretreatment has been strikingly successful for facilitating allograft acceptance of endocrine tissues. Work in the mid 1970s indicated that pretreatment of thyroid tissues in 95% O_2 culture would facilitate long-term graft acceptance in nonimmunosuppressed, allogeneic recipient mice *(21)*. This technique later was applied for the modification of pancreatic islet allograft immunogenicity *(22)*. Grafting experimentally induced diabetic mice with untreated islet allografts results in an initial return to euglycemia followed by a rapid return to hyperglycemia owing to graft rejection. Following organ culture in 95% O_2 for 7 d, islet allografts survive and function indefinitely in recipient mice *(22)*. Application of 95% O_2 culture has also allowed successful islet allografting in rats *(23)* and even in outbred mice *(24)*, though short-term immunosuppression with Cyclosporine A was necessary for long-term graft survival in this later study.

Table 1
Approaches to Successful Islet Allografting Through Modulation of Islet Tissue Immunogenicity

Tissue pretreatment	Reference
High O_2 culture	*22*
Low temperature (24°C) culture	*26*
Ultraviolet irradiation	*25*
Low pH Culture	*30*
Anti-class II or anti-dendritic cell antibodies	*27–29*
Perinatal islet harvesting	*31*

A variety of other tissue pretreatment techniques have likewise led to long-term islet allograft acceptance (Table 1). Graft pretreatment with ultraviolet irradiation *(25)*, low temperature culture *(26)*, anti-Ia, or dentritic cell antibodies *(27–29)*, and low pH media *(30)* have all facilitated islet allograft acceptance. Hegre and coworkers *(31)* have shown that perinatal rat islets isolated by in vitro cultivation are accepted in nonimmunosuppressed, allogeneic recipients. Further, appropriate graft pretreatment techniques have led to prolonged graft acceptance of a variety of tissues, including thyroid and parathyroid *(21,32,33)*, ovarian tissue *(34)*, and keratinocytes *(35)*. Taken together, a wide range of techniques with a variety of donor-recipient strain combinations indicate that allograft acceptance can be facilitated by appropriate pretreatment of the graft.

Antigenicity vs Immunogenicity of MHC Alloantigens

A key question centers on the mechanism whereby pretreated tissues survive in immunocompetent, allogeneic recipients. Is the immunogenicity of cultured grafts altered by the modulation of graft antigens *(36,37)*, or the elimination/inactivation of passenger leukocytes (S+ cells)? This issue has become important because of the finding that hyperbaric oxygen culture of thyroid tissue leads to reduced antigen expression of the graft *(32,38)*. Studies by Hullet et al. *(32)* show that thyroid grafts cultured in hyperbaric oxygen survive even in recipient mice primed against donor antigens. These results indicate that the regulation of graft antigen expression may play a role in subsequent graft survival. Although antigen modulation may occur during some forms of organ culture, a number of studies indicate that this modulation in not *necessary* for allograft acceptance. That is, loss of immunogenicity does not require a loss of antigenicity in the graft.

Experiments from Batchelor's laboratory studied the role of antigen expression in long-term kidney allograft survival. These investigators demonstrated that kidney grafts would survive in immunologically enhanced, allogeneic recipient rats. When such long-surviving kidney allografts were transplanted from the primary to a secondary recipient of the same haplotype, the kidney did not elicit alloimmunity in the untreated, secondary recipient *(39)*. Significantly, the failure of long-surviving kidney grafts to activate a rejection response could not be attributed to a lack of either class I or class II antigen expression in the graft *(40)*, leading these investigators to conclude that the effect resulted from a loss of donor-derived passenger leukocytes in the graft while in the primary recipient. They later showed that immunization with donor strain dendritic cells (a source of S+ cells) in very low numbers would trigger rejection of the established kidney graft *(40)*. Clearly, the antigens of the grafted kidney could not elicit alloimmunity but could serve as a target of immune destruction once the animal was primed.

Islet allografts cultured in 95% O_2 also are vulnerable to rejection by active immunization of the recipient *(41)*. Challenge of the recipient animal with donor-type S+ cells during the immediate post-transplant period triggers acute rejection of the established islet graft. Active immunization of the host also triggers the rejection of established cultured thyroid *(42)* and keratinocyte *(35)* allografts. These results illustrate the distinction between graft antigenicity and immunogenicity; the cultured graft cannot trigger allograft immunity but can serve as a target for immune destruction.

The issue of class II MHC immunogenicity was elegantly examined by Markmann et al. *(43)*. These investigators studied the response to fetal pancreas grafts from trangenic mice expressing a class II MHC alloantigen (I-E) under control of the insulin promoter (ins-I-E), leading to tissue-specific, ectopic expression of the I-E molecule on the surface of pancreatic islet β-cells. Importantly, the I-E class II MHC molecule was expressed on islet parenchymal cells and not on hematopoietic (S+) cells *(44)*. Despite high expression of the transgene on the β-cell surface, such fetal pancreas grafts did not trigger allommunity in I-E$^-$ parental strain mice. However, immunizing recipient mice with I-E+ spleen cells (a source of S+ cells) triggered prompt rejection of the ins-I-E graft, indicating that the ins-I-E fetal pancreas could serve as a target for immune destruction. What these experiments clearly demonstrated was that class II MHC antigen was not inherently immunogenic and so was not sufficient to trigger allograft immunity.

La Rosa *(38)* tested the relationship between donor antigen expression and the survival of cultured thyroid allografts. In these experiments thyroid grafts were cultured in 95% O_2 to reduce tissue immunogenicity. These cultured thyroid grafts were then grafted directly or were pretreated with γ-interferon (γ-IFN) to induce high levels of class I MHC antigen expression on the graft. Whereas fresh (uncultured) thyroid grafts were uniformly rejected, the acceptance of cultured grafts was not altered with γ-IFN treatment of the graft. That is, acceptance of the cultured graft was not owing simply to the alteration of antigen expression. Our own experiments using γ-IFN-treated cultured islet allografts also indicate that the enhanced expression of class I MHC molecules on islet tissue does not increase the rejection response (unpublished observations).

Taken together, these varied studies indicate that neither class I nor class II MHC alloantigens are the primary barrier to allografting. Given that the goal of islet transplanation is to eliminate or reduce the immunosuppression of the recipient, tissue pretreatment aimed at eliminating S+ cells from the graft may, at least in part, be a useful tool in future clinical islet allografting.

Pancreatic Islet Xenografting: The Xenograft Paradox

A major dilemma facing clinical organ and tissue grafting is the shortage of donor tissue for transplantation. This problem requires the consideration of tissues from other species (xenografts) as a potential source of donor material. The classification by Calne *(45)* denoted xenografts as discordant or concordant based on the presence or absence, respectively, of preformed or natural antibodies against the donor. Such natural antibodies correlate with the phylogenetic disparity between species and are thought to be responsible for the initiation of hyperacute rejection that occurs between discordant species combinations *(46,47)*. Although hyperacute rejection presents a major barrier to the survival of anastomosed solid-organ xenografts, neovascularized xenografts—such as skin and cellular transplants—generally do not appear sensitive to hyperacute rejection but rather involve cellular immunity *(46,48)*. The relative lack of vulnerability of cellular xenografts to hyperacute rejection is probably owing to the fact that the graft vasculature is of *host* rather than *donor* origin; donor vascular endothelium appears to be a major target of antibody-mediated hyperacute rejection *(46,47)*. A variety of evidence indicates that cellular immunity to xenogeneic tissues can be *qualitatively* distinct from the response to allogeneic tissues.

Understanding of the cellular immune response to xenogeneic tissues is less clear than is understanding of the allograft response as illustrated by an important paradox concerning xenoreactivity: Although cellular xenograft immunity in vivo—apart from hyperacute rejection—is generally more vigorous than allograft rejection *(46,48,49)*, the intensity of the T-cell-dependent response to xenogeneic antigen presenting cells in vitro tends to *decrease* as the phylogenetic disparity between stimulating and responding species increases *(48–52)*. This hyporeactivity of the interspecies T-cell-APC interaction in vitro could be attributed to three primary defects in the response:

1. Low precursor frequency. The view that the T-cell receptor (TcR) repertoire is positively selected in the thymus using the MHC of the species as a template *(53)* would leave the possibility that the frequency of xenoreactive T-cells might be quite low relative to the high precursor frequency of alloreactive T-cells. This possibility would account for the low xenoreactive precursor frequency on a quantitative basis.
2. Species-specific accessory/coreceptor molecule interactions. A number of cell surface molecules, in addition to the antigen-specific TcR, facilitate T-cell activation. For example, the CD4 and CD8 coreceptor molecules, which characterize T-cell subsets, interact with conserved regions of class I and class II MHC molecules, respectivley *(54)*. Importantly, the interaction of these accessory/coreceptor molecules with their respective ligands can display species-specificity. The interaction of CD4 and CD8 with MHC molecules from different species can be quite weak. Although human CD4 is capable of functionally associating with mouse class II *(55)* the reciprocal binding of

mouse CD4 to human class II is quite weak *(56,57)*. Further, the association of CD8 with the α3 domain of class I MHC also displays species-specificity between human and mouse *(58,59)*.

3. Species-specificity of cytokines required for T-cell activation. A number of cytokines exhibit species specificity/preference such that cytokines necessary for T-cell activation may not function across particular species barriers *(50,51)*. Studies addressing these issues have found that reconstitution of xenoreactivity in vitro can occur through restoring appropriate accessory/coreceptor molecule interactions *(57–60)* or by the addition of the relevant responder-type cytokines *(50,51)*. Such studies indicate that the potential frequency of xenospecific T-cells may be fairly high, with the lack of reactivity being a result of species-specific interactions that are secondary to the TcR repertoire.

"Direct" vs "Indirect" Antigen Presentation

In light of these deficiencies in the xenogeneic T-cell-APC interaction, a key question is: How does a low reactivity in vitro account for the violent reactivity in vivo? One solution to this paradox can be inferred by considering the consequence of two pathways of host sensitization by the graft, *direct* (donor APC-dependent), and *indirect* (host APC-dependent) presentation (Fig. 2). Direct antigen presentation would be the result of host T-cell recognition and activation by donor-derived APC. It is this pathway of activation that is expected to be sensitive to the species-specific interactions required for T-cell activation mentioned above. The indirect pathway would involve the processing and presentation of graft antigens by host APCs. Although this indirect (responder APC-dependent) pathway can occur in allorecognition *(61)*, some xenogeneic combinations may depend on this pathway for T-cell activation. The operation of the indirect pathway in xenoreactivity is shown by the observation that the mouse antihuman *(62)* and human-antimouse *(63)* responses in vitro require responder-type APCs. Allogeneic responses, or some xenogeneic combinations such as mouse antirat, do not require responder-type APCs *(49)*.

The function of the indirect (host APC-dependent) pathway may solve the xenograft paradox: Although the xenogeneic APC cannot activate responding T-cells via the direct pathway, the antigenic disparity of the xenograft relative to the host might favor a

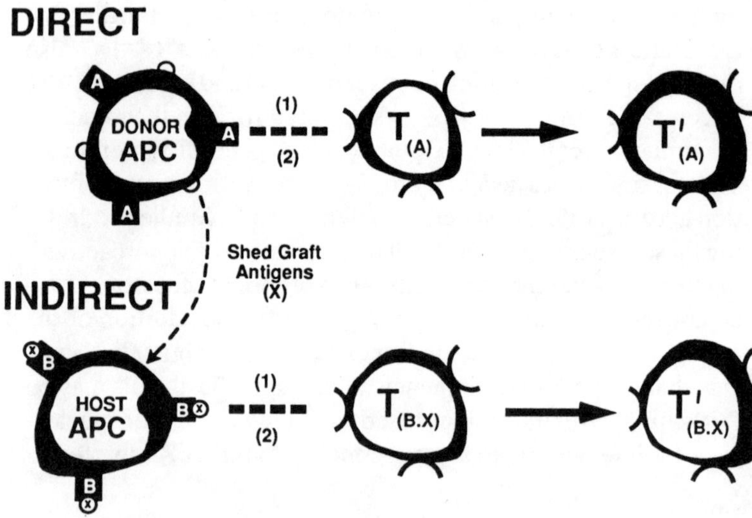

Fig. 2. Direct vs indirect antigen presentation. *Direct* Antigen Presentation: Donor-type APC of genotype ("A") to T-cells along with an appropriate second signal (costimulator) required for T-cell activation (T-cell specificity indicated by the parentheses). Such a T-cell will be specific for graft antigens directly on the surface of donor cells. *Indirect* Antigen Presentation: Graft antigens, generically termed "x," will be processed by host-type APC of genotype "B" and presented in association with class II MHC. Responsive T-cells will not be directly graft specific but rather specific for graft antigens in association with host class II MHC (specificity "B.x").

strong response to antigens processed by host APC. This form of xenopresentation would be expected to activate host CD4 T-cells specific for xenogeneic antigens in the context of self class II MHC. The function of this indirect pathway may explain why xenograft rejection is more dependent on CD4 T-cells than is allograft rejection in some cases *(64–66)*.

Role of T-Cell Subsets in Islet Graft Rejection: A Central Role for CD4 T-Cells

It is clear that both islet allograft *(67,68)* and xenograft *(65,66,69,70)* rejection are heavily dependent on the function of CD4 T-cells. However, this does not mean that the role of the CD4 cell is the same in each case. Three possible functions for the CD4 T-cell can be envisioned in the rejection process (Fig. 3):

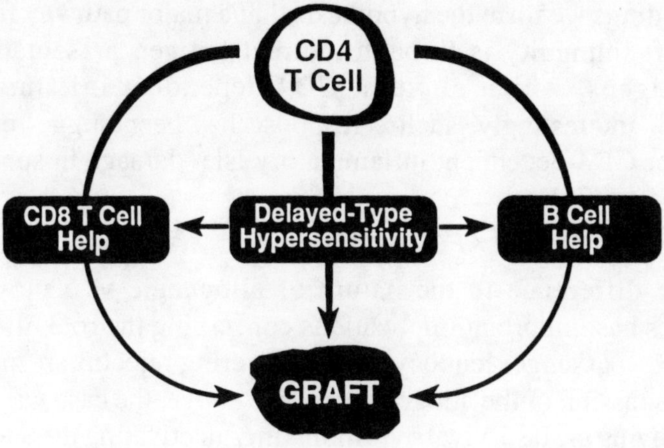

Fig. 3. Possible roles for class II MHC-restricted CD4 T-cells in the rejection response.

1. A helper cell for the activation of CD8 T-cells that in turn mediate graft destruction;
2. A helper cell for antibody-producing B-cells, leading to a graft-specific antibody response; or
3. An effector cell mediating islet graft destruction by direct interaction with the graft and/or through inflammatory tissue damage *(71,72)*.

A difference in the role of CD4 T-cells in islet xenograft vs allograft immunity is demonstrated by examining the requirement for other lymphocyte subpopulations in these responses. Unlike islet allograft immunity, xenograft immunity does not appear to require class I MHC-restricted CD8 T-cells *(66)*. Our cell transfer studies into severe-combined-immune-deficient C.B-17 SCID mice show that although CD4 T-cells are both necessary and sufficient to reconstitute these animals for islet xenograft immunity, islet allograft immunity requires both CD4 and CD8 T-cells (Gill et al.; in preparation). B-cells were not required for either response. Furthermore, other studies show that islet allografts from transgenic mice that are deficient in class I MHC expression enjoy prolonged survival as allografts but are acutely rejected as xenografts *(73)*. Taken together, these results indicate that neither CD8 T-cells nor their corresponding class I MHC target antigens are required for islet xenograft rejection. From these findings we form the hypothesis that a major pathway for islet xenograft immunity is through indirect antigen presentation of xenoantigens, which elicits a CD4-dependent inflammatory response. Interestingly, such a response has been suggested as a model for CD4-dependent inflammatory islet damage in spontaneous diabetes *(71)*.

The Role of Donor APCs in Allograft vs Xenograft Immunity

The difference in the nature of allogeneic vs xenogeneic responses has important implications concerning the role of donor-type APC (passenger leukocytes) in triggering rejection responses. In the discussion of the allograft response above, the case was made for improving graft survival by eliminating/inactivating the S+ APCs within the graft that were responsible for triggering host immunity. Implicit in this approach is the assumption that the indirect pathway, the presentation of graft antigens by host-type APC, is not a major pathway for eliciting a graft-destructive response (Fig. 2). Empirically, the observation that APC-depleted of islet allografts survive in nonimmunosuppressed recipients is consistent with this concept. The xenograft, however, represents a different situation. If the xenograft response is primarily a function of the indirect pathway of antigen presentation (Fig. 2), then the host response should be dependent on host-type, and not donor-type APC. This predicts that removal of APCs from islet xenografts should have little influence on the rejection response. This issue remains controversial in that our studies suggest that APC-depleted xenografts are rejected *(49)*, whereas other studies have shown a benefit to islet xenograft survival through tissue pretreatment *(69,70)*. Thus, a potential for pretreating xenogeneic tissues to reduce immunogenicity remains to be clarified.

Islet Xenografting in Autoimmune Diabetes

An important goal for islet xenotransplantation will be grafting in spontaneous, autoimmune diabetes. Previous studies show that the recurrence of disease in islet grafts in NOD mice is CD4 T-cell-dependent *(72)*. Combined with the finding that islet xenograft immunity is CD4 T-cell dependent, anti-CD4 therapy should facilitate xenograft survival in diabetic autoimmune NOD mice. This has been shown to be the case for fetal pig pancreas xenografts *(74,75)*. An important aspect of these results was that xenografts actually

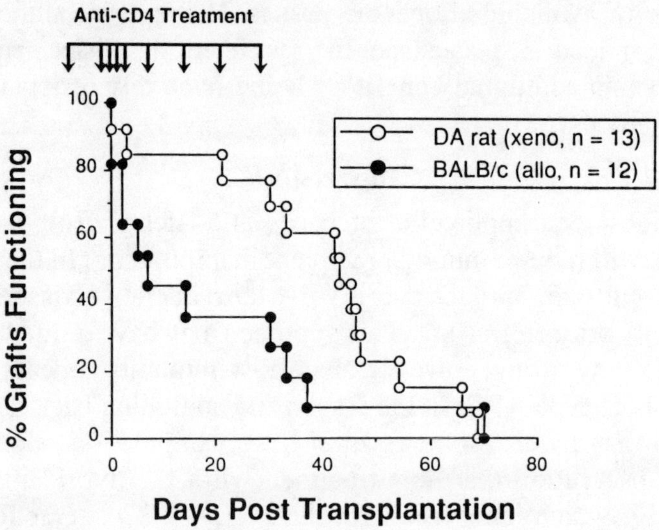

Fig 4. Allograft vs xenograft survival in anti-CD4 treated nonobese diabetic (NOD) mice. Spontaneously diabetic NOD mice were treated with a monoclonal anti-CD4 antibody (GK1.5; 10 mg/kg/d) on the indicated day relative to transplantation. Recipients were grafted with 450 untreated pancreatic islet allografts (Balb/c) or xenografts (DA rat) on d 0 and graft function assessed by the restoration of euglycemia. Rat xenograft survival was significantly longer ($p < .05$) than Balb/c allograft survival. All islet allografts and xenografts functioned for <8 d in untreated NOD mice (not shown).

showed superior survival relative to allografts in anti-CD4 treated NOD mice. We have generated similar results whereby rat islet xenografts show prolonged function relative to Balb/c islet allografts in anti-CD4-treated diabetic NOD mice (Fig. 4). On one hand, such results may reflect the fact that xenograft immunity is more exquisitely CD4-dependent than is allograft immunity. However, another hypothesis is that the disease process displays a degree of species-specificity; that is, islet reactive T-cells from NOD mice may preferentially recognize murine islet-associated antigens. This concept is supported by the finding by Haskins et al. that a panel of islet-reactive T-cell clones derived from NOD mice show little crossreactivity with islet antigens from differing species *(76)*. The key rationale for considering islet xenotransplantation has generally been to fill the shortage of available allogeneic tissues. However, if autoimmune diabetes indeed is species-specific/restricted, then islet xenografts may have an additional benefit by being relatively resistant to the disease process.

Conclusions

Widespread application of pancreatic islet grafting in type I diabetes will require minimal recipient manipulation. In the case of allografting, one approach may involve the reduction of tissue immunogenicity prior to grafting. This approach may have limited benefit for islet xenografting, however, since host immunity appears dependent on host-type APCs in the response. Facilitating islet xenograft survival may require some form of host manipulation, such as the recent observation that host treatment with the hybrid molecule CTLA4Ig, which interferes with the CTLA-4/B7 interaction, can result in long-term islet xenograft survival *(77)*. This result, along with other reports whereby long-term islet xenograft survival is accomplished by transient host treatment *(69,70,75,78,79)*, makes islet xenografting an exciting area of future study.

Acknowledgment

This work was supported in part by PHS grants R01 #DK45773 and DK33470.

References

1. Gray BN, Watkins E: Prevention of vascular complications of diabetes by pancreatic islet transplantation. *Arch Surg* 111:254–257, 1976.
2. Federlin KF, Bretzel RG: The effect of islet transplantation on complications in experimental diabetes of the rat. *World J Surg* 8:169–178, 1984.
3. Woehrle M, Spitzer D, Linn T, Federlin K, Bretzel RG: The effect of early islet transplantation on prevention of nephropathy in the spontaneously diabetic BB rat. *Transplant Proc* 22:819–820, 1990.
4. Warnock GL, Rajotte RV: Human pancreatic islet transplantation. *Transplant Rev* 6:195–208, 1992.
5. Sutherland DER, Sibley R, Xu XZ, Srikanta MS, Taub F, Najarian J, Goetz FC: Twin-to-twin pancreas transplantation: reversal and reenactment of the pathogenesis of type I diabetes. *Trans Assoc Am Phys* 97:80–87, 1984.
6. Terada M, Lennartz K, Mullen Y: Allogeneic and syngeneic pancreas transplantation in non-obese diabetic mice. *Transplant Proc* 19:960–961, 1987.
7. Naji A, Silvers WK, Kimura H, Anderson AO, Barker CF: Influence of islet and bond marrow transplantation on the diabetes and immunodeficiency of BB rats. *Metabolism* 32(Suppl1):62–68, 1983.

8. Calcinaro F, Wegmann DR, Lafferty KJ: Pathogenesis of Autoimmune Diabetes (in this volume).
9. Medawar PB: *The Uniqueness of the Individual* (2nd rev ed), Dover, New York, pp. 1–155, 1957.
10. Snell GD: The homograft reaction. *Ann Rev Microbiol* 11:439–458, 1957.
11. Batchelor JR, Welsh K, Burgos H: Transplantation antigens per se are poor immunogens within a species. *Nature* 273:54–56, 1978.
12. Lafferty KJ, Cunningham AJ: A new analysis of allogeneic interactions *Aust J Exp Biol Med Sci* 53:27–42, 1975.
13. Bretscher P, Cohn M: A theory of self-nonself discrimination. *Science* 169:1042–1049, 1970.
14. Talmage DW, Woolnough JA, Hemmingsen H, Lopez L, Lafferty KJ: Activation of cytotoxic T cells by nonstimulating tumor cells and spleen cell factor(s). *Proc Natl Acad Sci USA* 74:1610–1614, 1977.
15. June CH, Ledbetter JA, Linsley PS, Thompson CB: Role of the CD28 receptor in T-cell activation. *Immunol Today* 11:211–216, 1990.
16. Linsley PS, Brady W, Urnes M, Grosmarie LS, Damle NK, Ledbetter JA: CTLA-4 is a second receptor for the B cell activation antigen B7. *J Exp Med* 174:561–569, 1991.
17. Schwartz RH: Costimulation of T lymphocytes: the role of CD28, CTLA-4, and B7/BB1 in interleukin-2 production and immunotherapy. *Cell* 71:1065–1068, 1992.
18. Kamle NK, Klussman K, Linsley PS, Aruffo A: Differential costimulatory effects of adhesion molecules B7, ICAM-1, LFA-3, and VCAM-1 on resting and antigen-primed CD4+ T lymphocytes. *J Immunol* 148:1985–1992, 1992.
19. Nabavi N, Freeman GJ, Gault A, Godfrey D, Nadler LM, Glimcher LH: Signalling through the MHC class II cytoplasmic domain is required for antigen presentation and induces B7 expression. *Nature* 360:266–268, 1992.
20. Lafferty KJ, Prowse SJ, Simeonovic CJ: Immunobiology of tissue transplantation: a return to the passenger leukocyte concept. *Ann Rev Immunol* 1:143–173, 1983.
21. Lafferty KJ, Bootes A, Dart G, Talmage DW: Effect of organ culture on the survival of thyroid allografts in mice. *Transplantation* 22:138–149, 1976.
22. Bowen KM, Andrus L, Lafferty KJ: Successful allotransplantation of mouse pancreatic islets to nonimmunosuppressed recipients. *Diabetes* 29:98–104, 1980.
23. Haug CE, Gill RG, Babcock SK, Lafferty KJ, Bellgrau D, Weil RW III: Cyclosporine-induced tolerance requires antigens capable of initiating an immune response. *J Immunol* 139:2947–2949, 1987.
24. Simeonovic CJ, Prowse SJ, Lafferty KJ: Survival and function of islet allografts in outbred mice. *Transplant Proc* 18:316–318, 1986.
25. Lau H, Reemtsma K, Hardy MA: Prolongation of rat islet allograft survival by direct ultraviolet irradiation of the graft. *Science* 223:607–608, 1984.
26. Lacy PE, Davie JM, Finke EH, Scharp DW: Prolongation of islet allograft survival. *Transplantation* 27:171–174, 1979.

27. Faustman D, Hauptfeld V, Lacy P, Davie J: Prolongation of murine islet allograft survival by pretreatment of islets with antibody directed to Ia determinants. *Proc Natl Acad Sci USA* 78:5156–5159, 1981.
28. Morrow CE, Sutherland DER, Steffes MW, Najarian JS, Bach FH: Lack of donor-specific tolerance in mice with established anti-Ia-treated islet allografts. *Transplantation* 36:691–694, 1983.
29. Faustman DL, Steinman RM, Gebel HM, Hauptfeld V, Davie JM, Lacy, PE: Prevention of rejection of murine islet allografts by pretreatment with anti-dendritic cell antibody. *Proc Natl Acad Sci USA* 81:3864–3868, 1984.
30. La Rosa FG: Abrogation of mouse pancreatic islet allograft rejection by a four-day culture. *Transplantation* 46:330–333, 1988.
31. Hegre OD, Hickey GE, Marshall S, Serie JR: Modification of allograft immunogenicity in perinatal islets isolated and purified in vitro. *Transplantation* 37:227–233, 1984.
32. Hullett DA, Landry AS, Leonard DK, Sollinger HW: Enhancement of thyroid allograft survival following organ culture. *Transplantation* 47:24–27, 1989.
33. La Rosa FG, Talmage DW: The abrogation of thyroid allograft rejection by culture in acid medium. *Transplantation* 44:592, 1987.
34. Jacobs BB: Ovarian allograft survival. *Transplantation* 18:454–457, 1974.
35. Punit SR, Sharp RJ, Yeoman H, Stanley MA: The influence of MHC-compatible and MHC-incompatible antigen-presenting cells on the survival of MHC-compatible cultured murine keratinocyte allografts. *Transplantation* 48:676–680, 1989.
36. Woodruff MFA, Woodruff HG: The transplantation of normal tissues: with special reference to auto and homotransplants of thyroid and spleen in the anterior chamber of the eye, and subcutaneously, in guinea-pigs. *Phil Trans R Soc Lond* 234:560–583, 1950.
37. Jacobs BB, Huseby RA: Growth of tumors in allogeneic hosts following organ culture explantation. *Transplantation* 5:410–419, 1967.
38. La Rosa FG, Talmage DW: Major histocompatibility complex antigen expression on parenchymal cells of thyroid allografts is not by itself sufficient to induce rejection. *Transplantation* 49:605–609, 1990.
39. Batchelor J, Welsh K, Maynard A, Burgos H: Failure of long surviving, passively enhanced kidney allografts to provoke T-dependent alloimmunity. I. Retransplantation of (AS X AUG)F_1 kidneys into secondary AS recipients. *J Exp Med* 150:455–464, 1979.
40. Lechler RI, Batchelor JR: Restoration of immunogenicity to passenger cell-depleted kidney allografts by the addition of donor strain dendritic cells. *J Exp Med* 155:31–41, 1982.
41. Bowen KM, Prowse SJ, Lafferty KJ: Reversal of diabetes by islet transplantation: vulnerability of the established allograft. *Science* 213:1261, 1262, 1981.
42. Vesole DH, Dart GA, Talmage DW: Rejection of stable cultured allografts by active or passive (adoptive) immunization. *Proc Natl Acad Sci USA* 78:1626–1628, 1982.

43. Markmann J, Lo D, Naji A, Palmiter RD, Brinster RL, Heber-Katz E: Antigen presenting function of class II MHC expressing pancreatic beta cells. *Nature* 336:476–479, 1988.
44. Lo D, Burkly LC, Widera G, Cowing C, Flavell RA, Palmiter RD, Brinster RL: Diabetes and tolerance in transgenic mice expressing class II MHC molecules in pancreatic beta cells. *Cell* 53:159–168, 1988.
45. Calne RY: Organ transplantation between widely disparate species. *Transplant Proc* 2:550, 1970.
46. Auchincloss HJ: Xenogeneic transplantation: A review. *Transplantation* 46:1–20, 1988.
47. Platt JL, Bach FH: The barrier to xenotransplantation. *Transplantation* 52:937–947, 1991.
48. Sachs DH, Bach FH: Immunology of xenograft rejection. *Hum Immunology* 28:245–251, 1990.
49. Gill RG: The role of direct and indirect antigen presentation in the response to islet xenografts. *Transplant Proc* 24:642,643, 1992.
50. Lafferty KJ, Warren HS, Woolnough JA, Talmage DW: Immunological induction of T lymphocytes: role of antigen and the costimulator. *Blood Cells* 4:395–404, 1978.
51. Alter BJ, Bach FH: Cellular basis of the proliferative response of human T cells to mouse xenoantigens. *J Exp Med* 171:333–338, 1990.
52. Moses R, Winn HJ, Auchincloss H Jr: Evidence that multiple defects in cell-surface molecule interactions across species differences are responsible for diminished xenogeneic T cell responses. *Transplantation* 53:203–209, 1992.
53. Sprent J: The thymus and T cell tolerance. *Today's Life Sci* 3:14–20, 1991.
54. Swain SL: T cell subsets and the recognition of MHC class. *Immunol Rev* 74:129–142, 1983.
55. von Hoegen P, Miceli MC, Tourvieille B, Schilham M, Parnes JR: Equivalence of human and mouse CD4 in enhancing antigen responses by a mouse class II-restricted T-cell hybridoma. *J Exp Med* 170:1879–1886, 1989.
56. Clayton LK, Sieh M, Pious DA, Reinherz EL: Identification of residues affecting class II versus HIV-1 gp120 binding. *Nature* 339:548–551, 1989.
57. Barzaga-Gilbert E, Grass D, Lawrance SK, Peterson PA, Lacy E, Engelhard VHd: Species specificity and augmentation of responses to class II major histocompatibility complex molecules in human CD4 transgenic mice *J Exp Med* 175:1707–1715, 1992.
58. Irwin MJ, Heath WR, Sherman LA: Species-restricted interactions between CD8 and the α3 domain of class I influence the magnitude of the xenogeneic response. *J Exp Med* 170:1091–1101, 1989.
59. Kalinke U, Arnold B, Hammerling GJ: Strong xenogeneic HLA response in transgenic mice after introducing an a3 domain into HLA B27. *Nature* 348:642–644, 1990.
60. Greenstein JL, Foran JA, Gorga JC, Burakoff SJ: The role of T cell accessory molecules in the generation of class II-specific xenogeneic cytolytic T cells. *J Immunol* 136:2358–2363, 1986.

61. Golding H, Singer A: Role of accessory cell processing and presentation of shed H-2 alloantigens in allospecific cytotoxic T lymphocyte responses. *J Immunol* 133:597, 1984.
62. Yoshizawa K, Yano A: Mouse T lymphocytes proliferative responses specific for human MHC products in mouse anti-human xenogeneic MLR. *J Immunol* 132:2820–2829.
63. Brunswick M, Lake P: Functional interactions of human and murine lymphoid cells. *Cell Immunol* 103:441–454, 1986.
64. Pierson RN III, Winn HJ, Russell PS, Auchincloss H: Xenogeneic skin graft rejection is especially dependent on CD4+ T cells. *J Exp Med* 170:991–996, 1989.
65. Mandel TE, Koulmanda M, Loudovaris T, Bacelj A: Islet grafts in NOD mice: a comparison of iso-, allo-, and pig xenografts. *Transpl Proc* 21:3813,3814, 1989.
66. Gill RG, Coulombe M: Rejection of pancreatic islet xenografts does not require CD8+ T-lymphocytes. *Transplant Proc* 24:2877,2878, 1992.
67. Shizuru JA, Gregory AK, Chao CTB, Fathman CG: Islet allograft survival after a single course of treatment of recipient with antibody to L3T4. *Science* 237:278–280, 1987.
68. Hao L, Wang Y, Gill RG, Lafferty KJ: Role of the L3T4+ T cell in allograft rejection. *J Immunol* 139:4022–4026, 1987.
69. Lacy PE, Ricordi C, Finke EH: Effect of transplantation site and αL3T4 treatment on survival of rat, hamster, and rabbit islet xenografts in mice. *Transplantation* 47:761–766, 1989.
70. Ricordi C, Lacy PE, Sterbenz K, Davie JM: Low-temperature culture of human islets or in vivo treatment with L3T4 antibody produces a marked prolongation of islet human-to-mouse xenograft survival. *Proc Natl Acad Sci USA* 84:8080–8084, 1987.
71. Gill RG, Lafferty KJ: The role of islet transplantation in the treatment of insulin-dependent diabetes mellitus. *Immunol Allergy Clin North Am* 9:165–186, 1989.
72. Wang Y, Pontesili O, Gill RG, La Rosa FG, Lafferty KJ: The role of $CD4^+$ and $CD8^+$ T cells in the destruction of islet grafts by spontaneously diabetic mice. *Proc Natl Acad Sci USA* 88:527–531, 1991.
73. Desai NM, Bassiri H, Odorico JS, Koller BH, Smithies O, Naji A, Barker CF, Markmann JF: Pancreatic islet allograft and xenograft survival in $CD8^+$ T-lymphocyte-deficient recipients. *Transplant Proc* 25:961,962, 1993.
74. Mandel TE, Koulmanda M: The survival of xeno-, allo- and isografts in NOD mice and xenografts in other strains, after immunosuppression with anti-CD4 monoclonal antibody. *Diabetes Nutr Metab* 5(Suppl 1):91–96, 1992.
75. Simeonovic CJ, Wilson JD: CD4+ T-cell depletion in mice facilitates induction of tolerance to pig proislet xenografts: a comparison of NOD and CBA/H recipient models. *Diabetes Nutr Metab* 5(Suppl 1):133–138, 1992.

76. Haskins K, Portas M, Bergman B, Lafferty K, Bradley B: Pancreatic islet-specific T-cell clones from nonobese diabetic mice. *Proc Natl Acad Sci USA* 86:8000–8004, 1989.
77. Lenchow DJ, Zeng Y, Thistlethwaite JR, Montag A, Brady W, Gibson MG, Linsley PS, Bluestone JA: Long-term survival of xenogeneic pancreatic islet grafts induced by CTLA41g. *Science* 257:789–792, 1992.
78. Carel J-C, Schreiber RD, Falqui L, Lacy PE: Transforming growth factor b decreased the immunogenicity of rat islet xenografts (rat to mouse) and prevents rejection in association with treatment of the recipient with a monoclonal antibody to interferon g. *Proc Natl Acad Sci USA* 87:1591–1595, 1990.
79. Faustman D, Coe C: Prevention of xenograft rejection by masking donor HLA class I antigens. *Science* 252:1700–1702, 1991.

Chapter 4

Pathogenesis of Autoimmune Diabetes

Filippo Calcinaro, Dale R. Wegmann, and Kevin J. Lafferty

Introduction

Insulin-dependent diabetes mellitus (IDDM) results from damage to the insulin-producing tissue of the pancreas. Thus, any cure for this disease must involve replacement of damaged islet tissue, by grafting this tissue either as a free islet graft or in the form of pancreas transplantation. In the case of a disease like diabetes, which is not immediately life-threatening, the long-term use of antirejection drugs may not be justified; the risk of antirejection therapy could be more dangerous than diabetes itself.

The discovery of a way around the transplantation barrier without recourse to antirejection therapy *(1)* raised hopes that a cure for this disease might be at hand. However, studies carried out both in humans and in animal models demonstrate that the disease that destroyed the original islet tissue returns to attack the transplant. Any cure for this disease must involve control of the disease process itself in addition to the replacement of damaged islet tissue.

This chapter traces new developments in the understanding of this disease that provide new possibilities for disease control.

From: *Molecular Biology of Diabetes, Part I*
Edited by: B. Draznin and D. LeRoith © 1994 Humana Press Inc., Totowa, NJ

Genetics of Diabetes

Diabetes or, more correctly, the likelihood of developing this disease, is under genetic control; siblings of diabetic individuals have a 20-fold higher risk of developing diabetes than individuals drawn from the general population *(2)*. A recent study reported only 36% concordance for disease between identical twins of diabetic individuals, demonstrating that we are not dealing with a strictly genetically defined disease *(3)*. However, genetic factors do control the susceptibility of a particular individual to the development of disease.

Genes of the major histocompatibility complex (MHC)—genes initially described as controlling tissue rejection—play a major role in the control of diabetes susceptibility. At the population level, many studies since the 1970s have documented both positive and negative associations between type I diabetes and particular MHC haplotypes *(4)*. In family studies, it has been shown that one of six siblings who share both MHC alleles with a diabetic family member will develop type I diabetes, whereas fewer than 1 in 100 siblings who share neither MHC haplotype develop overt disease. Siblings with a single shared MHC haplotype have an intermediate risk of approx 1 in 20. Although susceptibility to diabetes is clearly regulated by genes that map to the MHC, animal breeding studies indicate that other genes outside of the MHC can also regulate susceptibility to diabetes, and that these genes can exert a protective effect. Although these genes have not been identified precisely at this time, breeding studies would appear to indicate that at least two protective alleles can be independently transmitted to offspring *(5)*.

Despite this complexity of genetic control, the major histocompatibility complex antigens, in particular class II MHC antigens, have been shown to play a critical role in the control of disease susceptibility. The Stanford group have provided evidence that resistance to diabetes is associated with the presence of aspartate at position 57 of the DQ β-chain of class II MHC antigen in Caucasians *(6)*. This situation also holds in the case of the NOD mouse, where diabetes-prone animals are non-Asp at position 57 of the class II β-chain *(7)*.

The involvement of class II MHC antigen in the development of diabetes is likely to operate at the immunological level. The MHC is a system of cell surface molecules that regulate immune function, both at the level of antigen presentation and in terms of shaping the reactive potential of each individual's immune system *(8)*. This contribution of the MHC to the development of autoimmunity (type I diabetes) could be expressed at either of these levels.

Activation of the Immune Process

Let us first consider the MHC contribution to antigen presentation. MHC antigens are of major importance in the regulation of the T-lymphocyte (T-cell) response, and diabetes in animal models is known to be a T-cell dependent disease *(see below)*.

T-cell activation is a two signal process requiring both engagement of the T-cell receptor by antigen, signal 1, and the provision of a second signal, the costimulator (CoS) (Fig. 1). CoS activity is provided by a metabolically active antigen presenting cell (Sc). Thus, T-cells do not respond directly to an immunizing antigen (Ag). This antigen is first broken down and processed by active antigen presenting cells (Fig. 1, Reaction A). Peptide components of the antigen (x) are then presented on the cell surface in association with MHC molecules (Fig. 1, Reaction B). On theoretical grounds we have proposed that this presentation as c.x, where c represents MHC antigen, is an absolute requirement for T-cell activation, because the complex acts as a control molecule regulating delivery of the CoS signal. That is, the only T-cells that can be activated must be of specificity defined by both c and x, where c represents MHC antigen (either class I or class II) on the antigen presenting cell and x is the peptide derivative of the immunizing antigen, Ag. It is this requirement for two signals in the process of T-cell activation that ensures T-cell responses are restricted by MHC antigens of the antigen presenting cell (Fig. 1, Reaction B).

One hypothesis, concerning how the antigen presenting cell function may regulate autoimmunity, is that the presence of the amino acid aspartate at position 57 of the class II β-chain causes a change in the conformation of this molecule (Fig. 2) so it no longer is capable of presenting the "autoantigen" in question—in this case, peptide β, the proposed initiating antigen in type I diabetes. Such a model of antigen presentation does not provide a complete solution to the autoimmunity problem. Although T-cell immunity of any kind

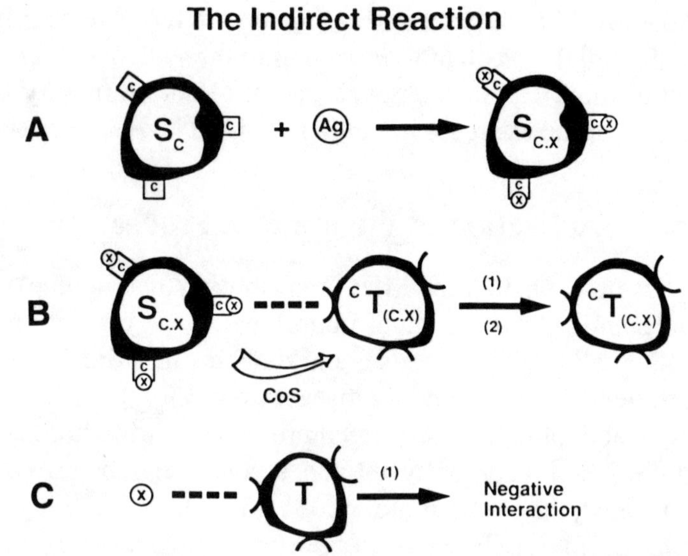

Fig. 1. The two signal model for T-cell activation is based on the function of a control molecule, c, which regulates release of the costimulator, the second signal in the process of T-cell activation. *Reaction A*, antigen (Ag) is taken up and processed by the stimulating cell, S_c, which carries a control molecule, c, on its surface. Processed antigen is converted to peptide structures, x, which are coupled to c and carried to the cell surface where the complex is presented as the complex c.x. *Reaction B*, antigen presented as c.x on the stimulating cell is recognized by a T-cell of specificity c.x (the left superscript denotes the T-cell genotype, the right subscript in parentheses denotes the T-cell specificity). This recognition provides signal 1 for the T-cell. Engagement of c.x on the surface of the stimulating cell activates release of the costimulator providing the second signal for T-cell induction. *Reaction C*, the interaction with the epitope x alone provides signal 1 for the T-cell, in absence of signal 2, resulting in a negative interaction.

requires appropriate antigen presentation, many self antigens are presented on the surface of active antigen presenting cells without leading to autoimmune responses. Presentation of self peptides is probably the normal rather than the abnormal situation. Some other element of immune regulation must be operating if we are to explain the development of autoimmunity.

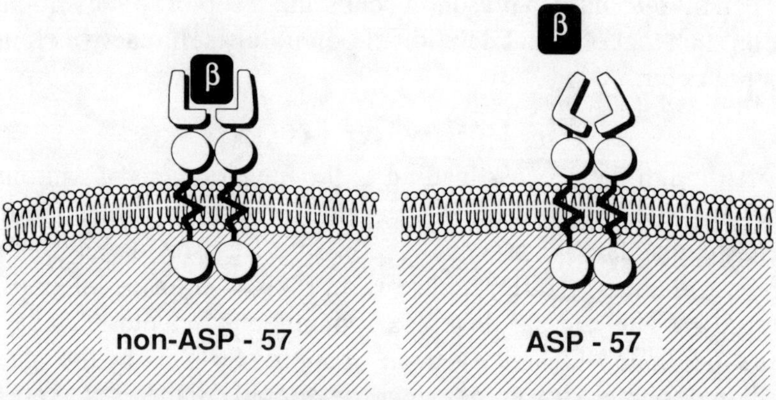

Fig. 2. The class II MHC antigen is a transmembrane protein made up of two chains (α- and β-chains). Both NOD mice and Caucasians that have the amino acid aspartate (ASP) at position 57 of the β-chain are resistant to the development of diabetes. Animals and individuals that are non-ASP at position 57 are susceptible to the development of diabetes. It has been proposed that resistance results from an inability of the ASP-containing molecule to present the β-cell antigen (β) involved in the development of diabetes.

MHC antigens also interact with T-cells during development of the T-cell repertoire in the thymus. Thymic maturation of T-cells matches the MHC of the individual with an appropriate range of T-cell receptor specificities. Positive selection in the thymus gives rise to a population of cells reactive to peptide derivatives (x) of antigens in association with self MHC molecules. This cell population, reactive to (self MHC + x) is not self reactive because (self MHC + x) is not equivalent to self. A process of negative selection resulting in the elimination of self reactive cells also occurs in the thymus *(9)*.

Although there is no direct evidence for a failure of clonal deletion in individuals susceptible to the development of type I diabetes, the assumed presence of self reactive T-lymphocytes causing pancreatic infiltration and islet damage could be accounted for if this process were defective in such individuals. It has been speculated that particular alterations in MHC molecule structure, such as that induced by substitution of serine for aspartate at position 57 of the class II molecule β-chain, could prevent normal interactions between thymic antigen presenting cells and receptors of developing T-cells such that efficient deletion of potentially self reactive clones does not occur.

The Destructive Process

Although the process leading to the development of "autoimmune" diabetes remains to be unraveled, we are on firmer ground when we discuss the process responsible for islet damage. The nonobese diabetic (NOD) mouse is an inbred strain developed in Japan *(10)*. This animal develops spontaneous diabetes. Diabetes occurs in female NOD mice at a rate of approx 80–85% by the age of 250 d; males have a lower incidence, developing diabetes at a rate of approx 35–40% by the same age. Microscopic examination of the pancreas shows the disease to commence as an inflammatory response adjacent to the pancreatic islet; the inflammation is focused primarily in the region adjacent to the islet that carries small pancreatic ducts and blood vessels (Fig. 3A). With the passage of time, this inflammation increases and spreads to invade the islet tissue itself (Fig. 3B).

The inflammatory lesion is made up of the full spectrum of immunological cells—T-cells, B-cells, and macrophages.

The disease process is very specific. Initially, β-cells (insulin producing cells), which make up the majority of cells in the islet, are intact and α-cells (glucagon producing cells) can be seen scattered neatly around the periphery of the islet. As the disease proceeds, β-cells are destroyed, whereas the α-cells, and other minority cells of the islet, remain intact. Eventually the islet collapses into what appears to be an "α-cell islet." That is, the disease process is the result of a very specific process leading to β-cell destruction while maintaining the integrity of other cellular components of the pancreatic islet.

T-Cell Involvement in the Disease Process

Both removal of the thymus at an early age, or T-cell depletion, can prevent the development of diabetes in rodent models of the disease *(11,12)*. The development of IDDM in animal models and man can be modified by immunosuppressive therapy with cyclosporine *(13,14)*. These findings suggest that diabetes is a T-cell-dependent disease.

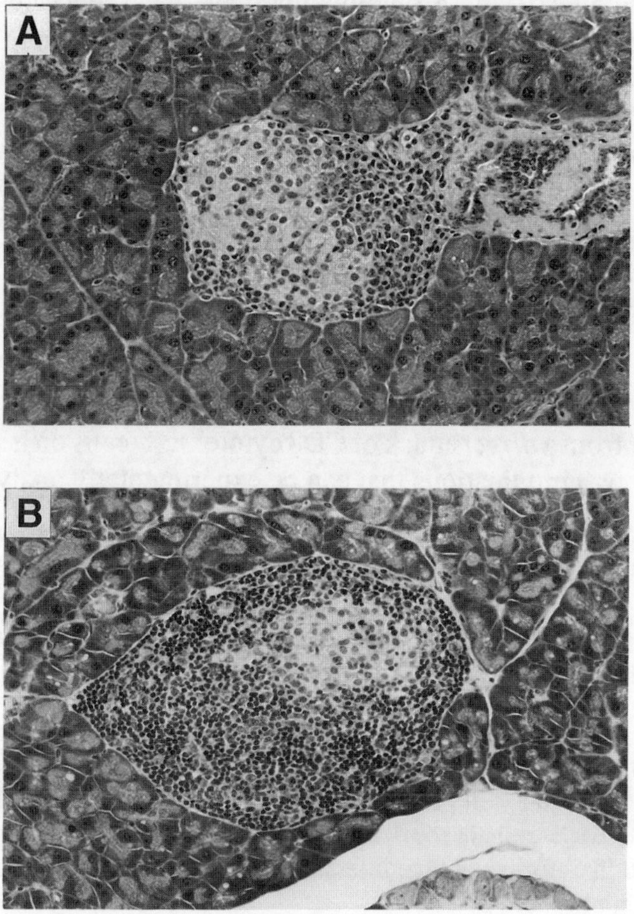

Fig. 3. (**A**) The early stage of islet inflammation is characterized by the accumulation of mononuclear cells around pancreatic ducts and small blood vessels adjacent to the islet (hematoxylin-eosin). (**B**) As the disease progresses the inflammation increases and spreads to invade the pancreatic islet tissue itself (hematoxylin-eosin).

The T-cell compartment of the immune system is made up of two major groups of cells, CD4 and CD8 T-cells. The CD4 T-cells are thought to be involved in inflammatory reactions and also exert helper function for both CD8 T-cells and B-cells. The CD8 T-cells are thought to play a role in direct cellular killing. Both CD4 and the CD8 subsets are required for the development of disease in diabetes prone

NOD mice *(15)*. These findings that have been reported independently by a number of groups have been interpreted in a classical immunological context as indicating that CD4 helper T-cells are required for the activation of CD8 cytotoxic cells and that β-cell damage results from specific CD8 T-cell-mediated killing of these targets. This model (Fig. 4, Direct reaction) would account for the specific destruction of β-cells seen in this disease process. However, when we test the major implications of the cytotoxic model, we find it to be in need of revision.

Implications of the Cytotoxic Model

The cytotoxic model (Fig. 4, Direct reaction) proposes diabetes to result from a *direct* attack of CD8 cytotoxic T-cells on islet β-cells and has two implications that can be experimentally analyzed:

1. The disease process that involves a direct interaction of T-cells with target β-cells, will be dependent on the activity of the CD8 cytotoxic subset.
2. The disease process will be restricted by MHC antigens expressed on the islet tissue (Fig. 4, Direct reaction). That is, allogeneic islet tissue (c1 genotype) will be resistant to "autoimmune" damage following transplantation to spontaneously diabetic animals (Fig. 4, Direct reaction); the allogeneic tissue will present c1.β on the cell surface, whereas the reactive T-cells in the diabetic animals will be specific for c.β, and therefore unable to interact effectively with the allogeneic target tissue.

Both these implications of the direct cytotoxic model have now been tested *(15)*.

Testing the Theoretical Models

T-Cell Requirement in the Disease Process

Let us examine the first implication of the *direct* cytotoxic model, namely, that the immunological effector cell responsible for β-cell destruction is the CD8 T-cell.

Using an antibody depletion protocol found to be effective in preventing disease transfer, we examined the T-cell requirement for disease recurrence observed when syngeneic (NOD) islets were grafted to spontaneously *diabetic* NOD mice (Fig. 5). In this study,

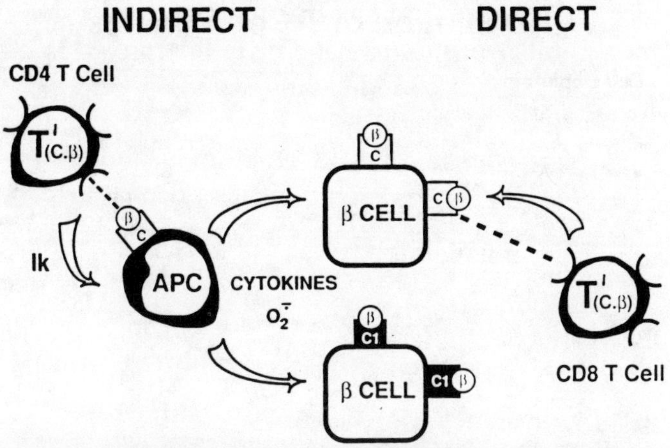

Fig. 4. Islet destruction may be the result of either an *indirect* or *direct* interaction of the immune system with target β-cells. In the case of the *indirect* reaction primed T-cells (T'[c.β]) interact with an islet-associated peptide (β) on the surface of the animal's antigen presenting cells (APC). This interaction leads to lymphokine production by the CD4 T-cell, activation of the APC, and possibly other inflammatory cells leading to the release of cytokines and oxygen radicals. Either or both of these agents then damage the target β-cell. In the case of the *indirect* reaction, both syngeneic and allogeneic islets are equally susceptible to damage.

The *direct* reaction results when a cytotoxic CD8 T-cell (T'[c.β]) interacts with the target β-cell expressing c.β on its surface and kills this cell by a cytotoxic mechanism. In the case of the *direct* reaction, the allogeneic islet expressing c1.β on its surface would be resistant to damage because the CD8 T-cell is specific for c.β and not c1.β, which is the complex expressed on the surface of the allogeneic β-cell.

disease was shown to be a CD4, and not a CD8, T-cell-dependent process. Depletion of the CD4 subset facilitated graft acceptance, and such islet grafts functioned for as long as the CD4 T-cells remained absent from the circulation. Depletion of CD8 T-cells, on the other hand, although shown previously to be quite effective in blocking the development of disease in *nondiseased* young NOD mice had no effect on disease recurrence to syngeneic islet tissue grafted to *already diabetic* animals *(15)*. In this latter situation, the grafted tissue was heavily infiltrated by inflammatory cells and failed to function. Examination of the lesion following CD8 depletion

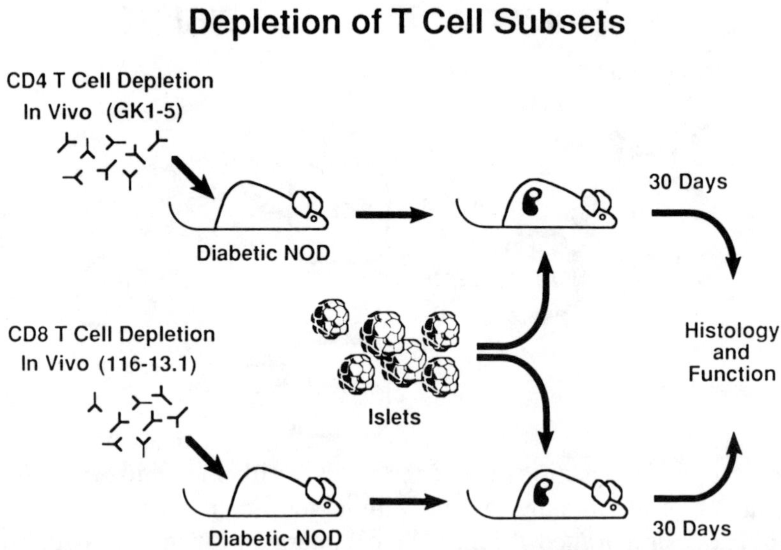

Fig. 5. Depletion of either CD4 or CD8 T-cell subsets was achieved by treating spontaneously diabetic NOD animals with monoclonal antibody reactive to either subset. These animals were then transplanted with islets obtained from nondiabetic NOD animals and the function of the grafted tissue was followed for 30 d posttransplantation. At the completion of the study, animals were sacrificed and the tissue was examined histologically. Depletion of the CD4 subset protected the grafted tissue from disease recurrence, whereas depletion of the CD8 subset did not prevent disease recurrence and the grafted tissue was destroyed.

showed large numbers of CD4 cells to be present in the damaged tissue and the complete absence of CD8 T-cells. Thus, although both CD4 and CD8 T-cells are required for the *initiation* of disease, the *expression* of disease is not a CD8 T-cell dependent process.

MHC Restriction of the Disease Process

We next set out to test the second implication of the cytotoxic damage model, namely, that destruction of islet β-cells is restricted by MHC antigen presented on the islet tissue.

As discussed earlier (Fig. 1), T-cell activation is a two signal event, therefore allograft reactions depend on the presence of antigen presenting cells capable of delivering CoS activity, signal 2, in conjunction with the engagement of the T-cell receptor, signal 1. As a

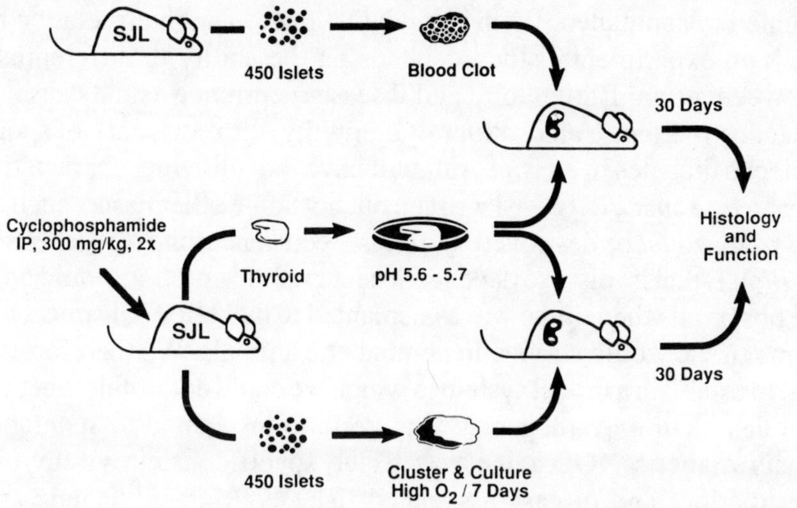

Fig. 6. Disease recurrence is not restricted by MHC antigens expressed on the islet tissue. In this experiment, both islets and thyroid were taken from allogeneic SJL donor mice, pretreated to eliminate tissue immunogenicity and then transplanted to spontaneously diabetic NOD animals. The cultured thyroid is used as a sentinel graft to demonstrate any development of an allograft response. In this study the islet tissue was heavily infiltrated and totally destroyed, whereas the thyroid tissue remained intact (*see also* Fig. 7) demonstrating tissue specificity of the disease process. The upper section shows the experimental design in which normal SJL islets, that is, islets that were not treated to reduce immunogenicity, were transplanted into diabetic NOD animals along with a precultured sentinel thyroid. In this case, both the islets and the thyroid were totally destroyed, indicating that the thyroid was an adequate monitor of the allograft response in the NOD animal.

consequence, a graft depleted of such cells will not elicit an allograft response; that is, it will not be immunogenic. Prolonged culture under special conditions has been shown to effectively remove antigen presenting cells from endocrine tissues so that such tissues can successfully be transplanted across major histocompatibility barriers without the need for immunosuppression *(1,16–19)*.

The model system used for these studies (Fig. 6) involves preculture of allogeneic (SJL) islet tissue in 95% oxygen to eliminate tissue immunogenicity. The cultured allogeneic tissue was then transplanted to spontaneously diabetic NOD mice. The interpretation of such an experimental study depends on the ability to differentiate between allograft immunity and disease recurrence as the cause of islet destruction. Unlike allograft immunity, the recurrence of spontaneous diabetes in an islet graft will have the following characteristics: *tissue specificity*—islet tissue but not some other tissue, such as thyroid, would be destroyed by disease recurrence; and *disease association*—that is, disease dependent islet graft destruction would only be observed when tissue was transplanted to diabetic NOD mice; the same tissue would survive in nondiabetic animals. We therefore set out to establish a model system in which we could determine whether the destruction of allogeneic islet grafts transplanted to spontaneously diabetic NOD mice was tissue specific (islets vs thyroid destruction) and disease associated (islet grafting in diabetic and nondiabetic NOD mice).

To test tissue specificity of the destructive process, cultured allogeneic islets or thyroid tissue was transplanted to spontaneously diabetic animals (Fig. 6). In this study, the thyroid graft acted as a sentinel to demonstrate any activation of the allograft response. Graft survival was determined by blood sugar control in the case of the islet graft, or by labeled iodine uptake by the thyroid. These measures of graft function were confirmed by microscopic examination of the tissues. The results of this study were clear cut. All cultured islet allografts were heavily infiltrated and damaged when transplanted to diabetic NOD mice (Fig. 7A), whereas the thyroid grafts transplanted at the same time remained intact in all recipients some 3–4 wk after grafting (Fig. 7B). Functional analysis showed the allogeneic thyroid grafts had the capacity to incorporate iodine at levels similar to control tissues. Control studies demonstrated the acute destruction of cultured allogeneic thyroid tissue following the grafting of cultured thyroid and uncultured (immunogenic) islet tissue from the same donor, demonstrating the capacity of the cultured thyroid graft to act as an immunological sentinel for the detection of the allograft response, when this is triggered. The comparison of allogeneic (SJL) islet tissue transplanted to nondiabetic and diabetic NOD animals showed that this destructive process was disease associated *(15)*.

These studies clearly demonstrate that disease recurrence in islet tissue grafted to spontaneously diabetic animals is not restricted

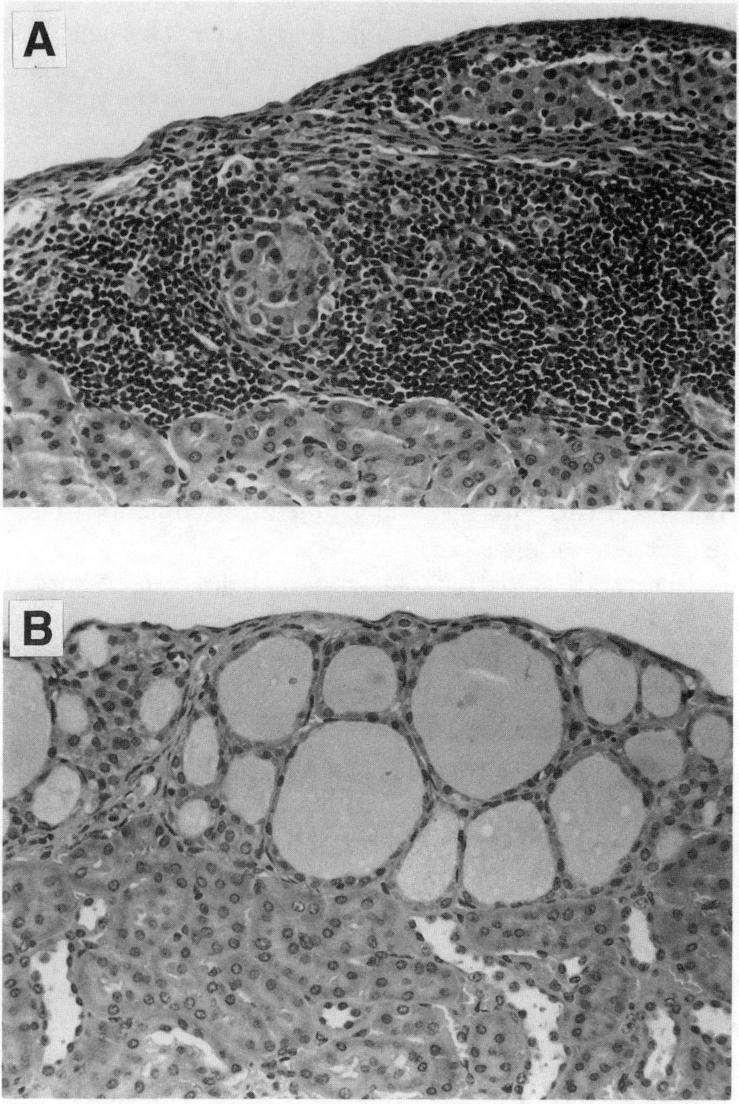

Fig. 7. Histological appearance of APC depleted islets and thyroid tissue (SJL) transplanted to spontaneously diabetic NOD mice. **(A)** Note the heavy infiltration and damage to the islet graft. **(B)** Note the normal appearance of thyroid tissue transplanted under the same kidney capsule of the NOD mouse. The tissue specificity of this reaction indicates we are not dealing with an allograft response. Thus, we conclude that disease recurrence occurs in allogeneic islets and therefore the disease process is not restricted by MHC antigens expressed on the islets.

by MHC antigens expressed on the grafted tissues. This lack of MHC restriction of the disease process by islet MHC antigens is not consistent with the direct killing hypothesis (Fig. 4, direct reaction).

T-Cell Cloning Studies

The experiments described earlier suggest that CD4 T-cells are sufficient to mediate the islet graft destruction observed in disease recurrence. If this is the case one would expect islet-specific CD4 T-cell clones to be capable of in vivo destruction of β-cells. This has been demonstrated by the capacity of islet-specific CD4 T-cell clones *(20,21)* to accelerate disease in young NOD mice *(22)* and initiate destruction of NOD islets grafted into (CBA x NOD) F1 mice *(23)*. In more recent experiments we have observed that adoptive transfer of diabetes is not affected by antibody mediated depletion of CD8 T-cells in recipient animals *(24)*.

Until recently, adoptive transfer of diabetes by islet-specific T-cell clones has been performed with immunocompetent recipients and it was therefore difficult to rule out contributions from host lymphocytes. Recently the NOD/SCID mouse, an ideal recipient animal for adoptive transfer experiments, has been developed. The NOD/SCID mouse was established by breeding the SCID defect onto the NOD background *(25)*. NOD/SCID mice have no detectable levels of mature T- or B-cells and thus do not develop insulitis or diabetes *(25)*. Adoptive transfer of diabetes to the NOD/SCID mouse is thus a more stringent test of the in vivo function of islet-specific T-cell clones than the use of conventional recipients. In experiments described below we have demonstrated that islet-specific CD4 T-cell clones are capable of adoptive transfer of diabetes to NOD/SCID mice.

In an effort to characterize the T-cells involved in islet graft destruction in the disease recurrence model we have established islet-specific T-cell lines. Destruction of islet grafts in the disease recurrence model is accompanied by lymphocytic infiltration of the grafts. It seemed likely that these infiltrating cells were responsible for graft destruction and would thus be a good starting source for isolation of T-cells that participate in graft destruction. Accordingly, we established islet-specific T-cell lines from islet graft infiltrates obtained from five individual recipient mice *(26)*. The infiltrating cells were isolated by explant of the infiltrated graft into in vitro culture. Islet-specific T-cell lines were established by antigenic stimulation of the cells that were recovered from these grafts. In this case the cells were stimulated with islet antigen, irradiated NOD spleen cells as a source of APCs, and lymphokines *(27)*. The T-cell lines that we established from graft infiltrating cells were essentially 100% CD4, with no detectable CD8 cells, and these lines proliferated vigorously in response to antigen in the form of NOD islet cells *(26)*.

Clones were established from one of the lines by limiting dilution cloning and, after expansion, the clones were tested for responsiveness to islet antigen. A number of clones, selected on the basis of strong proliferative responses to islet antigen, were tested for the capacity to mediate islet destruction on adoptive transfer into NOD/SCID recipients. The results of these experiments indicated that several of our islet-specific CD4 T-cell clones will induce diabetes in recipient NOD/SCID mice 30–50 d after injection *(26)*. These results demonstrate that CD4 T-cells are *sufficient* for induction of diabetes and that there is no requirement for CD8 cells in this process.

On the basis of the aforementioned observations, we find it necessary to abandon the direct cytotoxic hypothesis. Studies relating to the T-cell involvement in the initiation of the disease process indicate that both CD4 and CD8 T-cells are required to activate the disease. However, the immunological effector cell does not appear to be the CD8 T-cell. The dependence of the actual disease process on the CD4 T-cell leads us to propose that "autoimmune" diabetes is the result of CD4 T-cell-dependent inflammatory tissue damage (Fig. 4, reaction): A β-cell associated antigen is processed by an antigen presenting cell (APC) and presented, in the correct MHC complex, to a $CD4^+$ T-cell. This interaction would trigger cytokine release and oxygen radical production that, in turn, would generate an inflammatory focus at the site of the graft. According to this model, both syngeneic or nonsyngeneic islets would be equally exposed to the deleterious effects of inflammatory mediators, explaining why the disease process is not restricted by the MHC of the islet tissue.

One problem with this notion is the cellular specificity of the disease process. If damage is simply the result of inflammatory mediators, how do we account for specific β-cell destruction seen in this disease? Pancreatic islet β-cells are particularly sensitive to free radical damage *(28)*, and one possibility is that in the case of this

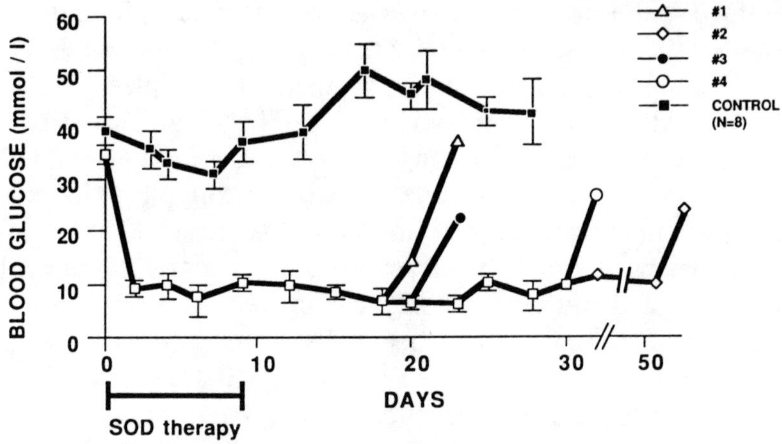

Fig. 8. Superoxide dismutase (SOD) therapy protects the islet allograft from disease recurrence following transplantation to spontaneously diabetic NOD mice. In the control study, APC depleted Balb/c islets were transplanted to spontaneously diabetic animals. All animals remained hyperglycemic for the length of the experimental study. Test animals were treated with SOD for 7 d following transplantation of APC depleted Balb/c islet tissue. All animals became normoglycemic within 24–48 h and remained normoglycemic for an extended period following cessation of SOD therapy. Disease recurrence was eventually seen in all animals following the cessation of SOD therapy. These studies show islet damage in the disease process is oxygen radical dependent.

disease we may be dealing with nonspecific inflammatory tissue damage that expresses itself as specific β-cell damage because of the target tissue's sensitivity to oxygen radicals.

Protection from Inflammatory Tissue Damage

Evidence for the involvement of oxygen radicals in the "autoimmune" diabetogenic process was obtained by examining the capacity of polyethylene glycol modified superoxide dismutase (PEG-SOD) to protect grafted islet tissue from damage in the diabetic animal (Fig. 8). In these studies, grafting of spontaneously diabetic NOD animals was effective in reversing diabetes only when the diabetic animals were treated with PEG-SOD for 10 d from the time of islet grafting *(29)*. The use of PEG-modified enzymes in these studies is required to reduce the immunogenicity of the bovine enzymes and to provide enzymic activity with a prolonged half life (approx 36 h) in the recipient animal.

The Disease Process in Humans

The data discussed above have been obtained from animal studies carried out mostly in the NOD mouse. Although this mouse develops spontaneous insulin-dependent diabetes that is clinically close to the human disease, we do have to keep in mind that what applies to this animal model may not apply to the human disease.

Little information is available on the pathogenesis of type I diabetes in humans because of several obvious limitations: heterogeneous genetic background, variation in environmental factors, and unavailability of pancreatic tissue for histology studies. However, there is evidence that the disease in humans also results from inflammatory tissue damage. If the human disease process involves an indirect attack (Fig. 4) it may be possible to detect and study cell-mediated immunity (CMI) in type I diabetes using xenogeneic islets as a target, by transferring unpurified mononuclear blood cells (MBCs), as a source of APCs and T-cells, from diabetic patients into immunodeficient mice. Under these conditions, human APCs (mainly monocytes and B-cells) could process an islet associated, human/murine cross reactive antigen, and display it in the correct MHC context to an islet reactive CD4 T-cell from the same donor. This interaction would trigger the release of cytokines, the generation of oxygen radicals, and, eventually, inflammation around the islet tissue, leading to islet specific damage. Such a reaction would be dependent on the use of crude white cell preparations as a source of APCs and MHC compatible T-cells.

In light of our animal studies, we therefore set out to test the hypothesis that islet specific damage can be transferred from IDDM subjects to the athymic nude mouse, a strain that lacks T-lymphocytes and T-cell-mediated immunity *(30)*.

Briefly, MBCs from 10 new onset diabetic patients (six tested positive for anti-islet cell antibodies, ICA) and from 10 control healthy subjects were injected intraperitoneally (ip) into groups of 2–4 nude mice. Plasma from the same individuals was also injected into additional groups of animals. Nonfasting blood glucose was monitored twice a week in all the test mice and oral glucose tolerance tests were carried out at weekly intervals. At the completion of the study, 4 wk after cell transfer, the animals were sacrificed for histological examination.

Even though we could not show any modification of the glycemic control of the injected mice, irrespective of the cell source, we were able to demonstrate that it is possible to transfer islet reactive CMI from type I diabetic patients to the nude mouse. In fact, MBCs, and not plasma, from six out of ten newly diagnosed patients induced significant damage in the pancreas of recipient nude mice (Fig. 9A–C); no damage was seen when mononuclear cells from ten normal control subjects were injected into nude mice under the same conditions ($p = 0.005$) (Fig. 9D). In all cases, a mononuclear cell infiltrate, of variable extent, was found focused on the islet tissue. Different degrees of insulitis and islet damage, ranging from β-cell degranulation to islet disruption, were observed (Fig. 9A–C) and not all islets in the recipient pancreas showed evidence of inflammation. Immunostaining for glucagon showed an unusual α-cell concentration among infiltrating mononuclear cells in many cases, suggesting β-cell death and islet collapse. Indirect immunofluorescence studies showed rare human leukocytes among the infiltrating cells. No inflammation was found in tissues other than islets, indicating the tissue specificity of the process. The finding that no animals in either the test or control group showed any impairment of blood glucose homeostasis probably results from the fact that only a fraction of the islets in the pancreas of recipient mice showed evidence of inflammation and only a proportion of the inflamed islets were damaged to the extent shown in Fig. 1C. The failure to consistently induce islet lesions in recipient mice and the variability in the extent of damage seen in different islets were probably owing to recirculation defects of the human blood cells in a murine environment.

The data presented here clearly show that pathology detected in this model system is islet specific and disease associated, providing us with a way to study human IDDM outside of the human. Moreover, these findings are consistent with the notion that the human disease is also the result of inflammatory tissue damage. New experimental systems are being developed to better characterize the disease process in humans.

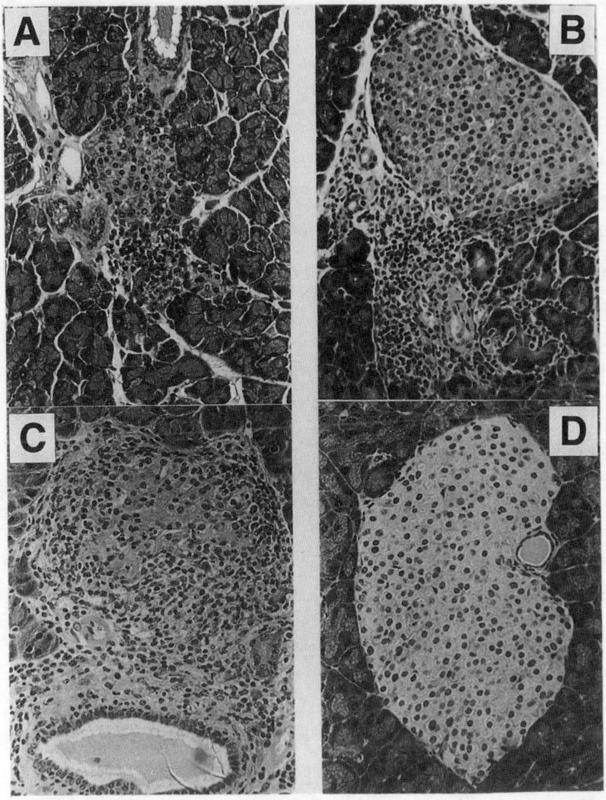

Fig. 9. Transfer of human MBCs to the nude mouse: pancreatic histology (hematoxylin-eosin). **(A–C)** MBCs from diabetic patients; **(D)** MBCs from control subject. (A) Bouin's fixative. Accumulation of infiltrating MBCs at a pole of the pancreatic islet. Note the absence of any infiltrating cells among the pancreatic exocrine cells. (B) Formalin fixative. Periductular mononuclear cell infiltrate in the process of surrounding a pancreatic islet that still appears relatively well preserved. (C) Formalin fixative. Impressive periductular mononuclear infiltrate that has filled the peri-islet space and is causing islet disruption. (D) Formalin fixative. Normal pancreatic islet appearance. No signs of inflammation.

Implications for Therapy

Evidence from animal models demonstrates "autoimmune" diabetes is dependent on T-cell function, and, in humans, suppression of T-cell activity with cyclosporine has been shown to arrest the development of this disease *(14)*. However, treatment of type I diabetics with immunosuppressive agents such as cyclosporine carries too many demonstrable and theoretical side effects to be useful as life-long therapy. The demonstrated effectiveness of superoxide dismutase in preventing the development of disease recurrence in transplanted pancreatic tissue suggests that agents directed at blocking inflammatory mediators, such as interleukins and oxygen radicals, may be effective in preventing damage to susceptible pancreatic β-cells.

Another approach may be to identify, by cloning procedures, the specific CD4 T-cell subsets in humans that are involved in pancreatic islet damage. Having identified such cells and the diversity of their expressed receptor it may be possible to design specific immunosuppressive therapies that "surgically" remove just these cells from the repertoire, so providing what is in effect antigen specific immunosuppression that would not carry with it the same lifetime risks of pan-immunosuppressive agents such as cyclosporine.

We now have the technology required for the grafting of islet tissue without the requirement of lifelong immune suppression. We can also use radical scavengers, or other agents, to regulate disease recurrence in the grafted tissue. The coming years will see attempts to transfer this technology to clinical trials.

Acknowledgment

This work was supported in part by US Public Health Service grants #DK46621 and #DK33470.

References

1. Prowse SJ, Steele EJ, Lafferty KJ: Islet allografting without immunosuppression: Reversal of insulitis-associated diabetes and a case of spontaneous juvenile onset diabetes in mice. *Aust J Exp Biol Med Sci* 60(6):619–627, 1982.
2. Gamble DR: An epidemiological study of childhood diabetes affecting two or more siblings. *Diabetologia* 19:341–344, 1980.
3. Thomson G, Robinson WP, Kuhner MK, Joe S, MacDonald MJ, Gottschall JL, Barbosa J, Rich SS, Betrams J, Baur MP, Partanen J, Tait BD, Schober E, Mayr WR, Ludvigsson J, Lindblom B, Farid NR, Thompson C, Deschamps I: Genetic heterogeneity, modes of inheritance, and risk estimates for a joint study of Caucasians with insulin-dependent diabetes mellitus. *Am J Hum Genet* 43:799–816, 1988.

4. Nerup J, Mandrup-Poulsen T, Molvig J: The HLA-IDDM association: implications for etiology and pathogenesis of IDDM. *Diabetes Metab Rev* 3(3):779–802, 1986.
5. Wicker LS, Miller BJ, Fischer PA, Pressey A, Peterson LB: Genetic control of diabetes and insulitis in the nonobese diabetic mouse; Pedigree analysis of a diabetic $H\text{-}2^{nod/b}$ heterozygote. *J Immunol* 142:781–784, 1989.
6. Todd JA, Bell JI, McDevitt HO: HLA-DQβ gene contributes to susceptibility and resistance to insulin-dependent diabetes mellitus *Nature* 329:599–604, 1987.
7. Acha-Orbea H, McDevitt HO: The first external domain of the non-obese diabetic mouse class I-A β chain is unique. *Proc Natl Acad Sci USA* 84:2435–2439, 1987.
8. Germain RG: Analysis of the expression and function of class–II major histocompatibility complex-encoded molecules by DNA-mediated gene transfer. *Ann Rev Immunol* 4:281–315, 1986.
9. Blackman M, Kappler J, Marrack P: The role of the T cell receptor in positive and negative selection of developing T cells. *Science* 248:1335–1341, 1990.
10. Makino S, Kunimoto K, Muraoka Y, Mizushima Y, Katagiri K, Tochino Y: Breeding of a non-obese, diabetic strain of mice. *Exp Anim* 29(1):1–13, 1980.
11. Ogawa M, Maruyama T, Hasegawa T, Kanaya T, Kobayashi F, Tochino Y, Uda H: The inhibitory effect of neonatal thymectomy on the incidence of insulitis in non-obese-diabetic (NOD) mice. *Biomed Res* 6(2):103–105, 1985.
12. Like AA, Anthony M, Guberski DL, Rossini AA: Spontaneous diabetes mellitus in the BB/W rat: effects of glucocorticoids, cyclosporin-A, and antiserum to rat lymphoctyes. *Diabetes* 32:326–330, 1983.
13. Like AA, Dirodi V, Thomas S, Guberski D, Rossini AA: Prevention of diabetes mellitus in the BB/W rat with Cyclosporin-A. *Am J Pathol* 117(1):92–97, 1984.
14. Dupre, J, Stiller CR, Gent M, Donner A, Von Graffenried B, Heinrichs D, Jenner M, Keown P, Mahon J, Martel R, Momah CI, Murphy G, Rodger NW, Wolfe BM: Clinical trials of Cyclosporin in IDDM. *Diabetes Care* 11(Suppl1):37–44, 1988.
15. Wang Y, Pontesilli O, Gill RG, La Rosa FG, Lafferty KJ: The role of CD4 and CD8 T cells in the destruction of islet grafts by spontaneously diabetic mice. *Proc Natl Acad Sci USA* 88:527–531, 1991.
16. Lafferty KJ, Cooley MA, Woolnough F, Walker KZ: Thyroid allograft immunogenicity is reduced after a period in organ culture. *Science* 188:259–261, 1975.
17. Lafferty KJ, Bootes A, Dart G, Talmage DW: Effect of organ culture on the survival of thyroid allografts in mice. *Transplantation* 22(2):138–149, 1976.
18. La Rosa FG, Talmage DW: The abrogation of thyroid allograft rejection by culture in acid medium. *Transplantation* 44(4):592, 1987.

19. La Rosa FG: Abrogation of mouse pancreatic islet allograft rejection by a four-day culture. *Transplantation* 46(1):330–333, 1988.
20. Haskins K, Portas M, Bradley B, Wegmann D, Lafferty KJ: T-lymphocyte clone specific for pancreatic islet antigen. *Diabetes* 37(10):1444–1448, 1988.
21. Haskins K, Portas M, Bergman B, Lafferty K, Bradley B: Pancreatic islet-specific T-cell clones from nonobese diabetic mice. *Proc Natl Acad Sci USA* 86:8000–8004, 1989.
22. Haskins K, McDuffie M: Acceleration of diabetes in young NOD mice with a CD4+ islet-specific T cell clone. *Science* 249:1433–1436, 1990.
23. Bradley BJ, Wang Y, Lafferty KJ, Haskins K: In vivo activity of an islet-reactive T-cell clone. *J Autoimmun* 3:449–456, 1990.
24. Bradley BJ, Haskins K, La Rosa FG, Lafferty KJ: CD8 T cells are not required for islet destruction induced by a CD4+ islet-specific T cell clone. *Diabetes* 41:1603–1608, 1992.
25. Prochazka M, Gaskins R, Shultz LD, Letter EH: The nonobese diabetic scid mouse: model for spontaneous thymomagenesis associated with immunodeficiency. *Proc Natl Acad Sci USA* 89:3290–3294, 1992.
26. Wegmann DR, Shehadeh N, Lafferty KJ, Norbury-Glaser M, Gill RG, Daniel D: Establishment of islet-specific T-cell lines and clones from islet isografts placed in spontaneously diabetic NOD mice. *J Autoimm* 6:517–527, 1993.
27. Glasebrook AL, Sarmiento M, Loken MR, Dialynas DP, Quintans J, Eisenberg L, Lutz CT, Wilde D, Fitch FW: Murine T lymphocyte clones with distinct immunological functions. *Immunol Rev* 54:225–266, 1981.
28. Malaisse WJ, Malaisse-Lagae F, Sener A, Pipeleers DG: Determinants of the selective toxicity of alloxan to the pancreatic B cell. *Proc Nat Acad Sci USA* 79:927–930,1982.
29. Nomikos IN, Wang Y, Lafferty KJ: Involvement of O_2 radicals in "autoimmune" diabetes. *Immunol Cell Biol* 67:85–87, 1989.
30. Calcinaro F, Hao L, Chase HP, Klingensmith G, Lafferty KJ: Detection of cell-mediated immunity in type I diabetes mellitus. *J Immunol* 5:137–147, 1992.

Molecular and Cellular Aspects of Insulin Synthesis and Secretion

Chapter 5

Insulin Gene Structure and Regulation

Michael S. German

Introduction

In the 70 years since Banting and Best extracted insulin from a dog's pancreas *(1)*, it has become the best studied of the peptide hormones. Insulin was the first protein for which the complete amino acid sequence was determined, and it was the first peptide hormone molecularly cloned. Insulin has been found throughout the animal world. It functions as a hormone in animals as divergent as sponges, flies, and humans, with very little sequence change over the one-and-a-half billion years this divergence represents.

In vertebrates, insulin signals the presence of nutritional substrates and stimulates uptake of these substrates, storage of energy, and growth. Conversely, a fall in insulin levels during fasting results in the release of stored energy and metabolism by the liver of the released amino acids and fatty acids to produce glucose and ketoacids. Dampening of the insulin signal by inadequate insulin secretion or altered insulin function results in the hyperglycemia, ketosis, growth retardation, and metabolic disarray that characterizes diabetes mellitus.

The cloning of the insulin gene permitted the production of human insulin in bacteria on a large scale, which allowed the now

From: *Molecular Biology of Diabetes, Part I*
Edited by: B. Draznin and D. LeRoith

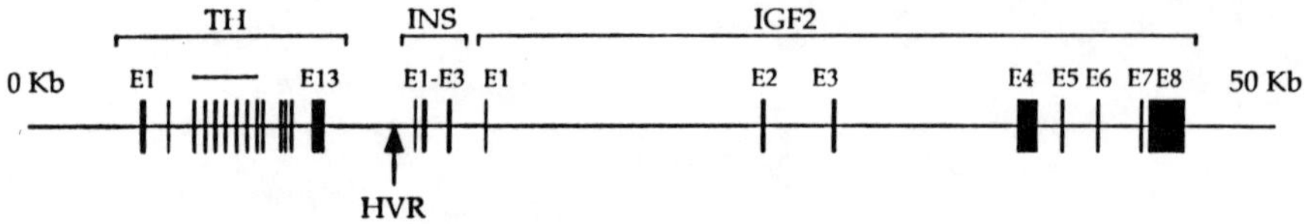

Fig. 1. The human insulin gene and surrounding loci on chromosome 11.

predominant use of human insulin for the treatment of insulin-requiring diabetic patients. Just as important, however, cloning of the insulin gene has led to new insights into how insulin is synthesized on a molecular level, how this synthesis is regulated, and what role the gene plays in the etiology of diabetes.

Insulin Gene Structure

A DNA copy (cDNA) of the preproinsulin messenger RNA (mRNA) was first cloned by Ullrich and colleagues *(2)* from a library of recombinant cDNAs made from rat islets. Shortly thereafter, both a human preproinsulin cDNA clone *(3)* and a chromosomal fragment containing the insulin gene (genomic clone) *(4)* were isolated. Insulin genomic and cDNA clones have since been isolated from a variety of animal species from primates to sponges.

The human insulin gene is located on chromosome 11 close between the tyrosine hydroxylase and IGFII genes (*see* Fig. 1). The gene contains three exons totaling 446 base pairs (bp) that form the mature preproinsulin mRNA. The two intervening sequences, or introns, between the exons are removed from the primary transcript during the process of RNA splicing and polyadenylation that occurs prior to export of the mRNA from the nucleus (Fig. 2). The first intron, IVS1, starts 42 bp downstream from the transcription start site, within the 5' untranslated sequence formed from exon 1 and the 5' end of exon 2. IVS2 splits the coding sequence for the C peptide between exons 2 and 3. When completely processed, the preproinsulin mRNA codes for the preproinsulin peptide, which includes a 20 amino acid prepeptide that is proteolytically removed prior to packaging of proinsulin. In addition, there are 59 bp on the 5' end and 73 bp on the 3' end of the mRNA and a long polyadenosine 3' tail that are not translated into protein.

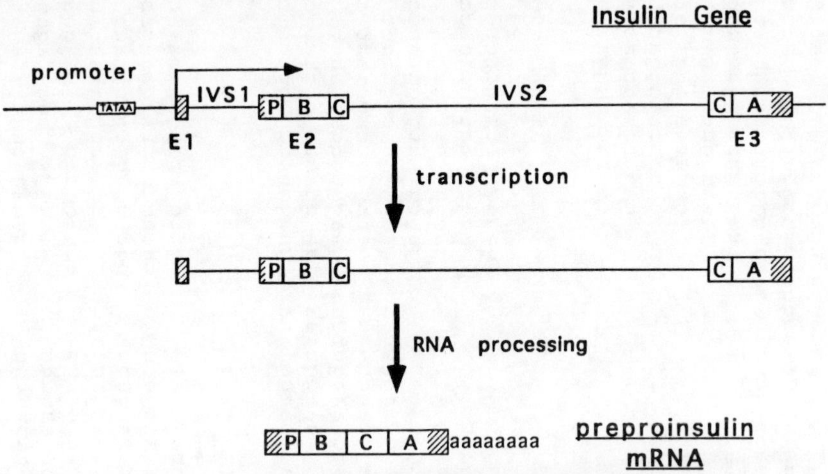

Fig. 2. An outline of the transcription, splicing, and polyadenylation of the preproinsulin mRNA.

The structure of the insulin gene has been remarkably well conserved throughout evolution. Most animals have a single copy of the insulin gene; the known exceptions are two tetraploid organisms, Arctic salmon and African clawed frog, and the murine species, rat and mouse. Apparently, the rat and mouse insulin gene duplication occurred in a murine ancestor and resulted from reverse transcription and reintegration of an incompletely processed RNA transcript of the original insulin gene (insulin gene II) *(5)*. The resulting duplicate gene (insulin gene I) lacks IVS2 but retains most of the structural features of the ancestral gene including untranscribed sequences on the 5' and 3' ends. All of the other known insulin genes have retained the same exon/intron structure with IVS1 in the 5' untranslated sequence and IVS2 invariably dividing the coding sequence for the C-peptide. The exact lengths and the internal sequences of both introns have not been conserved.

Evolutionary conservation of the insulin gene extends to the promoter sequence (*see* Fig. 3). The insulin promoter is defined as that portion of the insulin gene that lies immediately upstream, or 5' relative to the transcription start site. This DNA is not transcribed into RNA, but it is critically important for insulin expression as it

```
                                                                                  HVR
human                     ccatggcggcatcttgggccatccgggactgggg     (acaggggtgtgggg)n     acagcagcgcaa
chimpanzee                ctatggcggcatcttgggccatcagggactgggg    (acaggggtcctgggg)20    acagcggtgcaa
African green monkey      ccatggggcatcttgggcaaccagggactgagaacagggtcccaggacaggggtctggggactgtggtgcaa
owl monkey                ccatgggggcatctcgggcaaccagagatagaggg                 caggggtctggggacagcagcgtga
dog                                                                             cagggcccggg      cagaa
mouse II                                                                        cagtccaagggacaaagatacta
mouse I                                                                         cagtccaagggacatcaatatta
rat II                                                                          cagttcaagggacaaagttacta
rat I                                                                           cagttccagggacaaagatacca

    SP1                              CT3                                                          NRE
agagccccgcc  ctgcagcctccagctctcctgg  tctaatgtggaaa  gtggcccaggt          gaggg  ctttgctctcctggagaca
agagccccgcc  ctgcagcctccagctctcctgg  tctaatgtggaaa  gtggcccaggt          gacgg  ctttgctctcctggagaca
agagccctgcc  ctgcagcc ccagctctcctgg  tgtaatgtggaaa  gtgg gccggg          gaggg  ctttgctctgctggagaca
agagccccgcc  ctgcagcctcccgcactcctgg  tctaatgtggaaa  gtggcccagat          gaggg  ctttgctctcctggagaca
gaagccccag   ctctggcccccagctcccctgc  actaatgtggaaaatgtggctcaggcaaggcccacgtgagggggctctgcccccgtggggaca
ggt ccccaa   ctgcaac        ttcctggggaatgatgtggaaaaa tg ctcagccaaggacaaa  gaaagcatcacccact ctgg aaca
ggt ccctaacaactgcagt        ttcctggggaatgatgtggaaaa  tg ctcagccaaagatgaa  gaaggtctcaccttc   tgg gaca
ggtcccccaacaactgcagc        ctcctggggaatgatgtggaaaaa tg ctcagccaaggacaaa  gaaggcctcaccctct ctg agaca
ggt ccccaacaactgcaac        tttctgggaaatgaggtggaaaa  tg ctcagccaaggaaaaa  gagggccttaccctct ctgg gaca

                          IEB2                        CT2                                    CRE
tttg cccccagctgtgagcagggacaggtctggccaccggg  cccctggttaagactctaatgacc    cgctggtcctgaggaagaggtgctgac
tttggcccccagctgtgagcagggacaggtctggccaccggg  cccctggttaagactctaatgacc    cgctggccctaaggaagaggtgctgac
tttgcccccccagctgcgagcaggaacaggcctggccaccagg  ccctggttaagactctaatgacc    cgctggccctgaggaagaggtgctgac
tttg cccccagctgtgagcagggacaggactggccaccagcg   cctggttaagactctaatgaccacccctcccggccctgaggaagaggtgctgac
t tgcccccagctgccagc               ggccatcagg  cccctcgccaagactctaacgacc    ccgaggccc        ggggtgctgac
a tgtcccc tgctgtgaactggttcat  caggccatcaggg cccttgttaagactctaattacc      ctaggactaag tagaggtgttgac
a tgtcccc tgctgggaactggttcat  caggccatctgg  tcccttattaagactataataacc     ctaagactaag tagatgtgttgat
a tgtcccc tgctgtgaactggttcat  caggccacccaggagcccctcttaagactctaattacc      ctaaggctaag tagaggtgttgtt
a tgattg  tgctgtgaactgcttcat  caggccatctgg  ccccttgttaataatctaattacc     ctaggtctaag tagagttgttgac
```

```
 CCAAT                                          RIPE3B               IEB1
gaccaaggagatcttcccacagacccagcaccagggaaatggtccggaaattgcagcctcagccc  ccagccatctgccgaccc cccca ccccagg
gaccaaggagatcttcccacagacccagcaccagggaaatggtccggaaattgcagcctcagccc  ccagccatctgccgaccc cccca ccccagg
gaccaaga   tcttcccacagacccagcaccagggaaatgatctggaaattgcagcctcagccc  ccagccatctgctaaccc cccca ccccagg
gaccaaggagatattcccgcagacccagcagccgggaaatgatctggaaagtgcagcctcagccc  ccagccatctgccagccc ctgca cctcagg
gaccaaggagctcttcccgcagacccagcactgggaaatgatccagaaattgcagcctcagcct  ccggccatctgccacc
gtccaatgagcgctttctgcagacctagcaccagggaagtg tttggaaactgcagcttcagcccctctggccatctgctgacctaccccacctggagc
gtccaatgagtgctttctgcagacctagcaccaggcaagtg tttggaaactgcagcttcagcccctctggccatctgcctacccaccccacctggaga
gtccaatgagcactttctgcagacctagcaccaggcaagtg tttggaaactgcagcttcagcccctctggccatctgctgatccac
gtccaatgagcgctttctgcagacttagcactaggcaagtg tttggaaattacagcttcagcccctctcgccatctgcctacctacccctcctagagc
              ctgcagacccagcaccagggaaatgatccagaaattgcaacctcagcccc ctggccatctgctgatgc caccaccccaggt

 CT1                        GAGA                 TATAA                       -1
ccctaatggccaggcggcaggggttgacaggtaggggagatggctctgaga ctataaagccagcggggg cccagcagccctc  human
ccctaatggccgggcggcaggggttgacaggtaggggagatggctctgaga ctataaagccagcggggg cccagcagccctc  chimpanzee
ccctaat   cgggcagcaggggttggcaggctggggagatggctctgaga ctataaagccagtgggagcccagcagccctc  A.g. monkey
ccctaatggccaggcggcaa ggttggcaggtaggggagatggctctgggc ctataaagccagcaggga cccagcagccctc  Owl monkey
ccctcat ggccaggccg                      tgggctcgggag ctataaagc aggagggt  ccagcagccccc  dog
ccttaatgggtcaaacagcaaagtccagggggcagagaggaggtgctttggt  ctataaaggtagtgggga cccagtaaccacc  mouse II
ccttaatggccaaacagcaaagtccagggggcagagaggaggtactttgga  ctataaagctggtgggca tccagtaaccccc  mouse I
ccttaatgggacaaacagcaaagtccaggggtcaggggggggtgctttgga  ctataaagctagtgggga ttcagtaaccccc  rat II
ccttaatggccaaacggcaaagtccagggggcagagaggaggtgctttgga  ctataaagctagtggaga cccagtaactccc  rat I
ccctaatgggcctggtggcagagttt         gggaagatgggctcagggctatataaagtccacaagga cctaagagccccc  guinea pig
```

Fig. 3. Comparison of the 5' flanking sequences of the known mammalian insulin genes. Alignments are arranged to optimize identity with the human gene. Alignment of the rodent and primate promoters resumes 100 bp upstream of the HVR. The names for the human functional elements are shown above the gene with the exception that the E1, RIPE3B, and GAGA elements have been characterized only for the rat genes. Sources: human *(65)*, chimpanzee and African green monkey *(Ceropithecus aethiops) (9)*, owl monkey *(Aotus trivirgatus) (10)*, dog *(75,76)*, mouse *(77)*, rat *(5,78,79)*, and guinea pig *(80)*.

determines the transcription start site for RNA polymerase and regulates the rate of transcription initiation.

Although it has been suggested that changes have appeared in the 5' flanking sequence of the insulin gene at a neutral rate (i.e., free of selective pressure), close examination of the mammalian promoters reveals several highly conserved regions close to the transcription start site. In contrast to mammals, the chicken *(6)* and salmon *(7)* promoters do not show obvious sequence conservation, with the exception of the TATAA sequence. This lack of conservation could result from random drift in the promoter sequence or could reflect differences in the function and regional expression of the insulin gene in the nonmammalian chordates. Furthermore, if conserved sequence blocks are grossly repositioned, this change would hinder our ability to detect sequence alignment, without necessarily altering promoter function.

The human *(8)* and chimpanzee *(9)* insulin promoters contain a variable number of tandem repeats of a 14 bp sequence at –360 bp relative to the transcription start site (*see* Fig. 3). The old world primate African green monkey has two copies of the repeat *(9)* and the new world primate owl monkey has a single copy *(10)*. The rat and mouse genes each contain one-half repeat. Although this hypervariable region (HVR) of the insulin gene is useful for linkage studies *(see below)* and the G-rich top strand is known to form an unusual DNA structure *(11)* in vitro, its functional importance is unknown.

Insulin Gene Expression

Because of its central role in metabolic control, tight regulation of insulin production and release is critical. In adult mammals, insulin production is limited to a single cell type: the β-cell at the core of the islets of Langerhans in the pancreas. Careful examination of other adult tissues has never revealed evidence of the preproinsulin mRNA that would be necessary for insulin production.

Any cell, however, if altered to allow transcription of the insulin gene, can produce proinsulin *(12,13)*; and other endocrine cells, similarly altered, can even process, package, and secrete mature insulin in a regulated fashion *(14)*. Since non-β-cells can perform all subsequent steps, it is initiation of transcription that restricts insulin production to the β-cell.

Gittes and Rutter *(15)* demonstrated that insulin mRNA first appears in the developing gut of the mouse during the ninth day postcoitus (E9), prior to the earliest morphologic development of the pancreas. By E12, when the first lobules of the developing pancreas are evident, specific antisera can demonstrate the presence of the insulin peptide in a subset of cells *(16)*. Interestingly, these earliest insulin-positive cells often also express immunoreactive glucagon *(17)*. As the islets develop, insulin and glucagon segregate into the β- and α-cells, respectively.

The Insulin Promoter

Transcription of the insulin gene is regulated, at least in part, by its 5' flanking DNA—the promoter. Walker et al. demonstrated that the insulin promoter still functions in a cell-specific fashion when isolated from the remainder of the gene *(18)*. They removed approx 400 bp of the proximal promoters from the human insulin and rat insulin I genes and inserted these fragments into bacterial DNA plasmids upstream from the coding sequence of the bacterial gene for chloramphenicol resistance, chloramphenicol acetyltransferase (CAT) (*see* Fig. 4). When these hybrid DNA plasmids are inserted into cells, the insulin promoter regulates transcription of the linked CAT gene. The CAT enzyme activity in extracts from these cells is then an indirect estimate of the CAT mRNA level, transcription rate, and activity of the insulin promoter. Walker et al. found that introduction of the hybrid plasmid generated high levels of CAT enzyme activity in β-cells, but little or no functional CAT enzyme or CAT mRNA in non-β-cells.

Subsequently, Hanahan performed a similar experiment in transgenic mice *(19)*. By linking the rat insulin II promoter to the coding sequence for the Simian Virus 40 large T antigen, Hanahan developed a transgenic mouse line in which the insulin promoter directed expression of this potent viral oncogene. These mice expressed T antigen exclusively in their β-cells and inevitably developed β-cell hyperplasia and insulin-producing islet tumors, demonstrating the cell-specific function of the insulin promoter in vivo.

The insulin promoter is not a single functional unit; rather a number of distinct sequence elements interact to give the characteristic function of the intact promoter. These sequence elements are

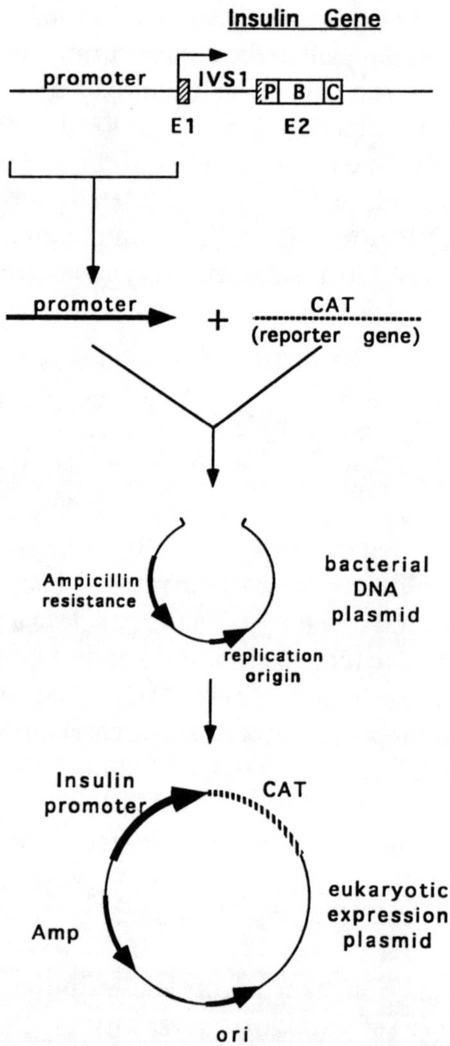

Fig. 4. Schematic representation of the construction of plasmids with the insulin promoter driving expression of the CAT gene.

cis-acting since they only regulate a gene to which they are physically linked; but the exact position of the *cis*-acting elements relative to the TATAA element or coding region can vary. When a large distal fragment of the insulin 5' flanking DNA was isolated and inserted upstream of a promoter from an unrelated gene, it enhanced the transcriptional activity of the heterologous promoter in β-cells *(20)*. This result led to the conclusion that the insulin gene 5' flanking DNA was formed from two distinct elements, both of which functioned in a tissue-specific fashion: an "enhancer" from approx –250 to –100 bp (relative to the transcription start site) that functioned independent of position or orientation, and a "promoter" from about –100 to –1 bp that functioned only in its native position *(20)*.

This distinction, however, may be misleading. The proximal "promoter" sequence also has enhancer-like properties when inverted and placed distal to a heterologous promoter *(20)*. The conceptual distinction between enhancer and promoter has become increasingly blurred; and in general usage now the term promoter signifies all of the 5' flanking DNA that regulates transcriptional activity. With the exception of the TATAA element, essentially all of the transcriptionally active sequences in the insulin promoter can function in the context of an enhancer as well.

It is now generally accepted that most of the *cis*-acting promoter elements act as recognition sequences for sequence-specific DNA binding proteins in the nucleus. These proteins, or transcription factors, interact with RNA polymerase and regulate transcription of the gene. The unique set of transcription factors in the nucleus determines the activity of the insulin promoter in that cell.

DNA binding proteins can be distinguished by their ability to bind a radiolabeled DNA fragment. Nuclear extracts of β-cells contain numerous distinct protein complexes that bind specific sequences on the insulin promoter. Many of these complexes are present in other cell types as well, but some are restricted to β-cells or a small subset of related cell types. Figure 5 shows the relative positions of some of the *cis*-acting sequence elements along the insulin promoter and some of the binding/transcription factors that bind these elements.

The IEB Elements

Initial analysis of truncated promoters linked to CAT and expressed in insulinoma cell lines revealed important sequences in the human and rat insulin promoters at approx –250 and –100 bp *(18,21,22)*. In the rat insulin I gene, two identical 8 bp sequences lie at these positions—the IEB2 and IEB1 elements, also called the Far and Nir elements. The IEB elements belong to a class of *cis*-acting

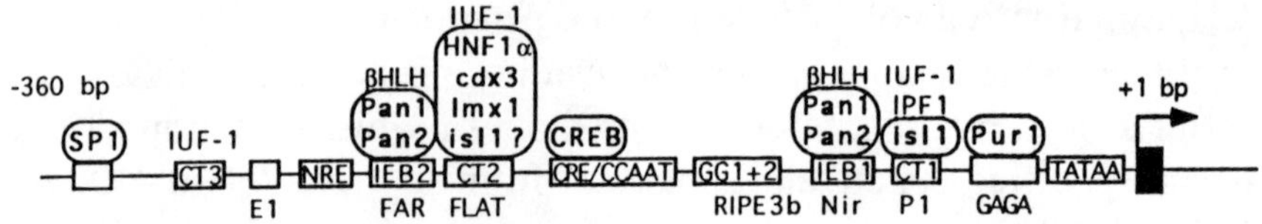

Fig. 5. The insulin promoter with known *cis*-acting elements and binding factors. The boxes represent characterized *cis*-acting functional elements and/or binding sites. Names for the human promoter elements are shown in the boxes, the names for the rat elements are shown below the boxes. Characterized binding factors are shown above the boxes, and the cloned factors are circled.

elements, E boxes, that share the common sequence CANNTG and regulate transcription of a wide array of genes in different cell types. When either of the rat insulin I IEB elements are mutated in an otherwise intact promoter, transcription falls tenfold; promoters with mutations in both IEB elements are essentially inactive in insulinoma cells *(23)*. The IEB1 element is similarly critical for the human insulin *(21)* and the rat insulin II *(22,24)* promoters.

The insulin promoter IEB elements bind a protein complex that is present in β-cell nuclei but is absent from non-endocrine cell nuclei *(25–29)*. We have cloned two cDNAs, Pan 1 and Pan 2 *(30,31)* whose protein products bind the IEB sites. The two cDNAs represent differential RNA splice products of the E2A gene *(32)* and are homologues of the human E12/E47 *(33)* and the mouse A1 *(34)* cDNAs. The proposed structures of these proteins based on their amino acid sequences predict a highly basic region immediately adjacent to a helix-loop-helix structure. Pan 1 and Pan 2 belong to a family of DNA binding proteins with this helix-loop-helix (HLH) structure. The HLH proteins dimerize via the HLH domain and different members of the family preferentially heterodimerize.

Antisera directed against the Pan proteins recognize the β-cell specific nuclear complex that binds the IEB sites *(25,28,30,35)*, despite the fact that the Pan proteins are expressed ubiquitously. Most likely, the cell-specific expression of the complex results from dimerization of the Pan proteins with another, β-cell specific, HLH protein. The size of this β-HLH has been predicted *(36)* but it has not yet been purified or cloned.

The CT Elements

Just downstream from both IEB1 and IEB2 are two similar sites, CT1 and CT2, respectively, with the core sequence CTAAT. Mutation of the rat insulin I CT2 element (also called FLAT) causes a marked loss of promoter activity, whereas mutation of the rat insulin CT1 site (or P1 element) causes only a modest reduction in activity *(23)*. The human promoter has an additional site, CT3, at approx -315 bp *(37)*. Similar elements have been described in two other β-cell specific promoters, islet amyloid polypeptide *(38)* and β-cell specific glucokinase *(38,39)*. All three sites from the human insulin promoter bind the same β-cell specific nuclear protein complex, insulin upstream factor 1 (IUF-1) *(37,40)*. The rat insulin I PI and FLAT sites, however, appear to bind different complexes *(25,38)*.

A cDNA clone, isl-1, encoding a FLAT and P1 element binding protein was cloned by Karlsson et al. *(41)*. Isl-1 was initially thought to be islet-specific (thus the name), but it has since been found in a variety of endocrine and nonendocrine cells *(42,43)*. Antisera to isl-1 do not recognize any of the FLAT or P1-binding nuclear complexes in β-cells *(25)*.

We have recently cloned two additional cDNAs, lmx-1 and cdx-3, that encode FLAT-binding proteins *(44)*. Both of these proteins and isl-1 share a common 61 amino acid domain, the homeodomain, that forms three alpha helices and binds DNA. A growing number of homeodomain proteins have been described from a variety of species and cell types. These proteins often play important roles in development, cell lineage determination, and gene transcription.

The lmx-1 and isl-1 proteins share an additional feature, a pair of cysteine-histidine rich regions in the amino-terminal end of the proteins. These regions, Lim domains, named after the first three Lim domain-containing proteins, Lin-11, isl-1, and mec-3, bind both zinc and iron-sulfur *(45)*.

The mRNA for cdx-3 can be found in the intestine and testes as well as the β-cell *(44)*, but so far lmx-1 mRNA or protein has only been recognized in β-cells. Both cdx-3 and lmx-1 bind to the FLAT element with much higher affinity than isl-1 and can activate the insulin promoter in non-β-cells *(44)*. It is not known if either lmx-1 or cdx-3 are the same as the previously described IUF-1 factor.

Another homeodomain containing protein, hepatocyte nuclear factor lα (HNF 1α) is expressed in β-cells and can bind to and activate the upstream half of the FLAT element in the rat insulin I promoter *(46)*. Since this binding site is not conserved in the other known insulin promoters, HNF 1α may not play an important role in the expression of these genes.

The GAGA Element

Just upstream from the TATAA element lies a 17 bp purine-rich sequence, the GAGA element. In primary cultured β-cells *(47)* and to a lesser extent insulinoma cells *(23)*, this element is critically important. Several nuclear complexes with different patterns of expression bind the GAGA element *(48)* in the rat insulin I promoter. Kennedy and Rutter *(48)* have cloned and characterized a ubiquitously expressed protein, Pur-1, that binds and activates the GAGA element. Pur-1 has six "zinc fingers," conserved cysteine-histidine containing structures that bind zinc. In many other proteins, including the steroid and thyroid hormone receptors, zinc fingers are known to bind DNA. When expressed in non-β-cells, Pur-1 activates the insulin promoter.

Negative Regulation

In addition to transcriptional activation by *cis*-acting elements and *trans*-acting transcription factors, some *cis*-acting sequences repress transcription, presumably through interaction with DNA binding proteins that interfere with activating transcription factors or that directly inhibit RNA polymerase. Such negative regulatory factors may contribute to the tight suppression of the insulin promoter in noninsulin producing cells. Nir et al. *(49)* showed that at least one negative trans-acting factor binds the rat insulin I proximal promoter in noninsulin-producing cells. *Cis*-acting negative regulatory elements that function in non-ß-cells have also been described in the human insulin promoter *(50)*, the distal rat insulin I 5' flanking DNA *(51)*, and the rat insulin II promoter *(24)*.

Boam et al. *(21)* have described a *cis*-acting negative regulatory element (NRE) that functions in both ß-cells and non-β-cells. They noted that deletion of the 5' end of human insulin promoter up to –258 bp caused a marked increase in promoter activity. The NRE sequence between bases –279 and –258 can also repress transcription when linked to a heterologous promoter, although this effect is much less dramatic and is dependent on exact position and orientation. The negative effects of the NRE may be dependent on the cell lines used or the surrounding sequences in the expression plasmid, because Walker et al. *(18)* did not see a similar effect of the –258 deletion. We also do not see activation with the –258 bp deletion in primary β-cells (German and Wang, unpublished data).

Other Cis-*Acting Elements*

Several less well-characterized *cis*-acting elements contribute to the activity of the insulin promoter. The human promoter contains a consensus sequence for ubiquitous Sp1 transcription factor at about 350 bp. Deletion of this site from the human insulin promoter results in a modest loss of activity *(52)*. The Sp1 site is not conserved in the nonprimate promoters.

A consensus binding site for a family of ubiquitous transcription of factors, the CCAAT sequence, is found in the rodent insulin promoters. Mutation of this region in the rat insulin II promoter causes a 5-fold reduction in activity *(22)*. Although mutation of the CCAAT element in the rat insulin I promoter does not affect promoter function in hamster insulinoma cells, it does reduce promoter activity in a mouse insulinoma cell line (L. Moss, personal communication).

At –310 bp in the rat insulin I promoter, between the positions of the CT3 and NRE elements in the human insulin promoter, mutation causes a large decrease in promoter activity *(23)*. This region, E1, binds a nuclear protein complex with limited tissue distribution *(25,53)*. It is not known if the homologous region in the human promoter has a similar function, but the sequence in this area is not well-conserved in the primate promoters.

Synergistic Interactions

The insulin promoter is more than the sum of its independent parts. Each *cis*-acting element with its cognate binding factors is not an independent unit but functions instead by interacting with the other elements along the promoter to activate transcription synergistically. The result is a promoter that can function properly only in the presence of a minimal set of transcription factors. This model explains the exquisite cell-type specificity of the insulin promoter, since deletion or substitution of any of these factors will drastically reduce promoter activity.

To avoid the complexity of these interactions in the intact promoter, we have studied a small fragment of the rat insulin I promoter including the IEB2 (Far) and the CT2 (FLAT) elements. When linked to a heterologous promoter, this Far-FLAT minienhancer dramatically activates transcription in a cell-type specific manner. Activation by the minienhancer requires both the Far and the FLAT elements. Minienhancers with either the Far or FLAT elements inactivated by mutation lose all activity and short minienhancers including just the Far or FLAT element also are inactive (*see* Fig. 6). Interestingly, the FLAT element contains two distinct binding sites; mutation of either site alone does not inactivate the FLAT element. This dual site architecture of the rat insulin I FLAT element is not conserved in the other insulin promoters (Fig. 3). The distal binding site, FLAT-F, is unique to the rat insulin I gene; but the proximal site, FLAT-E, corresponds to the conserved CT2 element *(38)*.

We assume that the synergy demonstrated by the Far-FLAT cooperativity results from interaction between the transcription factors that bind these sites. In fact, lmx-1 and the Pan proteins show just such a synergistic activation (*see* Fig. 7) *(44)*. When expressed at high levels in noninsulin-producing cells, Pan 1 causes no appreciable activation of the Far-FLAT minienhancer and lmx-1 only stimulates a modest tenfold rise in activity. When both proteins are expressed in the same cell, however, minienhancer-driven transcription rises approx 1000-fold.

The synergistic activation capacity of lmx-1 appears to map to the Lim domains, since truncated lmx-1 proteins without one or both of the Lim domains do not synergistically cooperate with Pan 1, although these truncated proteins still bind the FLAT element and activate transcription in the absence of Pan (basal activation). Removal of the carboxy-terminus of the protein causes the loss of basal activation, and of course removal of the homeodomain causes loss of DNA binding and all activation capacity (*see* Fig. 7b).

Other *cis*-acting elements in the insulin promoter demonstrate similar cooperativity. The rat insulin II promoter IEB1 element cooperates with a sequence element immediately upstream, the RIPE3B element *(28,54)*. Like the Far-FLAT interaction, both of these elements have minimal intrinsic activity, but together they function as

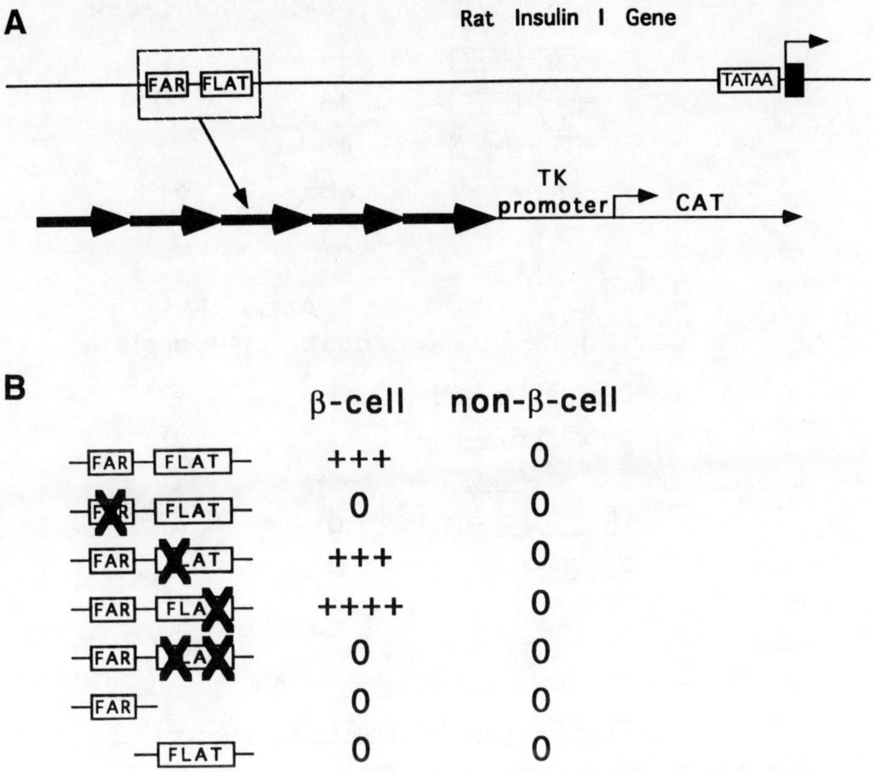

Fig. 6. Function of the Far-FLAT minienhancer. **(A)** The construction of minienhancer CAT plasmids is shown. Five copies of the minienhancer are linked in tandem to the herpes simplex virus thymidine kinase minimal promoter driving the CAT gene. **(B)** The relative transcriptional activities of mutant and partially truncated minienhancers in insulinoma cells and fibroblasts (non-β-cells) are shown (taken from ref. *38*).

a potent transcriptional activator. RIPE3B binds a β-cell specific nuclear complex *(28)* and may overlap GG2, a site in the human insulin promoter that has been shown to bind a ß-cell specific nuclear complex *(21)*. We have shown that the human and rat insulin I promoter equivalents of the RIPE3/IEB1 region function similarly (unpublished data). It is unknown if the IEB1 and CT1/P1 elements cooperate, but given the parallels with the Far-FLAT interaction, this seems likely as well.

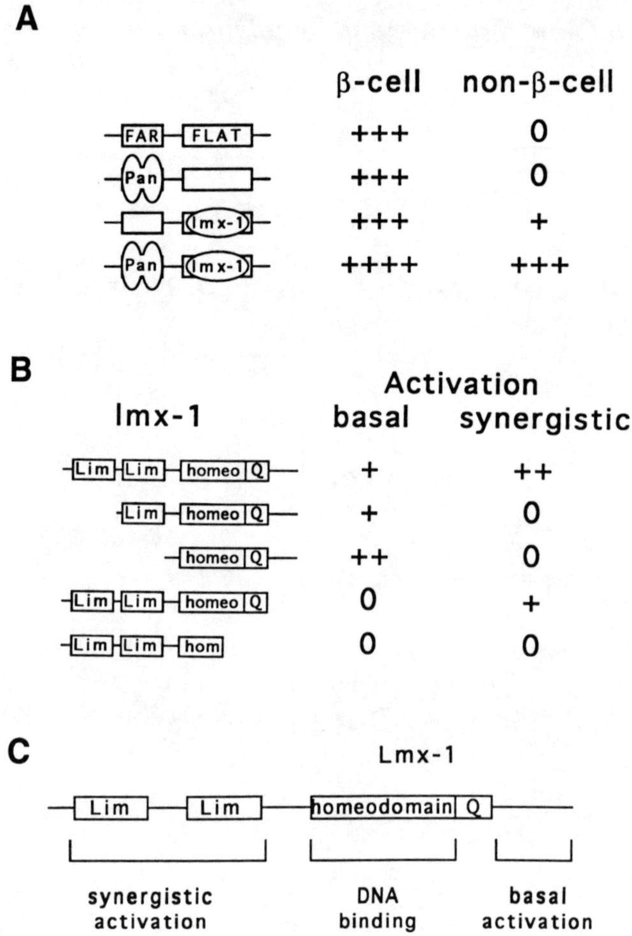

Fig. 7. Synergistic activation of the insulin promoter by Pan and lmx-1. **(A)** The Pan and lmx-1 cDNAs were expressed in insulinoma cells and fibroblasts, and the relative activity of the Far-FLAT minienhancer is shown. **(B)** Truncated lmx-1 cDNAs were co-expressed with Pan-1 and the Far-FLAT minienhancer driven CAT plasmid. The relative effects on basal and synergistic activation of transcription in insulinoma cells are shown. **(C)** The functional domains on lmx-1 are outlined (taken from ref. *44*).

Metabolic Regulation of the Insulin Promoter

The β-cell responds to rising glucose concentration by increasing insulin synthesis and secretion. Insulin mRNA levels rise in the β-cells of fed animals and fall during fasting *(55)*. Isolated islets show the same response to glucose and also to other metabolic substrates such as leucine and glutamine *(56,57)*. The rise in insulin mRNA levels results from the combined effects of an increased rate of transcription and a decreased rate of messenger RNA degradation *(58,59)*. Glucose selectively affects insulin mRNA levels, as the total mRNA level in islets increases only slightly in response to glucose stimulation.

The relative contribution of insulin gene transcription to the overall increase in insulin production and secretion in response to glucose has been difficult to estimate accurately. In the healthy individual with normal insulin sensitivity and regular activity and meals, changes in transcription and synthesis probably contribute little to the insulin secretory fluctuations. On the other hand, when insulin requirements increase, such as in noninsulin dependent diabetes mellitus (NIDDM), or when the total ß-cell mass decreases, such as in early insulin dependent diabetes mellitus (IDDM), either total insulin synthesis or insulin gene transcription may limit insulin secretory capacity. Animal models suggest that changes in mRNA level may be more important than changes in translation rate in this setting *(60)*.

We have shown that the insulin promoter contributes to the synthetic response to glucose *(61)*. When the insulin promoter-CAT hybrid plasmid (Fig. 4) is inserted into cultured β-cells, CAT enzyme activities and CAT mRNA levels fluctuate in response to the glucose concentration in the culture media. The entire promoter is not required for this response, as the Far-FLAT minienhancer linked to a nonresponsive heterologous promoter (Fig. 6A) can recapitulate the glucose response of the intact promoter *(61)*.

The Far element appears to be the predominant site of glucose regulation within the minienhancer since mutations of the Far element, but not of the FLAT element, ablate the Far-FLAT minienhancer's response to glucose, and the isolated Far element can respond to glucose. Furthermore, when the Pan 1 protein is overexpressed in β-cells, the Far-FLAT minienhancer and the isolated Pan element lose their ability to respond to glucose *(47)*. We have interpreted these results as showing that glucose stimulation modifies the Pan-βHLH transcription complex that in turn modulates transcription of the gene through binding and activation of the Far/IEB2 element and the identical Nir/IEB1 element (*see* Fig. 8).

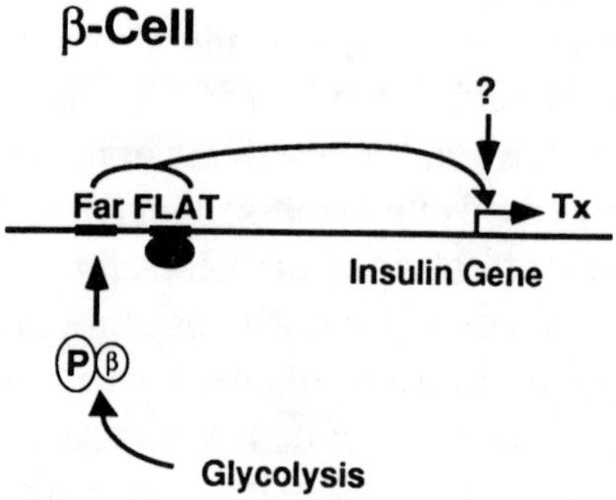

Fig. 8. A schematic outline of the effects of glucose on insulin gene transcription via the Far box.

Although these experiments demonstrate that the Far element can respond to glucose, we cannot rule out the possibility that the FLAT element contributes to the overall transcriptional response to glucose coded by the intact Far-FLAT minienhancer, because the FLAT element does not have any transcriptional activity on its own and therefore cannot be expected to respond to glucose on its own. Furthermore, an intact promoter with mutations in both the IEB elements can still respond to glucose, demonstrating that the insulin promoter contains additional glucose responsive *cis*-acting elements *(47)*.

Glucose stimulates insulin secretion indirectly through the end products of glycolysis and mitochondrial oxidation. The same is true for glucose stimulation of transcription. When glycolysis is accelerated in β-cells by expressing high levels of hexokinase I (the enzyme that catalyzes the rate-limiting step of glucose catabolism in β-cells), the insulin promoter responds to much lower glucose levels *(62)*. This response to glucose requires glycolysis and is mimicked by other sources of the glycolytic intermediates *(62)*.

Glucose metabolism in β-cells causes widespread changes in intracellular signaling systems. Because the insulin promoter contains consensus sequence for a cAMP response element (CRE), it has been suggested that cAMP might be the signal that activates the promoter in response to glucose. Although the rat insulin I gene is activated by cAMP through the CRE *(61,63)*, we have found that the transcriptional response to glucose is unaffected by cAMP agonists or antagonists *(61)*, and the glucose responsive Far-FLAT minienhancer lacks a CRE. On the other hand, calcium channel blockers decrease the transcriptional response to glucose, suggesting that calcium influx—the critical signal for insulin secretion—may also play a critical role in transcription.

Insulin Gene Expression and Diabetes Mellitus

The role of the insulin gene in the etiology of diabetes mellitus remains unclear. Although mutations in the coding portion of the insulin gene that result in mutant insulin molecules are sometimes associated with NIDDM, these coding mutations are rare, only a minority of individuals who inherit the mutations develop diabetes, and the disease is usually mild (for a review, *see* Vinik and Bell *[64]*). There is indirect evidence, however, that alterations in insulin gene expression may contribute to the more common forms of diabetes mellitus.

Insulin Gene Polymorphisms and IDDM

The human insulin gene varies slightly in sequence from one individual to the next. The most striking of these variations, or polymorphisms, is the variable-sized insert (HVR) at –360 bp in the promoter. Most HVR inserts fall into one of two size classes, less than 600 bp (class 1 allele) and greater than 1600 bp (class 3 allele). HVRs between 600–1600 bp in size (class 2 allele) are rare except in African and African American populations.

The size of the HVR can be used as a genetic marker to study the association of this region of chromosome 11 with clinical evidence of disease. There are several statistical means for testing for an association, the simplest being population association studies. Analysis of the relative frequency of HVR size classes among diabetic patient and nondiabetics reveals a significantly higher number of HVR class 1 alleles in patients with IDDM *(65)*. A weak and inconsistent association has been noted between the class 3 allele and NIDDM *(66,67)*. Although population studies are subject to misinterpretation if there are unrecognized allele and disease frequency variations in subpopulations, a higher risk of IDDM in individuals with class 1 alleles has since been demonstrated in several distinct populations, increasing the probability that this association is real. One exception has been the Japanese population in which the class 3 allele is extremely rare, making statistically significant analysis difficult *(68)*.

Family studies of direct linkage between genetic markers and disease states are statistically more informative than population association studies. Analysis of affected sib pairs with IDDM initially did not demonstrate a linkage between the HVR/insulin locus and IDDM. Recently, however, Julier et al. *(69)* in a study of French, American, and North African families demonstrated a statistically significant linkage between the class 1 allele and risk of IDDM by limiting their analysis to families with heterozygous parents. Interestingly, this linkage was strongest when the class 1 allele was inherited from the father and when the affected family member was HLA-DR4 positive. Linkage was seen also for 6 other polymorphic genetic markers within the insulin locus and one marker in IVS3 of the IGF2 gene, but not for markers in the distal IGF2 gene or the tyrosine hydroxylase gene. The HVR/insulin linkage to IDDM has since been noted in Belgian *(70)*, English *(71)*, and Norwegian *(71)* families, but these studies did not find an association between the insulin locus polymorphisms and HLA-DR haplotype.

Although these studies have conclusively demonstrated linkage between the HVR/insulin/IGF2 locus and IDDM, the molecular mechanisms of this disease association remain obscure. There are three possible explanations. First, the HVR and other polymorphic loci could be in linkage disequilibrium with differences in the insulin or the IGF2 gene coding sequences that result in abnormal gene products. No such mutations have been found in the insulin genes of individuals with IDDM, and the 19 kb limits of genetic linkage outlined by Julier et al. do not include the coding portion of the IGF2 gene *(69)*. Second, some portion of a previously unrecognized gene may lie within the 19 kb linkage region. Finally, polymorphisms in this region could directly affect expression of insulin, IGF2, TH, or other nearby genes.

Because of its location immediately adjacent to critical *cis*-acting elements in the insulin promoter and the large size difference between class 1 and class 3 alleles, it seems likely that the HVR itself could affect gene expression. Although previous experiments with a class 1 HVR in hamster insulinoma cells did not support this model *(18)*, the intact gene in normal β-cells may function differently—especially during fetal development and childhood when the risk of developing IDDM is highest.

In addition, the HVR could affect the nearby TH and IGF2 promoters. The IGF2 gene is subject to parental imprinting: The maternal copy of the IGF2 gene is suppressed, and only the paternal gene is expressed *(72)*. The insulin gene is not subject to similar imprinting. Individuals who inherit two copies of the paternal IGF2 gene develop islet hyperplasia, hyperinsulinema, and hypoglycemia along with other abnormalities (Beckwith-Weidemann syndrome *[73]*). The paternal linkage of the HVR with IDDM suggests that the HVR may be linked to differences in IGF2 expression, specifically in the β-cell, resulting in differences in islet development, expression of islet antigens, or ability to respond to β-cell damage.

Gene Expression and NIDDM

NIDDM is most likely a multigenic (results from independent alterations in several different genes) and/or polygenic (results from the interaction of several altered genes) disease, which makes the demonstration of association with individual genetic markers within a diverse population difficult. Most patients with NIDDM have some degree of peripheral resistance to insulin action, but similar levels of resistance are common in nondiabetics as well, demonstrating that development of frank NIDDM requires a β-cell defect in stimulated insulin secretion as well. Despite the lack of a strong association between NIDDM and the HVR/insulin locus, inherited defects in insulin gene expression might be expected to limit stimulated insulin secretion and predispose individuals to NIDDM.

Olansky et al. *(74)* found an 8 bp repeat inserted at -315 bp in the insulin promoter in ~5% of African Americans and Mauritius creoles (also of African descent) with NIDDM. The incidence of this insertion in non-diabetics from the same populations was significantly lower. The inserted bases, TGGTCTAA, occur within the CT3 elements, but recreate two CT3 sites. The net result is apparently deleterious to promoter function: The variant promoter has less than 50% of the transcriptional activity of the normal promoter when linked to a reporter gene and expressed in insulinoma cells. Because the affected individuals have one copy of the normal gene, only a modest net reduction (about 75% of normal) in insulin gene expression would be expected. Whether this reduction in insulin gene expression alone predisposes these individuals to NIDDM is unknown.

Progress in understanding the regulation of insulin gene expression has led to a new set of genes, the transcription factor genes, whose proper function is essential for insulin production. The availability of the cloned insulin gene transcription factors will allow us to look for defects in their respective genes in NIDDM. These β-cell transcription factors regulate not only the insulin gene but also other β-cell genes whose products control the critical β-cell processes of metabolic sensing and insulin secretion. Defects in the transcription factor genes could explain the multiple β-cell defects recognized in NIDDM.

References

1. Banting FG, Best CH: The internal secretion of the pancreas. *J Lab Clin Med* 7:251–266, 1922.
2. Ullrich A, Shine J, Chirgwin J, Pictet R, Tischer E, Rutter WJ, et al.: Rat insulin genes: Construction of plasmids containing the coding sequences. *Science* 196:1313–1319, 1977.
3. Bell GI, Swain WF, Pictet RL, Cordell B, Goodman HM, Rutter WJ: Nucleotide sequence of a cDNA clone encoding human preproinsulin. *Nature* 282:525–527, 1979.
4. Bell GI, Pictet RL, Rutter WJ, Cordell B, Tischer E, Goodman HM: Sequence of the human insulin gene. *Nature* 284:26–32, 1980.
5. Soares MB, Schon E, Henderson A, Karathanasis SK, Cate R, Zeitlin S, et al.: RNA-mediated gene duplication: the rat preproinsulin I gene is a functional retroposon. *Mol Cell Biol* 5:2090–2103, 1985.
6. Perler F, Efstratiadis A, Lomedico P, Gilbert W, Kolodner R, Dodgson J: The evolution of genes: the chicken preproinsulin gene. *Cell* 20:555–566, 1980.
7. Koval AP, Petrenko AI, Kavsan VM: Sequence of the salmon *(Oncorhynchys keta)* preproinsulin gene. *Nucleic Acids Res* 17:1758, 1989.
8. Bell GI, Selby M, Rutter WJ: The highly polymorphic region near the human insulin gene is composed of simple tandemly repeating sequences. *Nature* 295:31–35, 1982.
9. Seino S, Bell GI, Li WH: Sequences of primate insulin genes support the hypothesis of a slower rate of molecular evolution in humans and apes than in monkeys. *Mol Biol Evol* 9:193–203, 1992.
10. Seino S, Steine DF, Bell GI: Squence of a new world primate insulin having low biological potency and immunoreactivity. *Proc Natl Acad Sci USA* 84:7423–7427, 1987.
11. Hammond-Kosack MCU, Dobrinski B, Lurz R, Docherty K, Kilpatrick M: The human insulin gene linked polymorphic region exhibits an altered DNA structure. *Nucleic Acids Res* 20:231–236, 1992.
12. Laub O, L Rall, Bell GI, Rutter WJ: Expression of the human insulin gene in an alternate mammalian cell and in cell extracts. *J Biol Chem* 258:6037–6042, 1983.

13. Laub O, Rutter WJ: Expression of the human insulin gene and cDNA in a heterologous mammalian system. *J Biol Chem* 258:6043–6050, 1983.
14. Moore HPH, Walker MD, Lee F, Kelly RB: Expressing a human proinsulin cDNA in a mouse ACTH-secreting cell. Intracellular storage, proteolytic processing and secretion of stimulation. *Cell* 35:531–538, 1983.
15. Gittes G, Rutter WJ: Onset of cell-specific gene expression in the developing mouse pancreas. *Proc Natl Acad Sci USA* 89:1128–1132, 1992.
16. Teitelman G, Lee JK, Alpert S: Cell lineage analysis of pancreatic exocrine and endocrine cells. *Cell Tissue Res* 250:435–439, 1987.
17. Alpert S, Hanahan D, Teitelman G: Hybrid insulin genes reveal a developmental lineage for pancreatic endocrine cells and imply a relationship with neurons. *Cell* 53:295–308, 1988.
18. Walker MD, Edlund T, Boulet AM, Rutter WJ: Cell-specific expression controlled by the 5' flanking regions of the insulin and chymotrypsin genes. *Nature* 306:557–581, 1983.
19. Hanahan D: Heritable formation of pancreatic β-cell tumors in transgenic mice expressing recombinant insulin/simian virus 40 oncogenes. *Nature* 315:115–122, 1985.
20. Edlund T, Walker MD, Barr PJ, Rutter WJ: Cell-specific expression of the rat insulin gene: evidence for the role of two distinct 5' flanking sequences. *Science* 230:912–916, 1985.
21. Boam D, Clark A, Docherty K: Positive and negative regulation of the insulin gene by multiple *trans*-acting factors. *J Biol Chem* 265:8285–8296, 1990.
22. Crowe DT, Tsai M-J: Mutagenesis of the rat insulin II 5'-flanking region defines sequences important for expression in HIT cells. *Mol Cell Biol* 9:1784–1789, 1989.
23. Karlsson O, Edlund T, Moss JB, Rutter WJ, Walker MD: A mutational analysis of the insulin gene transcription control region: expression in β-cells is dependent on two related sequences within the enhancer. *Proc Natl Acad Sci USA* 84:8819–8823, 1987.
24. Whelan J, Poon D, Weil PA, Stein R: Pancreatic β-cell-type-specific expression of the rat insulin II gene is controled by positive and negative cellular transcription elements. *Mol Cell Biol* 9:3253–3259, 1989.
25. Aronheim A, Ohlsson H, Park CW, Edlund T, Walker MD: Distribution and characterization of helix-loop-helix enhancer-binding proteins from pancreatic β-cells and lymphocytes. *Nucleic Acids Res* 19:3893–3899, 1991.
26. Moss LG, Moss JB, Rutter WJ: Systematic binding analysis of the insulin gene transcription control region: insulin and immunoglobulin enhancers utilize similar transactivators. *Mol Cell Biol* 8:2620–2627, 1988.
27. Ohlsson H, Karlson O, Edlund T: A β–cell-specific protein binds to the two major regulatory sequences of the insulin enhancer. *Proc Natl Acad Sci* 85:4228–4231, 1988.
28. Sheih S, Tsai M: Cell-specific and ubiquitous factors are responsible for the enhancer activity of the rat insulin II gene. *J Biol Chem* 266:16,708–16,704, 1991.

29. Whelan J, Cordle SR, Henderson E, Weil PA, Stein R: Identification of a pancreatic β-cell insulin gene transcription factor that binds to and appears to activate cell-type-specific expression: its possible relationship to other cellular factors that bind to a common insulin gene sequence. *Mol Cell Biol* 10:1564–1572, 1990.
30. German MS, Blanar MA, Nelson C, Moss LG, Rutter WJ: Two related helix-loop-helix proteins participate in separate cell-specific complexes that bind to the insulin enhancer. *Mol Endocinol* 5:292–299, 1991.
31. Nelson C, Shen L-P, Meister A, Fodor E, Rutter WJ: Pan: a transcriptional regulator that binds chymotrypsin, insulin, and AP-4 enhancer motifs. *Genes Dev* 4:1035–1043, 1990.
32. Sun XH, Baltimore D: An inhibitory domain of E12 transcription factor prevents DNA binding in E12 homodimers but not in E12 heterodimers. *Cell* 64:459–470, 1991.
33. Murre C, McCaw PS, Baltimore D: A new DNA binding and dimerization motif in immunoglobulin enhancer binding, daughterless, MyoD, and *myc* proteins. *Cell* 56:777–783, 1989.
34. Walker, MD, Park CW, Rosen A, Aronheim A: A cDNA from a mouse pancreatic β-cell encoding a putative transcription factor of the insulin gene. *Nucleic Acids Res* 18:1159–1166, 1990.
35. Cordle SR, Henderson E, Masuoka H, Weil PA, Stein R: Pancreatic β-cell-type-specific transcription of the insulin gene is mediated by basic helix-loop-helix DNA-binding proteins. *Mol Cell Biol* 11:1734–1738, 1991.
36. Park CW, Walker MD: Subunit structure of cell-specific E box-binding proteins analyzed by quantitation of electrophoretic mobility shift. *J Biol Chem* 267:15,642–15,649, 1992.
37. Boam DSW, Docherty K: A tissue-specific nuclear factor binds to multiple sites in the human insulin-gene enhancer. *Biochem J* 264:233–239, 1989.
38. German MS, Moss LG, Wang J, Rutter WJ: The insulin and islet amyloid polypeptide genes contain similar cell-specific promoter elements that bind identical β-cell nuclear complexes. *Mol Cell Biol* 12:1777–1788, 1992.
39. Shelton KD, Franklin AJ, Khoor A, Beechem J, Magnuson MA: Multiple elements in the upstream glucokinase promoter contribute to transcription in insulinoma cells. *Mol Cell Biol* 12:4578–4589, 1992.
40. Scott V, Clark AR, Hutton JC, Docherty K: Two proteins act as the IUF1 insulin gene enhancer binding factor. *FEBS Letts* 290:27–30, 1991.
41. Karlsson O, Thor S, Norberg T, Ohlsson H, Edlund T: Insulin gene enhancer binding protein isl-1 is a member of a novel class of proteins containing both a homeo- and a cys-his domain. *Nature* 344:879–882, 1990.
42. Dong J, Asa SL, Drucker DJ: Islet cell and extrapancreatic expression of the LIM domain homeobox gene isl-1. *Mol Endocrinol* 5:1633–1641, 1991.
43. Thor S, Ericson J, Brannstrom T, Edlund T: The homeodomain LIM protein isl-I is expressed in subsets of neurons and endocrine cells in the adult rat. *Neuron* 7:1–9, 1991.
44. German MS, Wang J, Chadwick RB, Rutter WJ: Synergistic activation of the insulin gene by a LIM-homeodomain protein and a basic helix-loop-

helix protein: building a functional insulin minienhancer complex. *Genes Dev* 6:2165–2176, 1992.
45. Li PM, Reichert J, Freyd G, Horvitz HR, Walsh CT: The LIM region of a presumptive *Caenorhabditis elegans* transcription factor is an iron-sulfur- and zinc-containing metallodomain. *Proc Natl Acad Sci USA* 88:9210–9213, 1991.
46. Emens LA, Landers DW, Moss LG: Hepatocyte nuclear factor 1α is expressed in a hamster insulinoma line and transactivates the rat insulin I gene. *Proc Natl Acad Sci USA* 89:7300–7304, 1992.
47. German MS, Wang J: The insulin gene contains multiple transcriptional elements that respond to glucose. *Mol Cell Biol,* in press.
48. Kennedy GC, Rutter WJ: Pur-1, a zinc-finger protein that binds to purine-rich sequences, transactivates an insulin promoter in heterologous cells. *Proc Natl Acad Sci USA* 89:11,498–11,502, 1992.
49. Nir U, Walker MD, Rutter WJ: Regulation of rat insulin 1 gene expression: evidence for negative regulation in nonpancreatic cells. *Proc Natl Acad Sci USA* 83:3180–3184, 1986.
50. Takeda J, Ishii S, Seino Y, Imamoto F, Imura H: Negative regulation of human insulin gene expression by the 5'-flanking region in non-pancreatic cells. *FEBS Letts* 247:41–45, 1989.
51. Laimins L, Holmgren-Konig M, Khoury G: Transcriptional "silencer" element in rat repetitive sequences associated with the rat insulin 1 gene locus. *Proc Natl Acad Sci USA* 83:3151–3155, 1986.
52. Docherty K: The regulation of insulin gene expression. *Diabetic Med* 9:792–798, 1992.
53. Ohlsson H, Edlund T: Sequence-specific interactions of nuclear factors with the insulin gene enhancer. *Cell* 45:35–44, 1986.
54. Hwung Y, Gu Y, Tsai M: Cooperativity of sequence elements mediates tissue specificity of the rat insulin II gene. *Mol Cell Biol* 10:1784–1788, 1990.
55. Giddings SJ, Chirgwin J, Permutt MA: Effects of glucose on proinsulin mRNA in rats in vivo. *Diabetes* 31:624–629, 1982.
56. Brunstedt J, Chan SJ: Direct effect of glucose on the preproinsulin mRNA level in isolated pancreatic islets. *Biochem Biophys Res Commun* 106:1383–1389, 1982.
57. Welsh M, Scherberg N, Gilmore R, Steiner DF: Translational control of insulin biosynthesis. *Biochem J* 235:459–467, 1986.
58. Nielsen DA, Welsh M, Casadaban MJ, Steiner DF: Control of insulin gene expression in pancreatic β-cells and in an insulin–producing cell line, RIN-5F cells. *J Biol Chem* 260:13,585–13,589, 1985.
59. Welsh M, Nielsen DA, MacKrell AJ, Steiner DF: Control of insulin gene expression in pancreatic β-cells and in an insulin-producing cell line, RIN-5F cells. *J Biol Chem* 260:13,590–13,594, 1985.
60. Orland MJ, Chyn R, Permutt MA: Modulation of proinsulin mRNA after partial pancreatectomy in rats. Relationships to glucose homeostasis. *J Clin Invest* 75:2047–2055, 1985.

61. German MS, Moss LG, Rutter WJ: Regulation of insulin gene expression by glucose and calcium in transfected primary islet cultures. *J Biol Chem* 265:22,063–22,066, 1990.
62. German M: Glucose sensing in pancreatic islet beta cells: the key role of glucokinase and the glycolytic intermediates. *Proc Natl Acad Sci USA* 90:1781–1785, 1993.
63. Philippe J, Missotten M: Functional characterization of a cAMP-responsive element of the rat insulin I gene. *J Biol Chem* 265:1465–1469, 1990.
64. Vinik A, Bell G: Mutant insulin syndromes. *Horm Metabol Res* 20:1–10, 1988.
65. Bell GI, Horita S, Karam JH: A polymorphic locus near the human insulin gene is associated with insulin-dependent diabetes mellitus. *Diabetes* 33:176–183, 1984.
66. Hitman GA, Jowett NI, Williams LG, Humphries S, Winter RM, Galton DJ: Polymorphisms in the 5'-flanking region of the insulin gene and non-insulin-dependent diabetes. *Clin Sci* 66:383–388, 1984.
67. Rotwein PS, Chirgwin J, Province M, Knowler WC, Pettitt DJ, Cordell B, et al.: Polymorphisms in the 5' flanking reion of the human insulin gene: a genetic marker for non-insulin dependent diabetes mellitus. *N Eng J Med* 308:65–67, 1983.
68. Takeda J, Seino Y, Fukomoto H, Koh G, Otsuka A, Ikeda M, et al.: The polymorphism linked to the human insulin gene: its lack of association with either IDDM or NIDDM in Japanese. *Acta Endocrinol* 113:268–271, 1986.
69. Julier C, Hyer RN, Davies J, Merlin F, Soularue P, Briant L, et al.: Insulin-IGF2 region on chromosome 11p encodes a gene implicated in HLA-DR4-dependent diabetes susceptibility. *Nature* 354:155–159, 1991.
70. van der Auwera BJ, Heimberg H, Schrevens AF, Van Waeyenberge C, Flament J, Schuit FC: 5' insulin gene polymorphism confers risk to IDDM independently of HLA class II susceptibility. *Diabetes* 42:851–854, 1993.
71. Bain SC, Prins JB, Hearne CM, Rodrigues NR, Rowe BR, Pritchard LE, et al.: Insulin gene region-encoded susceptibility to type I diabetes is not restricted to HLA-DR4-positive individuals. *Nature Genet* 2:212–215, 1992.
72. DeChiara TM, Robertson EJ, Efstratiadis A: Parental imprinting of the mouse insulin-like growth factor II gene. *Cell* 64:849–859, 1991.
73. Henry I, Bonaiti-Pellie C, Chehensse V, Beldjord C, Schwartz C, Utermann G: Uniparental paternal disomy in a genetic cancer–predisposing syndrome. *Nature* 351:665–667, 1991.
74. Olansky L, Welling C, Giddings S, Adler S, Bourey R, Dowse G, et al.: A variant insulin promoter in non-insulin-dependent diabetes mellitus. *J Clin Invest* 89:1596–1602, 1992.
75. Kwok SM, Chan SJ, Steiner DF: Cloning and nucleotide sequence analysis of the dog insulin gene: Coded amino acid sequence of canine preproinsulin predicts an additional C-peptide fragment. *J Biol Chem* 258:2357–2363, 1983.
76. Steiner DF, Chan SJ, Welsh JM, Kwok SCM: Structure and evolution of the insulin gene. *Ann Rev Genet* 19:463–484, 1985.

77. Wentworth BM, Schaefer IM, Villa-Komaroff L, Chirgwin JM: Characterization of the two nonallelic genes encoding mouse preproinsulin. *J Mol Evol* 23:305–312, 1986.
78. Cordell B, Bell G, Tischer E, DeNoto FM, Ullrich A, Pictet R, et al.: Isolation and characterization of a cloned rat insulin gene. *Cell* 18:533–543, 1979.
79. Lomedico P, Rosenthal N, Efstratiadis A, Gilbert W, Kolodner R, Tizard R: The structure and evolution of the two nonallelic rat preproinsulin genes. *Cell* 18:545–558, 1979.
80. Chan SJ, Episkopou V, Zeitlin S, Karathanasis SK, MacKrell A, Steiner DF, et al.: Guinea pig preproinsulin gene: an evolutionary compromise? *Proc Natl Acad Sci USA* 81:5046–5050, 1984.

Chapter 6

Molecular Engineering of Glucose-Regulated Insulin Secretion

Christopher B. Newgard, Sarah Ferber, Christian Quaade, John H. Johnson, and Steven D. Hughes

Introduction

Rapid advances in the technology of gene transfer into mammalian cells have been made in recent years. These improvements in methodology have allowed investigators to begin to use molecular strategies for testing hypotheses about the role of certain genes in the process of fuel-mediated insulin release *(1)*. To this point, most of the work has focused on genes that regulate the acute insulin secretory response to glucose. Interest in the glucose response is naturally motivated by the fact that its loss is an early event in the etiology of both major forms of diabetes *(2,3)*. In this chapter, recent studies employing molecular approaches for dissecting the relative contributions of glucose transport and glucose phosphorylation in the control of glucose-stimulated insulin release will be reviewed.

From: *Molecular Biology of Diabetes, Part I*
Edited by: B. Draznin and D. LeRoith

The Biochemistry of Glucose-Stimulated Insulin Release

The metabolic fuel glucose exerts a powerful stimulatory effect on insulin release from the pancreatic islet β-cell and mediates a synchronous decrease in release of the counterregulatory hormone glucagon from the α-cell. The mechanisms involved in the β-cell glucose response have been investigated and debated for several decades. Early discussion centered on the issue of whether glucose signaling occurs through binding of the metabolite to a receptor, the so-called "regulator site" hypothesis, vs the "substrate-site" hypothesis, in which glucose metabolism within the β-cell represents the triggering event for insulin exocytosis (reviewed in refs. *4,5*). Over time, evidence in favor of a primary role for β-cell glucose metabolism in regulating the insulin secretory response to the sugar has accumulated to the point where the substrate site concept is now commonly accepted *(4–10)*. Examples of experiments supporting the role of glucose metabolism include those showing that nonmetabolizable analogs of glucose such as 3-*O*-methyl- and 2-deoxyglucose fail to cause insulin release and others demonstrating that inhibitors of glucose metabolism, such as glucosamine or mannoheptulose are capable of blocking the glucose response *(4–7)*. Glucose metabolism can generally not be dissociated from the secretory effects of the sugar, but the possibility remains that glucose metabolism is necessary, but not sufficient for the response. In other words, it is still conceivable that glucose signaling occurs through a combination of the regulatory site and substrate site models. This concept will be elaborated upon below with reference to recent studies from our laboratory showing differential effects of GLUT-2 vs GLUT-1 in inducing insulin release in transfected cells that are independent of the rates of glucose metabolism *(11)*.

The curves describing the glucose concentration dependence of insulin secretion on the one hand, and of glucose metabolism in islet β-cells on the other are virtually superimposable *(6,7)*. The identity of the metabolic signal or signals that link(s) glucose flux to insulin release has to this date not been clearly established, despite decades of intensive investigation. One widely quoted hypothesis holds that glucose metabolism increases the β-cell ATP:ADP ratio, resulting in inhibition of ATP-sensitive K^+ channels, leading to membrane depolarization and activation of voltage-gated Ca^{2+} channels. Several aspects of this model are undoubtably correct. ATP-sensitive K^+ channels are clearly expressed in β-cells and are closed upon glucose administration *(12,13)*. Glucose also markedly enhances Ca^{2+} entry into islet β-cells, and blocking of β-cell voltage gated Ca^{2+} channels with agents such as nitrendipine markedly reduces or eliminates the glucose-stimulated insulin secretory response *(8,9)*. On the other hand, Henquin and coworkers have demonstrated that administration of diazoxide, an agent that specifically opens ATP-sensitive K^+ channels, does not prevent glucose-stimulated insulin secretion *(14)*. Also, recent measurements show that the whole-islet ATP:ADP ratio is not altered in response to glucose administration *(15)*, suggesting either that signaling to ion channels occurs through a nucleotide-independent pathway or that significant alterations in ATP:ADP ratio occur only in localized microenvironments within individual cells. In light of these seemingly conflicting pieces of information, it seems important to continue to investigate the potential role of other metabolic events that could be influenced by glucose flux, such as the redox potential, the levels of various mitochondrial metabolites, phospholipid turnover, and the relative activities of the fatty acid oxidation and esterification pathways *(4–10,16)*.

Downstream of ionic events, the exocytotic process is thought to be triggered by the action of one or more protein kinases. Possible participants include members of the Ca^{2+}/calmodulin class of kinases, which are thought to associate with components of the β-cell cytoskeleton *(17)*. Similarly, recent studies have demonstrated a clear translocation of protein kinase C from the cytosol to the plasma membrane in response to glucose administration, an effect that appears to be dependent on glucose metabolism *(18)*. Glucose was also found to increase the phosphorylation of the protein kinase C substrate Myristolated Alanine-Rich Protein C Kinase Substrate (MARCKS) *(19)*. Although the precise function of MARCKS is not understood, it too appears to associate with cytoskeletal elements; phosphorylation of MARCKS appears to cause disruption of these interactions. In sum, protein kinases may affect the secretory process

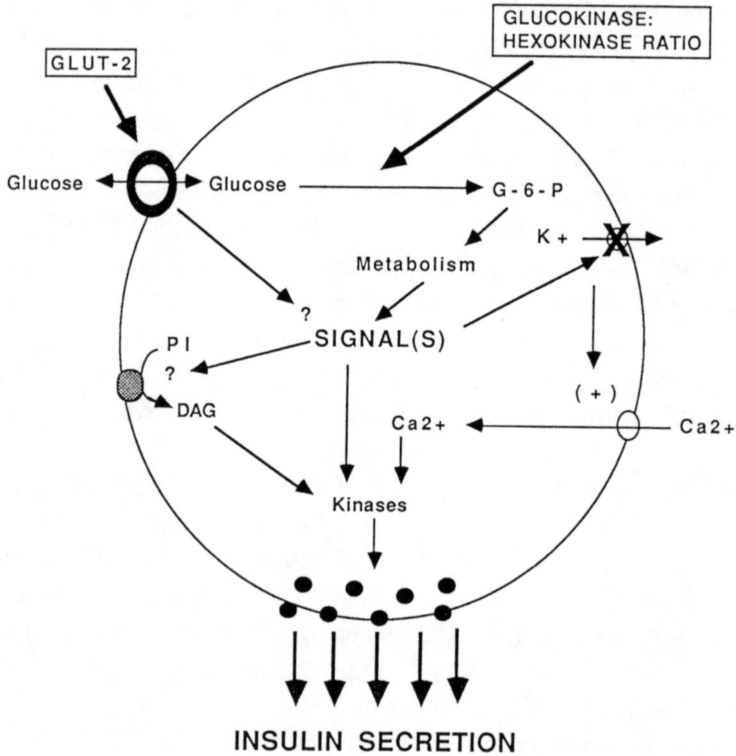

Fig. 1. Schematic summary of biochemical events involved in glucose-regulated insulin release. The amount of insulin release is thought to be proportional to the rate of glucose metabolism. Changes in extracellular glucose concentration are translated into changes in the rate of glucose metabolism through the combined action of GLUT-2 and glucokinase in the normal β-cell. In insulinoma cells, the glucose response threshold is probably determined by the glucokinase:hexokinase ratio.

by controlling the movement of secretory granules along their relevant cytoskeletal elements. Invoking participation of protein kinase C is also attractive in that activation of this enzyme by diacylglycerol may represent the link between enhanced phospholipid metabolism in response to glucose and exocytotic events *(9)*. Further investigation will be required to fully validate these intriguing concepts. A schematic summary of the events described in the foregoing summary is presented in Fig. 1.

The Role of Glucose Transport and Phosphorylation in Regulation of Glucose-Stimulated Insulin Secretion

The Role of Glucose Phosphorylation

A rate-controlling role for the glucose phosphorylating enzyme glucokinase in β-cell glycolysis and hence glucose-stimulated insulin release was first suggested by the groups of Matschinsky and Randle in the 1960s *(20,21)*. Subsequently, these laboratories provided most of the detailed experimental evidence supporting the notion that glucokinase is the metabolic pace-setter for β-cell glycolysis (*see* refs. *7,22,23* for review). Key observations linking glucokinase activity and glucose-stimulated insulin release include:

1. Glucokinase is clearly expressed in the islets, but at levels that are substantially lower than other potential glycolytic regulatory enzymes such as phosphofructokinase and pyruvate kinase, supporting a rate-limiting role for the glucose phosphorylation step *(24)*;
2. The curve describing the glucose concentration dependence of glucose metabolism in intact islets is virtually superimposable on that describing the glucose concentration dependence of glucokinase activity in islet cell extracts *(6,7)*; and
3. Alloxan *(25)* and mannoheptulose *(26)*, inhibitors of glucokinase activity, are capable of blocking β-cell glycolysis and glucose-stimulated insulin release.

Glucokinase has a K_m for glucose of approx 8 m*M*, a feature which allows large alterations in the enzyme's activity in response to modest increments in glucose concentration over the physiological range (4–9 m*M*). Interestingly, the low K_m glucose phosphorylating enzyme hexokinase (K_m for glucose of approx 50 μ*M [27]*) is expressed in islets at levels similar to glucokinase, yet islets metabolize glucose inefficiently at submillimolar concentrations and exhibit no insulin secretory response to low concentrations of the sugar. The most logical explanation for these observations is that hexokinase is kept in an inhibited state in intact islet β-cells, possibly by its allosteric effector glucose-6-phosphate, thus preventing metabolism-induced secretion at subphysiological glucose concentrations *(24,28)*.

Dramatic evidence for the involvement of glucokinase in normal glucose-stimulated insulin release and glucose homeostasis has recently appeared in the form of genetic studies on individuals with a form of NIDDM known as Maturity-Onset Diabetes of the Young or MODY (*see* the chapter by G. Bell in this volume for complete review). Frougel and colleagues were the first to report a strong association between a polymorphic dinucleotide repeat located near the glucokinase gene and disease in French families *(29)*. Subsequently, a series of studies have demonstrated that many MODY families are heterozygous at the glucokinase locus, with one normal allele and one mutant allele containing a mutation within the protein coding region *(30–32)*. Expression of the cDNA versions of a number of the mutant alleles in bacteria and kinetic analysis of the purified protein products reveals compromised enzymatic activity in all mutants, with effects ranging from very mild changes in K_m or V_{max} to complete abolition of activity *(32)*. Studies on patients from four different MODY families with glucokinase mutations revealed a reduced insulin and C-peptide release in response to a glucose challenge, especially in the second prolonged phase of the secretory response *(33)*. These data have been used to argue for a gene-dosage effect, in which the absence of all or part of the activity from one allele is sufficient to reduce the insulin secretory response to glucose *(32)*. Such a model may not completely explain the fact that alleles encoding either severely compromised or modestly affected glucokinase enzymes are both associated with disease phenotype. This concept will be discussed further below.

The Role of Glucose Transport

The role of glucose transport in mediating the glucose-stimulated insulin secretory response is less well understood. Glucose transport has been traditionally perceived as in excess relative to the glycolytic rate of the β-cell. This perception relies largely on two studies. The first of these described experiments with inhibitors of glucose transport showing that large decreases in glucose uptake had negligible effects on glucose metabolism or on stimulated insulin release in mouse islets *(34)*. The second study found that extracellular and intracellular glucose concentrations were nearly identical in isolated islets cultured over a wide range of glucose concentrations, suggesting that equilibration of the sugar across the plasma membrane of islet cells is rapid *(21)*. Whereas this study did not discriminate between glucose uptake in β-cells vs non-β-cells, subsequent work showed that the rapid equilibration is largely a property of the β-cell, since isolated α-cells were shown to reach equilibrium only very slowly *(35)*. Rapid equilibration of glucose across the β-cell plasma membrane at physiological glucose concentrations can now be understood in terms of the molecular biology of facilitated glucose carriers. The major glucose transporter of the islet β-cell is GLUT-2, as originally demonstrated by Thorens et al *(36)*. This isoform is both functionally and structurally distinct from other members of the facilitated glucose transporter gene family, with a higher K_m and V_{max} for glucose uptake *(37)*. It also appears to be expressed constitutively at the cell surface of cells in which it is expressed *(38)*, as opposed to GLUT-4, which is stored in intracellular vesicles and recruited to the cell surface in response to the binding of insulin to its receptor.

The pairing of GLUT-2 with glucokinase in both the liver and islets suggests that the transporter may be important for the normal functioning of the enzyme, and that the two proteins operate in tandem as the "glucose sensing apparatus" of the β-cell. In such a model, glucokinase would still be considered the rate-limiting step, but the kinetic features of GLUT-2 could also come into play if it were the only glucose transporter isoform that could ensure rapid equilibration of the extracellular and intracellular glucose concentrations over the physiological range, or, as discussed below, if it participates directly in the signaling process. In support of this concept, several laboratories have demonstrated that the loss of glucose-stimulated insulin release that occurs in rodent models of noninsulin dependent diabetes mellitus (NIDDM) is accompanied by underexpression of GLUT-2 (reviewed in *39*). Johnson et al. showed that GLUT-2 expression was inversely correlated with the severity of hyperglycemia in Zucker Diabetic Fatty (ZDF) rats *(40)*. The loss of GLUT-2 in this model did not appear to be secondary to hyperglycemia, since lowering of blood glucose with acarbose did not prevent GLUT-2 underexpression *(41)*. Furthermore, chronic infusion of glucose into normal rats increases rather than decreases GLUT-2 mRNA in the islets *(42)*. In an elegant study, Thorens et al. demonstrated that loss of GLUT-2 expression is induced by the diabetic environment

(43). Islets isolated from normoglycemic db/+ mice were transplanted into db/db mice, a model of NIDDM, or into streptozotocin diabetic db/+ animals, a model of IDDM; in both cases, near-complete loss of immunodetectable GLUT-2 expression was observed. The effect of the diabetic environment seemed to be reversible, since transplantation of GLUT-2 deficient db/db islets into normoglycemic db/+ animals was shown to restore GLUT-2 expression. From these and the foregoing studies, the authors concluded that the loss of GLUT-2 expression is not caused by hyperglycemia or the levels of insulin, but rather by some as yet unidentified factor in diabetic animals.

The parallelism between loss of GLUT-2 expression and the β-cell dysfunction that accompanies hyperglycemia in a wide variety of rodent models is remarkable. These studies seem to point to GLUT-2 expression as a critical determinant of normal glucose-stimulated insulin secretion. Any such conclusion must include a cautionary note, however, in light of the following points:

1. GLUT-2 is the only gene that has been studied in detail in the wide variety of rodent models, and it remains possible that altered expression of several genes involved in islet glucose sensing could contribute to the diabetic phenotype. In support of this notion, Malaisse and coworkers have recently shown that the low-dose streptozotocin-injected neonatal rat, a model of β-cell dysfunction that is characterized by a sharp reduction in expression of GLUT-2 *(44)*, also has a severe decrease in glycerol-phosphate dehydrogenase activity (the glycerol phosphate "shuttle") and a consequent decrease in the capacity for transfer of reducing equivalents into the mitochondria that may be more directly responsible for the secretory defect *(45)*;
2. The relationship of the observed underexpression of GLUT-2 in the various rodent models to human NIDDM is currently unknown; and
3. Experiments resulting in altered expression of GLUT-2 in islets or other insulin secreting cells have produced conflicting pictures of the importance of GLUT-2 in the glucose-stimulated insulin secretion pathway, as will be discussed further below.

In sum, a great deal of correlative evidence has accumulated implicating glucokinase and GLUT-2 as important controlling elements in glucose-stimulated insulin secretion. With the recent application of the powerful tools of molecular biology to cloning genes that are expressed in the islets of Langerhans, it is now possible to design and implement experiments that directly test their role in glucose sensing. Our review of molecular strategies for testing the relative importance of glucose transport and glucose phosphorylation will be divided into two sections, studies performed on insulin-secreting cell lines, and studies done directly on islets, either in vitro or *in situ*.

Molecular Manipulations of Glucose Transporter Expression and Glucose Phosphorylation in Insulin-Secreting Cell Lines

Insulin-Secreting Cell Lines Derived from Islet β-Cells

A number of insulin-secreting cell lines are available that are derived from islet β-cells of rodents or other small animals. These are generally produced by one of three methods:

1. Induction of islet cell tumors with X-irradiation and culturing of cells (RIN cells are an example of lines produced by this approach *[46]*);
2. Viral transformation of isolated islets to produce cell lines (HIT cells for example *[47]*); or
3. Creation of β-cell tumors by expression of oncogenes in transgenic mice, using the insulin promoter for targeted transformation (examples include the β-TC or MIN cell lines *[48,49]*).

The currently available lines exhibit a wide range of phenotypes with regard to glucose-stimulated insulin release. RINm5F cells are completely lacking in glucose responsiveness *(50,51)*. Interestingly, measurements of the rate of glucose metabolism in these cells indicate that their maximal rate of metabolism is equivalent to that of islets, but that the full rate is reached at subphysiologic glucose concentrations *(50,51)*. In keeping with the predominance of high affinity glucose usage, RIN m5F cells are found to express high levels of GLUT-1 and hexokinase and very little, if any GLUT-2 or glucokinase *(36,51)*. Other RIN lines, such as RIN1046-38 *(52)* exhibit a robust glucose-stimulated insulin secretion response, but with maximal secretion occurring at subphysiological glucose concentrations (≤0.5 m*M* glucose, as compared to the threshold for response of islet β-cells at 5 m*M* glucose). Furthermore, RIN1046-38 cells lose their glucose responsiveness with time in culture, such that cells kept beyond 35 passages are completely unresponsiveness *(52)*. While low passage RIN 1046-38 cells express both GLUT-2 and glucokinase at high levels, expression of these genes is lost in parallel with the passage-dependent loss of glucose sensing *(53)*. Like RIN 1046-38 cells, the SV40-transformed hamster insulinoma cell line HIT exhibits a glucose-stimulated insulin secretion response that is maximal at subphysiological glucose concentration *(54)*. Culturing of HIT cells at various glucose concentrations changes the levels of GLUT-2 mRNA and activity in parallel with changes in the magnitude of the glucose-stimulated insulin secretion response, suggesting that glucose transport may be a rate-limiting step for glycolysis in this line *(54)*.

In recent years, application of transgenic technology has yielded a number of interesting insulinoma lines, some of which have near-normal glucose regulation of insulin secretion. The general strategy has been to utilize a vector containing the insulin promoter driving T-antigen expression to produce β-cell tumors from which cell lines are derived. The first transgenically derived β-cell line, βTC-1, had a phenotype very similar to that of low passage RIN1046-38 cells in that these cells exhibited a glucose-stimulated insulin secretion response that was maximal at subphysiological glucose concentrations *(48)*. Subsequent studies have shown that the subphysiologic glucose dose responsiveness of βTC-1 cells *(55)*, or the related βTC-3 line *(56)* is correlated with a left-shifted glucose concentration dependence for glucose usage. More recently, new lines have been described that exhibit near-normal glucose dose responsiveness, at least in a transient sense. The first of these to emerge was the MIN-6 cell line *(49)*. These cells were found to express high levels of GLUT-2 and to exhibit a tenfold increase in insulin secretion in response to 25 m*M* glucose compared to secretion at 5 m*M* glucose *(49)*. Interestingly, another line (MIN-7) isolated by the same group from transgenic animals injected with the identical insulin promoter/T-antigen construct expressed GLUT-1 rather than GLUT-2 as its major glucose transporter and was found to be completely glucose unresponsive *(49)*. The stability of the near-physiologic dose response profile of the MIN-6 line as a function of prolonged time in culture has not yet been reported. Experience with a new, well-differentiated βTC line, βTC-7 *(57)*, may provide insights into this issue. This line was produced by crossing the original transgenic founder strain *(48)* with another mouse strain to yield a new line with β-cell tumors. Several resulting cell lines, including βTC-7, initially exhibited a glucose dose-responsiveness that is similar to the normal islet β-cell. This differentiated phenotype was correlated with a glucokinase:hexokinase ratio similar to that of the normal islet and a predominant expression of GLUT-2. With time in culture, glucose-stimulated insulin release was retained, but the dose response shifted such that maximal effects were now achieved at low, subphysiologic glucose concentrations. This left-shifted response was accompanied by no discernible change in expression in GLUT-2 or GLUT-1, a twofold increase in glucokinase activity, and perhaps most importantly, a fourfold increase in hexokinase enzymatic activity. The authors suggested that the dominance of hexokinase in βTC-7 cells of higher passage might be responsible for the shift in glucose concentration dependence *(57)*.

Insulin-Secreting Cell Lines Derived from Non-β-Cell Neuroendocrine Tissue

Neuroendocrine cells lines derived from tissues other than β-cells could potentially serve as interesting vehicles for studies on engineering of glucose-stimulated insulin secretion. This concept was brought to the fore with the establishment of the AtT-20ins cell line, which is derived from ACTH-secreting corticotrophs of the anterior pituitary gland, and which has been stably transfected with a viral promoter driving expression of the human proinsulin cDNA *(58)*. Remarkably, these cells secrete the mature insulin polypeptide and very little proinsulin or processing intermediates *(58,59)*. This fact is now understood in light of recent studies showing that the peptidases known as PC2 and PC3 that are thought to process proinsulin to insulin in the islets are also expressed in AtT-20ins cells *(60,61)*. We have shown that AtT-20ins cells are completely lacking in glucose-stimulated insulin secretion despite their expression of the islet or "β" isoform of glucokinase *(62)*. These cells contain low levels of glucokinase enzymatic activity, consistent with their expression of a mixture of intact glucokinase mRNAs and cryptically deleted transcripts that lack a portion of the second exon *(62)*. Expression of this deleted product and another glucokinase transcript of liver that contains an insertion in combination with the same deletion in exon two *(63)* in bacteria demonstrated that the deleted transcripts do not encode active glucokinase enzymes *(64)*. In work from other laboratories, the expression of glucokinase mRNA in anterior pituitary cells and in an AtT-20 cell line was confirmed, but in the hands of these investigators no intact transcripts or glucokinase enzymatic activity was found in AtT-20 cells *(65)*. The explanation for this difference in results may lie in the use of cell lines from different sources, although this has not yet been investigated. Unlike liver or islets, which coexpress glucokinase and GLUT-2, AtT-20ins cells are completely devoid of GLUT-2 expression, and instead appear to preferentially express GLUT-1 *(62)*.

Molecular Engineering of Glucose Sensing in Insulin-Secreting Cell Lines

A general conclusion from the studies cited above is that a glucose-stimulated insulin secretion response that mimics that of the normal islet β-cell is either absent or only transiently retained in currently available cell lines. This has led our laboratory to investigate the use of stable gene transfer for the dual purposes of investigating the relative importance of genes in the glucose sensing mechanism and to determine whether stable expression of relevant genes confers glucose responsiveness that is retained with time in culture *(1)*. The general strategy that we have used is depicted in schematic form in Fig. 2. We have focused to date on stable transfection of insulin secreting cell lines that lack a glucose response with GLUT-2 and/or glucokinase in an effort to determine whether expression of these genes is necessary or sufficient for conferring a response. At the time that we began contemplating these studies, it was suspected that the GLUT-2 and glucokinase gene products expressed in the islet might be different from those that had been characterized in liver. Consistent with this notion, we had observed differential regulation of glucokinase gene expression in islets and liver in response to fasting and refeeding. In the islet, no change in glucokinase mRNA or protein was seen in response to fasting or refeeding, whereas very large changes in glucokinase mRNA and a

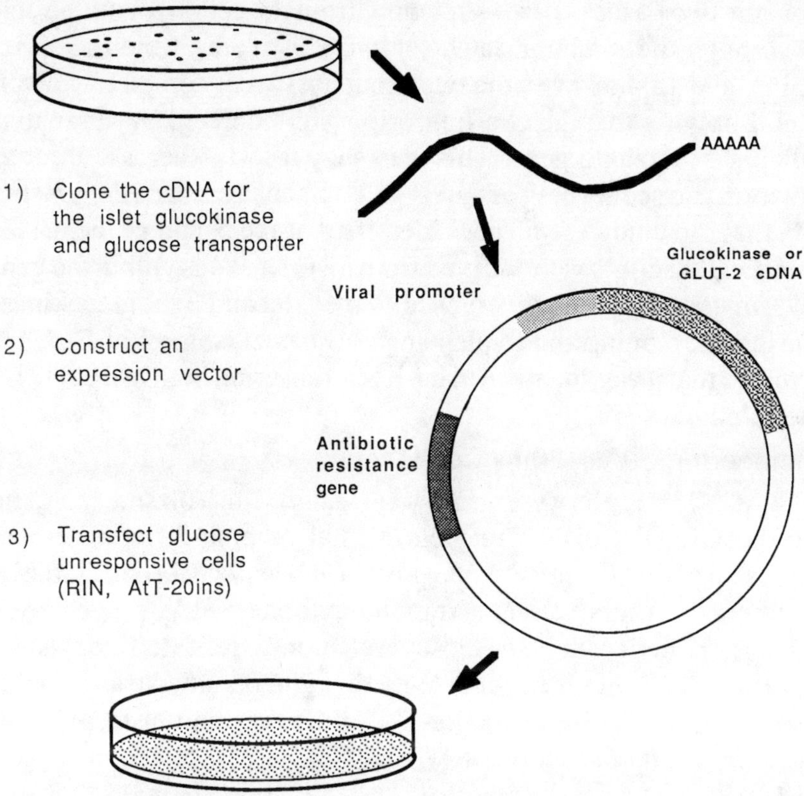

Fig. 2. General strategy for engineering of glucose-stimulated insulin secretion in clonal cells. The figure is reprinted from Newgard et al. *(92)*, with permission.

lesser change in protein levels was consistently observed in liver in response to such a regimen *(66)*. Using the cloned hepatic glucokinase cDNA *(67)*, we also noticed that the glucokinase mRNA in islets was distinctly larger than that in liver, whereas that for GLUT-2 was identical in size in the two tissues *(66,68)*. To address this issue in more detail, we constructed a cDNA library from normal rat islets and used it to clone the islet GLUT-2 and glucokinase gene products *(37,62,68)*. Cloning of the glucokinase cDNA from our islet cDNA library *(62,68)* and from an insulinoma library by Magnuson and Shelton *(69)* and comparison to the previously published liver glucokinase cDNA sequence *(70)* revealed exact identity in the clones from the two tissue sources stretching from the codon for amino acid 15 through the 3' untranslated region. Upstream of the codon for amino acid 15, however, the two sequences were completely divergent, implying that the two transcripts were derived by alternative splicing of a single gene. This was shown to be the case through isolation and sequencing of the rat glucokinase gene, and demonstration that the unique sequences identified at the 5' end of the tissue-specific transcripts were derived from distinct exons within the gene *(69)*. In contrast to the divergence of the islet and liver glucokinase transcripts, cloning and sequencing of the islet isoform of GLUT-2 revealed that it was identical to the liver transcript, both in the rat *(37)* and in humans *(71)*.

Engineering of AtT-20ins Cell Lines

AtT-20ins cells were stably transfected with a plasmid containing the GLUT-2 cDNA to yield a total of nine different clones expressing GLUT-2 mRNA and protein at levels easily detectable by Northern blot analysis and immunocytochemistry, respectively *(11,72)*. Kinetic analysis of several clones revealed consistent increases in K_m and V_{max} for 3-*O*-methyl glucose uptake as a consequence of GLUT-2 transfection *(72)*. Whereas untransfected cells had a K_m of 1 m*M* and a very low V_{max} of 0.5 mmol/min/L cell space, GLUT-2 transfection increased these values to 18–20 m*M* and 17–25 mmol/min/L cell space, respectively, values that are nearly identical to the kinetics of glucose uptake into normal islets *(37)*. GLUT-2 transfection conferred a clear glucose-stimulated insulin secretion response in AtT-20ins cells *(11,72)*. Static incubation studies demonstrated that the cells are hypersensitive to glucose, with a maximal insulin secretion response realized at 10–50 μ*M* concentrations of the sugar. Although static incubation measurements are useful for screening of cell lines and for establishing glucose dose-responsiveness, they do not provide a measure of the moment-to-moment dynamics of insulin release in response to a given secretagog. This can instead be achieved with perifusion studies, in which the cells are grown in liquid culture either on gelatin beads or on polyester discs, allowing easy transfer into a column. Studies of this type *(11)* revealed that GLUT-2 transfected cells released insulin within 2 min of exposure to glucose, and that in some cases, a biphasic response reminiscent of normal islets was observed, as shown in the example

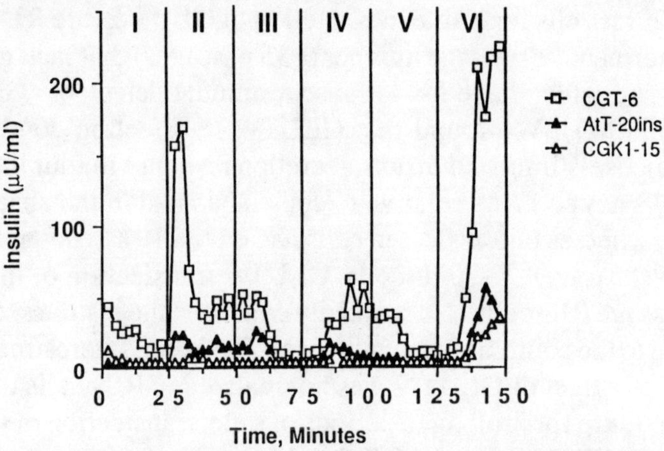

Fig. 3. Glucose-stimulated insulin secretion response from representative AtT-20ins clonal cell lines. Cells were grown in liquid culture on Matrigel-coated beads, and 50–100 × 10^6 cells were loaded into a Pharmacia P10/10 column for perifusion studies. Cells were perifused with the following; Phase I, Hank's Balanced Salt Solution (HBSS) with no supplements; Phase II, HBSS + 5 m*M* glucose; Phase III, HBSS with no supplements; Phase IV, HBSS + 5 m*M* glucose; Phase V, HBSS with no supplements; Phase VI, HBSS with 5 m*M* glucose + 5 µ*M* forskolin. Shown are a GLUT-2 transfected line (CGT-6), a GLUT-1 transfected line (GT1-15), and the untransfected parental cells (AtT-20ins). Data are reprinted from Hughes et al. *(11)*, with permission.

in Fig. 3. Furthermore, switching back to a buffer lacking glucose resulted in a cessation of stimulated insulin secretion. In addition to its direct stimulatory effects, glucose has a clearly enhanced potentiating effect in GLUT-2 transfected AtT-20ins cells relative to untransfected cells on forskolin, IBMX, dibutryl cAMP, and amino acid-induced insulin release *(11,72)*.

Engineering of Insulinoma Cell Lines

The effects of GLUT-2 transfection on AtT-20ins cells are not necessarily instructive for glucose sensing mechanisms that are operative in islets or islet-derived cells. It was therefore important to determine whether enabling effects of GLUT-2 gene transfer could also be observed in glucose unresponsive insulinoma cells. To this end, we have recently utilized the same plasmid used for transfection of AtT-20ins cells for stable introduction of GLUT-2 into RIN1046-38 of intermediate passage number (≈35 passages) that lack glucose sensing and which have low or absent immunodetectable GLUT-2 expression *(53)*. We found that GLUT-2 transfection conferred a mean glucose-stimulated insulin secretion response in four independent cell lines of 170% relative to cells incubated in the absence of glucose, whereas untransfected cells had only a 10% response to the sugar *(53)*. As in AtT-20ins cells, GLUT-2 transfection of intermediate passage RIN cells also markedly enhanced the insulin secretion response to the combination of glucose + forskolin. Interestingly, the "enabling" effect of GLUT-2 was not realized in RIN cells that had been in culture for prolonged periods of time; transfection of cells of passage number ≥90 with GLUT-2 did not result in any improvement in the glucose-stimulated insulin secretion response in four independent clonal lines *(53)*. These results suggest that in addition to the passage-dependent loss of GLUT-2 and glucokinase expression, other elements of the differentiated glucose response machinery are lost with time in culture and are not restored by GLUT-2 transfection. Constant presence of GLUT-2 may delay these events, but probably does not prevent them, since the glucose-stimulated insulin secretion response is reduced in magnitude after culturing of GLUT-2 transfected intermediate passage lines for an additional 30 passages (cells reaching passage 60–65 without reduction in GLUT-2 expression). The response is restored to its full magnitude by implantation of GLUT-2 transfected higher passage cells into nude rats and growth of the cells as a solid tumor (Ferber S, Schnedl W, and Newgard CB, unpublished observations). The latter results are consistent with those of Madsen et al., who found that the insulinoma cell line MSL-G2 gradually shifts from an insulin secreting cell line to one secreting primarily glucagon and CCK with time in culture in vitro; with in vivo passage, the line reverts to its differentiated, insulin-secreting phenotype *(73)*. The specific mediators of this tonic differentiating effect of the in vivo environment are not understood but could represent a valuable area for future study.

Transfection of RIN 1046-38 cells, but not AtT-20ins cells with GLUT-2 causes a fourfold increase in glucokinase enzymatic activity *(53,72)*. As was the case for glucose-stimulated insulin release, the activating effect of GLUT-2 was confined to cells of intermediate passage number, and was not observed in GLUT-2 transfected high passage cell lines *(53)*. The mechanism by which GLUT-2 gene transfer induces increased glucokinase activity is currently under investigation. It is worth noting that there is growing evidence that glucokinase activity can be modulated in cells without the need for changes in glucokinase gene expression. Our studies in collaboration with Iynedjian and coworkers showed that glucokinase mRNA and protein levels do not change in islets in response to fasting and refeeding *(58)*, even though glucokinase enzyme activities are sharply reduced by fasting and restored upon refeeding in this tissue *(74,75)*. Furthermore, Liang et al. have shown that culturing of islets at high glucose concentrations causes dramatic increases in glucokinase activity relative to islets cultured at low glucose, but that these changes are accompanied by no change in glucokinase mRNA and changes in glucokinase protein levels that do not fully account for the changes in activity *(76)*. Finally, a recent study has shown that infusion of 50% glucose into rats causes an increase in islet glucokinase enzymatic activity that is only partially accounted for by an increase in immunodetectable glucokinase protein *(77)*. Possible mediators of the increased activity at the posttranslational level could include:

1. The glucokinase regulatory protein, a recently discovered protein that either inhibits or activates glucokinase depending on the level of specific sugar phosphates in the cell *(78)*;
2. Modulation of glucokinase activity by covalent modification or allosteric effectors *(79)*; or
3. A direct interaction between glucokinase and GLUT-2 *(68)*.

This last concept is attractive but lacks direct experimental support. Furthermore, if a GLUT-2/glucokinase interaction were the only operative mechanism, an increase in glucokinase activity would have been expected in GLUT-2 transfected AtT-20ins cells as well.

The increased glucokinase activity in GLUT-2 expressing RIN cells led us to investigate whether these cells exhibit a more physiologic glucose dose responsiveness. Two independent lines were studied over a range of glucose concentrations from 10 μ*M* to 20 m*M* and were both found to exhibit a maximal response at 50 μ*M* glucose *(53)*. This is so despite the fact that glucokinase enzymatic activity exceeds that of the normal islet in GLUT-2 transfected RIN cells and represents nearly half of the total glucose phosphorylating activity. It should be pointed out, however, that the hexokinase activity of the RIN lines is also much higher than found in normal islets. Furthermore, the high affinity glucose usage profile of many RIN cell lines *(50,51)* suggests that hexokinase activity is in a less inhibited state in cell lines compared to normal β-cells, a finding that could be explained by the degree to which the enzyme is associated with the mitochondria in the various cell types. In fact, a large percentage of hexokinase is clearly associated with mitochondria in RIN cells *(80)* where it would be less susceptible to glucose-6-phosphate inhibition *(27)*. Thus, our data, as well of those of Efrat et al. *(57)* are consistent with a dominant effect of hexokinase on glucose metabolism in insulin secreting cell lines, even when glucokinase levels are high. This would suggest that engineering of the "correct" threshold for glucose response in the clonal lines under study will require down-regulation of hexokinase enzymatic activity *(1,72)*. We have recently tested this hypothesis by preincubating GLUT-2 transfected RIN cell lines with 2-deoxyglucose prior to measuring glucose-stimulated insulin release *(53)*. The rationale for this experiment is that 2-deoxyglucose will enter the cell and accumulate as 2-deoxyglucose-6-phosphate, a potent inhibitor of hexokinase, but not glucokinase. Pretreatment with 2-deoxyglucose resulted in a shift of two orders of magnitude in the maximal glucose response from 50 μ*M* in the untreated cells to 5 m*M* in the treated cells *(53)*. This experiment therefore provides encouragement for difficult experiments that are now underway in our laboratory aimed at reducing hexokinase by antisense or gene knockout strategies. It should be pointed out, however, that the glucose responsiveness of 2-deoxyglucose treated RIN cells, while shifted to the right, is still clearly different from that of the β-cell, which only begins to be stimulated by glucose at concentrations of ≈5 m*M*. This difference could be due to incomplete inhibition of hexokinase by the glucose analog, or alternatively, could mean that other regulated steps in glycolysis or mitochondrial metabolism come into play when hexokinase is inhibited. This point will clearly require further study.

New Insights into the Role of GLUT-2 in Glucose Sensing from Studies with Engineered Cells

If hexokinase is the dominant glucose phosphorylating enzyme, and the enabling effect of GLUT-2 on glucose-induced insulin release in transfected RIN and AtT-20ins cells is simply due to enhanced glucose entry, then one would predict that transfection of these lines with any facilitated glucose transporter isoform that enhances glucose uptake would reproduce the effects of GLUT-2. To test this hypothesis, we have recently transfected AtT-20ins cells with GLUT-1 instead of GLUT-2 *(11)*, and have found, as shown in the example in Fig. 3 (cell line GT1-15), that GLUT-1 does not confer glucose-stimulated insulin release in AtT-20ins cells. The enabling effect of GLUT-2 and lack of effect of GLUT-1 are consistently observed in 9 and 6 independently transfected clonal lines, respectively *(11)*. In an effort to understand this result, we have formulated three potential models that might explain the divergent effects of the transporter isoforms, as summarized in Fig. 4. The first of these postulates that our GLUT-2 transfection experiment was simply more effective than our GLUT-1 transfection experiment. If this were the case, then the glucose responsiveness of the GLUT-2 transfected lines would be explained by a greater number of GLUT-2 transporters than GLUT-1 transporters and a consequent enhanced rate of glucose uptake that might impact the overall metabolic rate and the magnitude of the insulin secretion response. Although this possibility seems unlikely in light of the very high levels of GLUT-1 mRNA and immunodetectable protein in the GLUT-1 transfected lines *(11)*, it can not yet be ruled out. The second model assumes that the number of glucose transporters expressed is the same for both the GLUT-2 and GLUT-1 transfection experiments, but that GLUT-2 has a higher intrinsic activity than GLUT-1. As in the first model, the explanation for the enabling effect of GLUT-2 would be enhanced glucose uptake into GLUT-2 transfected cells compared to those transfected with GLUT-1. The last of the three proposed models would hold that GLUT-2, but not GLUT-1 is capable of interacting with other components of the glucose sensing system to directly stimulate insulin release.

If either of the first two models is correct, this should be reflected in a clear difference in the kinetics of glucose uptake in GLUT-2 vs

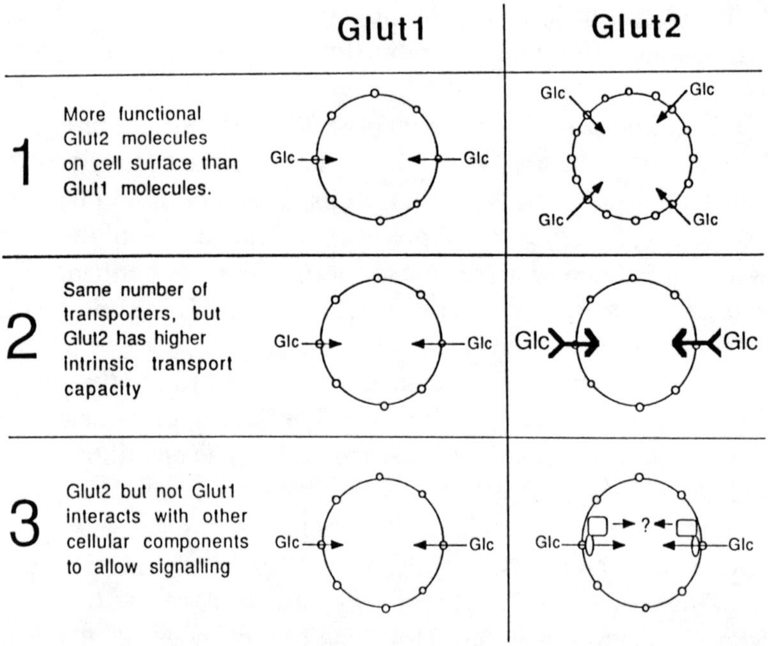

Fig. 4. Models directed at explaining the fact that transfection of AtT-20ins cells with GLUT-2, but not GLUT-1 confers glucose-stimulated insulin release. Reprinted from Hughes et al. *(11)*, with permission.

GLUT-1 transfected AtT-20ins cells. To address this point, we measured 3-*O*-methyl glucose uptake into two representative clones of each type. Overexpression of GLUT-1 in AtT-20ins cells caused only a slight increase in K_m relative to untransfected cells from 2 to 4 m*M*, whereas V_{max} was increased by tenfold from 0.5 to 5–6 mmol/min/L cell space. Transfection with GLUT-2, in contrast, caused an increase in K_m from 2 to 18–20 m*M*, and a 40-fold increase in V_{max} from 0.5 to 17–25 mmol/min/L of cell space *(11,72)*. Thus, at first glance, there appears to be a significant advantage in glucose transport capacity in GLUT-2 transfected cells compared to GLUT-1 transfected cells that could explain the glucose-stimulated insulin secretion response of the former cells. Glucose metabolism appears to be required to stimulate insulin release in GLUT-2 transfected AtT-20ins cells, since nonmetabolizable analogs of glucose such as 3-*O*-methyl or 2-deoxyglucose do not stimulate insulin release or potentiate the effect of forskolin *(11)*. In light of these results, one

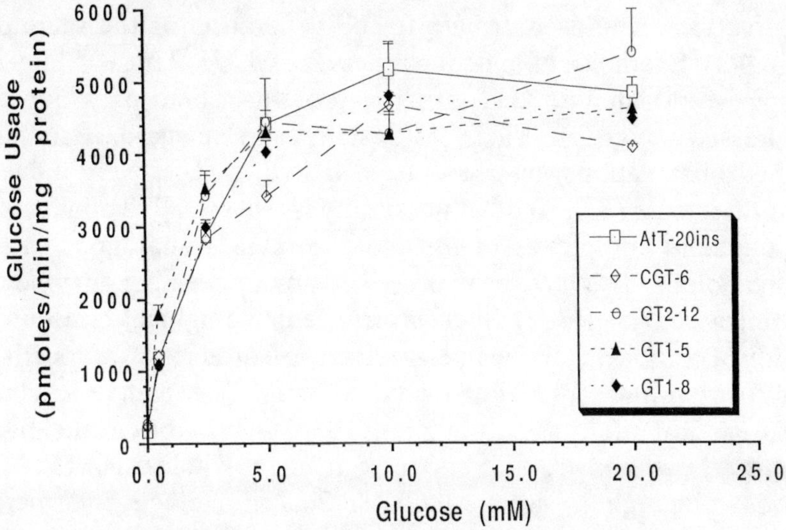

Fig. 5. Glucose usage in AtT-20ins cell lines. Glucose usage was determined by measuring the rate of generation of ^3H_2O from [5-^{3}H] glucose. The AtT-20ins cell lines assayed were as follows: untransfected, parental AtT-20ins cells (AtT-20ins); GLUT-2 transfected lines CGT-6 and GT2-12; GLUT-1 transfected lines GT1-5 and GT1-8. The symbol legend is provided at the right of the figure. Each data point represents the mean ± SEM for four independent experiments. Data are reprinted from Hughes et al. *(11)*, with permission.

would expect to observe elevated rates of glucose metabolism in GLUT-2 transfected cells coinciding with the increased capacity for glucose uptake, as suggested in either model I or model II. In fact, as seen in Fig. 5, measurement of glucose usage with [5-^{3}H]-glucose reveals that untransfected, GLUT-1 transfected, and GLUT-2 transfected cell lines metabolize glucose at similar rates, with half maximal activities achieved at 2.5, 1.6, and 1.9 m*M* glucose, respectively *(11)*. Thus, glucose metabolism does not appear to be limited by glucose uptake in AtT-20ins cells, but is instead controlled by a low K_m step or steps, possibly including hexokinase. These data argue against models I or II and suggest instead that GLUT-2 provides a necessary but not sufficient signal for insulin secretion that requires glucose metabolism for transmission. Embodied in such a model (model III) is the concept that GLUT-2 might engage in physical interactions with other cellular proteins or structures, and that such interactions would contribute to the generation of the secretory signal(s). Examples of logical partners for GLUT-2 in such interactions would include GTP-binding proteins, some of which are expressed at high levels in islets (Sestak A and Newgard CB, unpublished observations) and have been linked to secretagog-induced insulin release *(81)*. Another possibility is that GLUT-2 might serve to nucleate complexes of metabolic enzymes analogous to the "metabolons" that have been described among member enzymes of the citric acid cycle *(82)*. Such an arrangement might allow accumulation of certain metabolic intermediates and products in a "localized microenvironment" (ATP in the vicinity of ATP-sensitive K^+ channels, for example), possibly helping to explain how ion channel function can be altered in the absence of a change in whole cell ATP:ADP ratios. Although the notion of GLUT-2 as an interactive partner in glucose sensing is inherently attractive, direct experimentation involving construction of GLUT-2/GLUT-1 chimeric glucose transporters, or other, more directed approaches will be required before such a concept can be accepted. It should also be pointed out that other investigators have shown that downregulation of GLUT-2 expression in islets expressing a modified, oncogenic HRAS protein *(83)* or in islets cultured at various glucose concentrations in vitro *(84)* does not diminish glucose-stimulated insulin release. These findings might be reconciled with our own data if low levels of GLUT-2 expression are sufficient for effective interactive signaling, or if loss of GLUT-2 expression is minimal in subpopulations of β-cells that are particularly competent for glucose-stimulated insulin release *(85,86)*.

Potential Use of Engineered, Insulin-Secreting Cell Lines for Cell-Based Insulin Delivery in IDDM

Insulin-dependent diabetes mellitus (IDDM) is a disease precipitated by autoimmune destruction of the insulin producing β-cells of the pancreatic islets of Langerhans. Administration of insulin by injection is clearly a lifesaving intervention for patients devoid of β-cells, but this approach falls short of the remarkable titration of insulin delivery and consequent control of glucose levels achieved in patients with normally functioning islets. Islet or pancreas transplantation has been investigated intensively for the past several decades as a potential alternative to insulin injection *(87)*. The progress made in recent years in the protocols for large scale islet isolation and cryopreservation coupled with the development of biocompatible, perm-selective devices for protection of transplanted islets has been significant *(87–91)*. Many believe that large-scale islet transplantation may represent the ultimate alternative to insulin injection therapy, since islets will provide the missing moment-to-moment titration of insulin delivery in response to varying metabolic needs. There is little doubt that successes can be achieved with individual patients, but the scale of applicability of this approach is called into doubt by the cost and difficulty associated with procuring islets and the issue of inconsistency of performance of isolated islets on a batch-to-batch basis. It is for these reasons that engineered cells, which can be grown in essentially unlimited quantity at relatively low cost, might represent a new strategy for cell-based insulin delivery in IDDM *(1,92)*.

A number of sizable obstacles remain to be overcome before this vision can be realized. First, the subphysiological threshold of the glucose response must be shifted into the physiological range. As discussed in detail above, this will likely require the establishment of a new glucokinase:hexokinase ratio. In RIN cells, the spontaneous increase in glucokinase activity achieved upon GLUT-2 transfection *(53)* suggests that further elevations in glucokinase may not be required; in AtT-20ins cells, in contrast, GLUT-2 transfection does not increase the low cellular levels of glucokinase *(72)*, suggesting that molecular enhancement of this activity will be required to produce therapeutically useful AtT-20ins lines. For both AtT-20ins and RIN cell lines, reduction in hexokinase activity will likely be required for physiologically relevant glucose sensing. This can theoretically be accomplished by application of antisense technology or by gene knockout. The second major hurdle is to eliminate secretion of undesirable products from the engineered cells. AtT-20ins cells have an advantage in that they are programmed for expression of human insulin. Although early AtT-20ins lines such as CGT-6 secreted <1% of the insulin secreted from islets, more recent lines approach 20% of the islet's insulin producing capacity *(93)*. Multiple strategies could be employed to increase insulin secretion even further, possibly even to the point where insulin output from engineered cells could exceed the insulin producing capacity of the islet. Although

AtT-20ins cells express human insulin, their major secreted product is ACTH (corticotrophin). Profound alterations in adrenal gland morphology and steroid metabolism (Cushing's syndrome) occur under conditions of ACTH overproduction; expression of the hormone will clearly have to be sharply reduced or eliminated in order for the AtT-20ins lines to be useful for therapy. RIN cells do not express ACTH, but do express rat insulin instead of human insulin. It will therefore likely be necessary to replace the rat insulin gene with that for human insulin by homologous recombination in RIN cells that have been engineered for physiologically relevant glucose sensing. Clearly, achieving multiple stable molecular manipulations in the cell lines under study will represent a major challenge. Recent advances in gene transfer technology described below may improve our chances for success in this area.

Molecular Engineering of Normal and Glucose Insensitive Islets

Traditional Approaches

Until recently, gene transfer into the islets of Langerhans was mainly accomplished either by relatively inefficient physical techniques such as electroporation *(94,95)*, or by the creation of transgenic animals in which genes were targeted to the islet β-cells *(96,97)* or α-cells *(98)*, using the insulin or glucagon promoters, respectively. Some of these experiments have provided important information about the relative importance of glucose phosphorylation in dictating the magnitude and dose dependence of glucose-mediated effects on insulin expression and release. For example, German has used electroporation for transient transfection of fetal islets with hexokinase I *(95)*, a technique that generally allows for a transfection efficiency of approx 10–20% of cells. Introduction of the hexokinase I gene into fetal islets resulted in a reduced glucose concentration threshold for activation of a cotransfected chimeric gene consisting of the rat insulin I promoter linked to chloramphenicol acetyl transferase (CAT) *(95)*. In normal fetal islets, glucose activation of CAT expression commences at 4–5 m*M* glucose and is maximal at >15 m*M* glucose, while in islets transfected with hexokinase, insulin promoter function is maximal at 1 m*M* glucose. Further support for a major role for hexokinase in mediating the change in glucose dose response was achieved by preincubation of transfected islets with 2-deoxyglucose, resulting in a return of the threshold for glucose stimulation to the physiologic range *(95)*. Since only a relatively small subset of cells actually receive the gene of interest with the transient transfection approach that was utilized, the effects of hexokinase expression on the acute glucose-stimulated insulin secretion response can not yet be measured. It is also unwise to assume that all elements of the pathways leading from glucose to insulin gene transcription on the one hand and insulin release on the other are identical, although there will surely be common elements. In another study of interest, yeast hexokinase driven by the rat insulin I promoter was expressed in β-cells of transgenic mice *(97)*. These animals were found to exhibit an enhanced insulin secretion response to glucose, both in terms of a lower glucose concentration threshold and in the magnitude of the response *(97)*. Mice obtained by crossing transgenic animals expressing hexokinase with animals made diabetic by transgenic expression of calmodulin exhibited better glucose control than animals derived from crosses of normal and calmodulin-expressing mice, suggesting that enhanced glucose phosphorylation in islets is sufficient to provide a better insulin secretory capacity *(97)*. It should be noted that yeast hexokinase is distinct from mammalian hexokinases in that it is not inhibited by glucose-6-phosphate. Thus, it is unclear that overexpression of mammalian hexokinase to a similar extent would have the same effect, since the mammalian enzyme that is normally present in islets is apparently in an allosterically inhibited state *(24,28)*.

New Approaches for Cellular Engineering

As detailed above, development of insulin secreting cell lines with potential therapeutic value will likely require simultaneous modulation of several genes by molecular techniques. Another major challenge is to be able to efficiently introduce genes into the islets directly, either in vivo or in vitro. We have recently begun to utilize recombinant adenovirus as a means for approaching both of these issues. As shown schematically in Fig. 6, the technique involves cloning genes involved in β-cell glucose sensing or replication into a vector (pACCMV) containing a portion of the adenovirus genome which is recombined with a second vector (pJM17) consisting essentially of the viral genome interrupted by PBR sequence *(99)*, to pro-

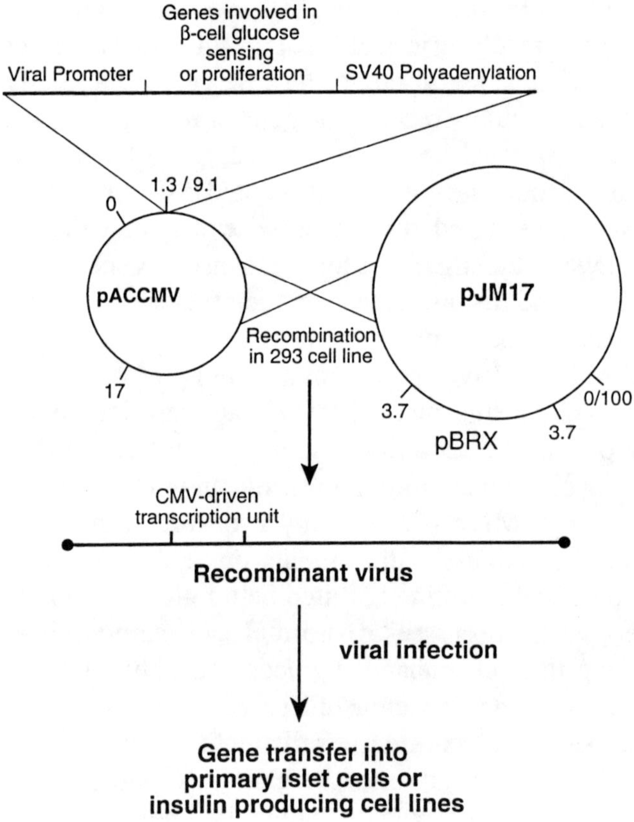

Fig. 6. General strategy for construction of recombinant adenoviruses to allow high efficiency gene transfer into islets or insulin-secreting cell lines.

duce a recombinant virus that is fully infection competent but replication defective. The efficacy of such recombinant viruses for gene transfer into nonreplicating cells was shown in a recent study in which the muscle glycogen phosphorylase cDNA was transferred into primary hepatoctyes with an efficiency of 86% *(100)*. Introduction of muscle phosphorylase into primary hepatocytes was found to confer a capacity for glycogenolytic responses that would otherwise not be apparent, suggesting that this approach may have applications for hepatic glycogen storage disorders *(100)*.

The remarkable efficiency of gene transfer with the adenovirus system in hepatocytes suggested that it may also be useful for metabolic engineering of islets or insulin-secreting clonal cells. In order to test the validity of this assumption, we have recently utilized a recombinant virus containing the β-galactosidase gene and a nuclear localization signal (AdCMV-βGal) for studies in isolated islets and insulin secreting cell lines. Freshly isolated rat islets were exposed to the AdCMV-βGal virus for 1 h and expression was scored by the presence of blue cells after incubation of the islets with X-gal, the chromogenic substrate for the enzyme, at 4, 6, and 14 d after infection. In two separate experiments an average of 70.3 ± 2.5% and 61.2 ± 1.1% of the islet cells were stained blue, respectively, with no detectable decrease in expression observed between 4 and 14 d (Becker T, Noel R, Johnson JH, and Newgard CB, manuscript in preparation). Furthermore, infected and uninfected islets showed near-identical insulin secretory responses to glucose, glucose + arginine, and glucagon-like peptide-1, showing that the virus per se has no detrimental effect on islet function. Finally, infection of RIN or AtT-20ins cells with recombinant adenoviruses allows gene transfer with near 100% efficiency. It should be pointed out, however, that adenovirus DNA integrates into genomic DNA only with low efficiency *(101)*, meaning that the introduced gene will not transfer as cells replicate, and will therefore ultimately be diluted. This issue is less of a concern in islets, since these cells are notorious for their slow rate of replication. We conclude that recombinant adenovirus is a highly efficient means for performing gene transfer into islets, and at least for short term experiments, into insulin secreting cell lines. Of particular relevance for the latter studies, we have recently constructed recombinant adenoviruses containing the cDNA encoding rat hexokinase I *(102)* in both the sense and antisense orientation.

Recombinant adenoviruses will likely be useful for the evaluation of candidate genes that may be involved in the β-cell dysfunction that is characteristic of NIDDM. For example, the controversy surrounding the issue of whether the reduction of GLUT-2 is the primary genetic lesion in the β-cell dysfunction of rodent models of NIDDM can now be directly addressed by restoring GLUT-2 expression to such islets via recombinant adenovirus. To this end we have recently prepared recombinant virus containing the GLUT-2 cDNA and demonstrated its efficacy for gene transfer into clonal cell lines *(53)*. The adenovirus system may also be useful for evaluating the impact of specific glucokinase mutations associated with MODY on glucose sensing function. It is intriguing that all MODY patients with glucokinase mutations are heterozygous, and that patients with alleles that predict severely compromised or near-normal glucokinase enzymes alike have some measure of disease phenotype *(32)*. These data suggest that some of the effect of mutant alleles is realized through a "dominant negative" effect, possibly involving interference with physical interactions between glucokinase and other components of the islet glucose sensing apparatus. This notion can now be tested by transferring normal and mutant glucokinase genes into normal islets for testing of their impact on glucose sensing. To this end, we have recently prepared recombinant adenoviruses containing normal as well as mutant glucokinases associated with MODY, and have demonstrated their utility for gene transfer into islets and cell lines (Becker T, Noel R, Johnson JH, Takeda J, Bell GI, and Newgard CB, unpublished observations).

Studies on the effect of candidate genes of NIDDM might initially be carried out on isolated islets. In vivo studies might be contemplated as well, assuming that the efficiency of gene transfer observed in lung and liver with the cystic fibrosis *(103)* and LDL receptor *(104)* genes, respectively, can be duplicated in the islets of Langerhans. Targeting of genes to the islets, and not to the exocrine pancreas via recombinant adenovirus might be anticipated because of the intense, fenestrated vasculature of the islet. More specific targeting to islet β-cells can probably be achieved by construction of viruses utilizing the insulin promoter to direct expression of the gene of interest. It should be clearly understood that the utility of the adenovirus system may be limited to short-term experimentation, since expression of a variety of genes in liver of virally infected animals begins to wane 2–3 wk after gene transfer (Gerard R, personal communication). Other related or derivative systems will likely be needed to achieve the longevity of expression required for gene therapy. Improvements in this area might be achieved with adeno-associated virus, a parvo virus that appears to integrate stably and with reasonable efficiency at a specific site in human chromosome 19 *(105)*. The intense investigation applied to understanding the safety and efficacy of retrovirus gene transfer systems in recent years must now be duplicated for the emerging DNA virus systems.

General Conclusions

Significant progress has been made in recent years in the area of cellular engineering for the purpose of studying the molecular basis of fuel-mediated insulin secretion. There is reason to hope that engineered cell lines that closely mimic the glucose-stimulated insulin secretion response of normal islets will eventually emerge. The therapeutic relevance of such lines will likely be dictated by the stability of their phenotype over time in the in vivo environment and by the extent to which such cells can be sensitized to the many other metabolic and hormonal signals that impact the β-cell. With the advent of new technologies such as the adenovirus system, one can envision the extrapolation of the approaches outlined for engineering of cell lines in culture to the level of gene therapy for syndromes of β-cell dysfunction. Many challenges remain, but the potential therapeutic implications of these approaches cannot be ignored.

Acknowledgments

Work in our laboratory relevant to this article has been supported by NIH grants R29-DK40734, PO1-DK42582, and RO1-DK46492, and grants from the Diabetes Research and Education Foundation and the Children's Liver Foundation.

References

1. Newgard CB: Cellular engineering for the treatment of metabolic disorders: prospects for therapy in diabetes. *Bio/Technology* 10:1112–1120, 1992.
2. Pfeiffer MA, Halter JB, Porte D Jr: Insulin secretion in diabetes mellitus. *Am J Med* 70:579–588, 1981.
3. Srikanta S, Ganda OP, Eisenbarth GS, Soeldner JS: Islet-cell antibodies and beta-cell function in monozygotic triplets and twins initially discordant for type I diabetes mellitus. *N Engl J Med* 308:322–325, 1983.
4. Hedeskov CJ: Mechanism of glucose-induced insulin secretion. *Physiol Rev* 60:442–508, 1980.
5. Ashcroft SJH: Metabolic controls of insulin secretion. In *The Islets of Langerhans*, Cooperstein SJ, Watkins D, eds, Academic, London, pp 117–148, 1981.
6. Malaisse WJ, Sener A, Herchuelz A, Hutton JC: Insulin release: The fuel hypothesis *Metabolism* 28:373–386, 1979.
7. Meglasson MD, Matschinsky FM: Pancreatic islet glucose metabolism and regulation of insulin secretion. *Diabetes Metab Rev* 2:163–214, 1986.

8. Prentki M, Matschinsky FM: Ca^{2+}, cAMP, and phospholipid-derived messengers in coupling mechanisms of insulin secretion. *Physiol Rev* 67:1185–1248, 1987.
9. Turk J, Wolf BA, McDaniel ML: The role of phospholipid-derived mediators including arachidonic acid, its metabolites, and inositoltrisphosphate and of intracellular Ca^{2+} in glucose-induced insulin secretion by pancreatic islets. *Prog Lipid Res* 26:125–181, 1987.
10. MacDonald MJ: Elusive proximal signals of β-cells for insulin secretion. *Diabetes* 39:1461–1466, 1990.
11. Hughes SD, Quaade C, Johnson JH, Ferber S, Newgard CB: Transfection of AtT-20ins cells with GLUT-2 but not GLUT-1 confers glucose-stimulated insulin secretion: relationship to glucose metabolism. *J Biol Chem* 268:15,205–15,212, 1993.
12. Cook DL, Hales CN: Intracellular ATP directly blocks K^+ channels in pancreatic B-cells. *Nature* 311:271–273, 1984.
13. Ashcroft FM, Harrison DE, Ashcroft SJH: Glucose induces closure of single potassium channels in isolated rat pancreatic islets. *Nature* 312:446–448, 1984.
14. Gembal M, Gilon P, Henquin J-C: Evidence that glucose can control insulin release independently from its action on ATP-sensitive K^+ channels in mouse B cells. *J Clin Invest* 89:1288–1295, 1992.
15. Ghosh A, Ronner P, Cheong E, Khalid P, Matschinsky FM: The role of ATP and free ADP in metabolic coupling during fuel-stimulated insulin release from islet β-cells in the isolated perfused pancreas. *J Biol Chem* 266:22,887–22,892, 1991.
16. Prentki M, Vischer S, Glennon MC, Regazzi R, Deeney JT, Corkey BE: Malonyl-CoA and long chain acyl-CoA esters as metabolic coupling factors in nutrient-induced insulin secretion. *J Biol Chem* 267:5802–5810, 1992.
17. Ashcroft SJH, Hughes SJ: Protein phosphorylation in the regulation of insulin secretion and biosynthesis. *Biochem Soc Trans* 18:116–118, 1990.
18. Ganesan S, Calle R, Zawalich K, Greenawalt K, Zawalich W, Shulman GI, et al.: Immunocytochemical location of α-protein kinase C in rat pancreatic β-cells during glucose-induced insulin secretion. *J Cell Biol* 119:313–324, 1992.
19. Calle R, Ganesan S, Smallwood JI, Rasmussen H: Glucose-induced phosphorylation of myristoylated alanine-rich C kinase substrate (MARCKS) in isolated rat pancreatic islets. *J Biol Chem* 267:18,723–18,727, 1992.
20. Coore HG, Randle PJ: Regulation of insulin secretion studied with pieces of rabbit pancreas incubated in vitro. *Biochem J* 93:66–78, 1964.
21. Matschinsky FM, Ellerman JE: Metabolism of glucose in the islets of Langerhans. *J Biol Chem* 243:2730–2736, 1968.
22. Matschinsky F M: Glucokinase as glucose sensor and metabolic signal generator in pancreatic β-cells and hepatocytes. *Diabetes* 39:647–652, 1990.
23. Randle PJ: Glucokinase and candidate genes for type 2 (non-insulin-dependent) diabetes mellitus. *Diabetologia* 36:269–275, 1993.

24. Trus MD, Zawalich WS, Burch PT, Berner DK, Weill VA, Matschinsky FM: Regulation of glucose metabolism in pancreatic islets. *Diabetes* 30:911–922, 1981.
25. Meglasson MD, Burch PT, Berner DK, Najafi H, Matschinsky FM: Identification of glucokinase as an alloxan-sensitive glucose sensor of the pancreatic β-cell. *Diabetes* 35:1163–1173, 1986.
26. Coore HG, Randle PJ: Inhibition of glucose phosphorylation by mannoheptulose. *Biochem J* 91:56–59, 1964.
27. Wilson JE: Regulation of mammalian hexokinase activity. In *Regulation of Carbohydrate Metabolism.* Beitner R, ed, CRC, Boca Raton, FL, pp 45–85, 1984.
28. Giroix M-H, Sener A, Pipeleers DG, Malaisse WJ: Hexose metabolism in pancreatic islets. *Biochem J* 223:447–453, 1984.
29. Frougel P, Vaxillaire M, Sun F, Vehlo G, Zouali H, Butel MO, et al.: Close linkage of glucokinase locus on chromosome 7p to early-onset non-insulin dependent diabetes mellitus. *Nature* 356:162–164, 1992.
30. Vionnet N, Stoffel M, Takeda J, Yasuda K, Bell GI, Zouali H, Lesage S, Velho G, Iris F, Passa P, Frouguel P, Cohen D: Nonsense mutation in the glucokinase gene causes early-onset non-insulin dependent diabetes mellitus. *Nature* 356:721,722, 1992.
31. Stoffel M, Froguel P, Takeda J, Zouali H, Vionnet N, Nishi S, et al.: Human glucokinase gene: Isolation, characterization, and identification of two missense mutations linked to early-onset non-insulin-dependent (type 2) diabetes mellitus. *Proc Natl Acad Sci USA* 89:7698–7702, 1992.
32. Gidh-Jain M, Takeda J, Xu LZ, Lange AJ, Vionnet N, Stoffel M, et al.: Glucokinase mutations associated with non-insulin-dependent (type 2) diabetes mellitus have decreased enzymatic activity: implications for structure/function relationships. *Proc Natl Acad Sci USA* 90:1932–1936,1993.
33. Vehlo G, Froguel P, Clement K, Pueyo ME, Rakotoambinina B, Zouali, H, et al.: Primary pancreatic beta-cell secretory defect caused by mutations in glucokinase gene in kindreds of maturity onset diabetes of the young. *Lancet* 340:444–448, 1992.
34. Hellman B, Lernmark A, Sehlin J, Taljedal I-B: Effects of phlorizin on metabolism and function of pancreatic β-cells. *Metabolism* 21:60–66, 1972.
35. Gorus FK, Malaisse WJ, Pipeleers DG: Differences in glucose handling by pancreatic A- and B-cells. *J Biol Chem* 259:1196–1200, 1984.
36. Thorens B, Sarkar HK, Kaback, HR, Lodish HF: Cloning and functional expression in bacteria of a novel glucose transporter present in liver, intestine, kidney, and beta-pancreatic islet cells. *Cell* 55:281–290, 1988.
37. Johnson JH, Newgard CB, Milburn JL, Lodish HF, Thorens B: The high K_m glucose transporter of islets of Langerhans is functionally similar to the low affinity transporter of liver and has an identical primary sequence. *J Biol Chem* 265:6548–6551, 1990.
38. Orci L, Thorens B, Ravazzola M, Lodish HF: Localization of the pancreatic beta cell glucose transporter to specific plasma membrane domains. *Science* 245:295–297, 1989.

39. Unger RH: Diabetic hyperglycemia: Link to impaired glucose transport in pancreatic β-cells. *Science* 251:1200–1205, 1991.
40. Johnson JH, Ogawa A, Chen L, Orci L, Newgard CB, Alam T, et al.: Underexpression of β cell high K_m glucose transporters in noninsulin-dependent diabetes. *Science* 250:546–549, 1990.
41. Orci L, Ravazzola M, Baetens D, Inman L, Amherdt M, Peterson RG, et al.: Evidence that downregulation of β-cell glucose transporters in non-insulin-dependent diabetes may be the cause of diabetic hyperglycemia. *Proc Natl Acad Sci USA* 87:9953–9957, 1990.
42. Chen L, Alam T, Johnson JH, Hughes S, Newgard CB, Unger RH: Regulation of β-cell glucose transporter gene expression. *Proc Natl Acad Sci USA* 87:4088–4092, 1990.
43. Thorens B, Wu Y-J, Leahy JL, Weir GC: The loss of GLUT-2 expression by glucose-unresponsive β-cells of db/db mice is reversible and is induced by the diabetic environment. *J Clin Invest* 90:77–85, 1992.
44. Thorens B, Weir G, Leahy J, Lodish HF, Bonner-Weir S: Reduced expression of the liver/beta cell glucose transporter isoform in glucose-insensitive pancreatic beta cells of diabetic rats. *Proc Natl Acad Sci USA* 87:6492–6496, 1990.
45. Giroix M-H, Rasschaert J, Bailbe D, Leclercq-Meyer V, Sener A, Portha B, et al.: Impairment of glycerol phosphate shuttle in islets from rats with diabetes induced by neonatal streptozotocin. *Diabetes* 40:227–232, 1991.
46. Gazdar AF, Chick WL, Oie HK, Sims HL, King DL, Weir GC, et al.: Continuous, clonal, insulin- and somatostatin-secreting cell lines established from a transplantable rat islet cell tumor. *Proc Natl Acad Sci USA* 77:3519–3523, 1980.
47. Santerre RF, Cook RA, Crisel RMD, Sharp JD, Schmidt RJ, Williams DC, et al.: Insulin synthesis in a clonal cell line of simian virus 40-transformed hamster pancreatic beta-cells. *Proc Natl Acad Sci USA* 78:4339–4343, 1981.
48. Efrat S, Linde S, Kofod H, Spector D, Delannoy M, Grant S, et al.: Beta-cell lines derived from transgenic mice expressing a hybrid insulin gene-oncogene. *Proc Natl Acad Sci USA* 85:9037–9041, 1988.
49. Miyazaki J-I, Araki K, Yamato E, Ikegami H, Asano T, Shibasaki Y, et al.: Establishment of a pancreatic β cell line that retains glucose-inducible insulin secretion: Special reference to expression of glucose transporter isoforms. *Endocrinology* 127:126–132, 1990.
50. Halban PA, Praz GA, Wollheim CB: Abnormal glucose metabolism accompanies failure of glucose to stimulate insulin release from a pancreatic cell line (RINm5F). *Biochem J* 212:439–443, 1983.
51. Shimizu T, Knowles BB, Matschinsky FM: Control of glucose phosphorylation and glucose usage in clonal insulinoma cells. *Diabetes* 37:563–568, 1988.
52. Clark SA, Burnham BL, Chick WL: Modulation of glucose-induced insulin secretion from a rat clonal β-cell line. *Endocrinology* 127:2779–2788, 1990.

53. Ferber S, BeltrandelRio H, Johnson JH, Noel R, Cassidy LE, Clark S, Becker TC, Hughes SD, Newgard CB: GLUT-2 gene transfer into insulinoma cells confers both low and high affinity glucose-stimulated insulin release: Relationship to glucokinase activity. *J Biol Chem,* in press.
54. Inagaki N, Yasuda K, Inoue G, Okamoto Y, Yano H, Someya Y, et al.: Glucose regulation of glucose transport activity and glucose-transporter mRNA in hamster β-cell line. *Diabetes* 41:592–597, 1992.
55. Whitesell RR, Powers AC, Regen DM, Abumrad NA: Transport and metabolism of glucose in an insulin-secreting cell line, bTC-1. *Biochemistry* 30:11,560–11,566, 1991.
56. D'ambra R, Surana M, Efrat S, Starr RG, Fleischer N: Regulation of insulin secretion from β-cell lines derived from transgenic mice insulinomas resembles that of normal β-cells. *Endocrinology* 126:2815–2822, 1990.
57. Efrat S, Leiser M, Surana M, Tal M, Fusco-Demane D, Fleischer N: Murine insulinoma cell line with normal glucose-regulated insulin secretion. *Diabetes* 42:901–907, 1993.
58. Moore H-P, Walker MD, Lee F, Kelly RB: Expressing a human proinsulin cDNA in a mouse ACTH-secreting cell intracellular storage, proteolytic processing, and secretion on stimulation. *Cell* 35:531–538, 1983.
59. Gross DJ, Halban PA, Kahn RC, Weir GC, Villa-Komaroff L: Partial diversion of a mutant proinsulin (B10 aspartic acid) from the regulated to the constitutive secretory pathway in transfected AtT-20 cells. *Proc Natl Acad Sci USA* 86:4107–4111, 1989.
60. Smeekens SP, Steiner DF: Identification of a human insulinoma cDNA encoding a novel mammalian protein structurally related to the yeast dibasic processing protease Kex2. *J Biol Chem* 265:2997–3000, 1990.
61. Hakes DJ, Birch NP, Mezey A, Dixon JE: Isolation of two complementary deoxyribonucleic acid clones from a rat insulinoma cell lin based on similarities to Kex2 and furin sequences and the specific localization of each transcript to endocrine and neuroendocrine tissues in rat. *Endocrinology* 129:3053–3063, 1991.
62. Hughes SD, Quaade C, Milburn JL, Cassidy LC, Newgard CB: Expression of normal and novel glucokinase mRNAs in anterior pituitary and islet cells. *J Biol Chem* 266:4521–4530, 1991.
63. Hayzer DJ, Iynedjian PB: Alternative splicing of glucokinase mRNA in rat liver. *Biochem J* 270:261–263, 1990.
64. Quaade C, Hughes SD, Coats WS, Sestak A L, Iynedjian PB, Newgard CB: Analysis of the protein products encoded by variant glucokinase transcripts via expression in bacteria. *FEBS Lett* 280:47–52, 1991.
65. Liang Y, Jetton T, Zimmerman EC, Najafi H, Matschinsky FM, Magnuson MA: Effects of alternate RNA splicing on glucokinase isoform activities in the pancreatic islet, liver, and anterior pituitary. *J Biol Chem* 266:6999–7007, 1991.
66. Iynedjian PB, Pilot P-R, Nouspikel T, Milburn JL, Quaade C, Hughes S, et al.: Differential expression and regulation of the glucokinase gene in liver and islets of Langerhans. *Proc Natl Acad Sci USA* 86:7838–7842, 1989.

67. Iynedjian PB, Ucla C, Mach B: Molecular cloning of glucokinase cDNA: Developmental and dietary regulation of glucokinase mRNA in rat liver. *J Biol Chem* 262:6032–6038, 1987.
68. Newgard CB, Quaade C, Hughes SD, Milburn JL: Glucokinase and glucose-transporter expression in liver and islets: implications for control of glucose homeostasis. *Biochem Soc Trans* 18:851–853, 1990.
69. Magnuson MA, Shelton KD: An alternate promoter in the glucokinase gene is active in the pancreatic β-cell. *J Biol Chem* 264:15,936–15,942, 1989.
70. Andreone TL, Printz RL, Pilkis SJ, Magnuson MA, Granner DK: The amino acid sequence of rat liver glucokinase deduced from cloned cDNA. *J Biol Chem* 264:363–369, 1989.
71. Permutt MA, Koryani L, Keller K, Lacy PE, Scharp DW, Mueckler M: Cloning and functional expression of a human pancreatic islet glucose-transporter cDNA. *Proc Natl Acad Sci USA* 86:8688–8692, 1989.
72. Hughes SD, Johnson JH, Quaade C, Newgard CB: Engineering of glucose-stimulated insulin secretion and biosynthesis in non-islet cells. *Proc Natl Acad Sci USA* 89:688–692, 1992.
73. Madsen OD, Andersen LC, Michelsen B, Owerbach D, Larsson L-I, Lernmark A, et al.: Tissue-specific expression of transfected human insulin genes in pluripotent clonal rat insulinoma lines induced during passage *in vivo*. *Proc Natl Acad Sci USA* 85: 6652–6656, 1988.
74. Malaisse WJ, Sener A, Levy J: The stimulus secretion coupling of glucose induced insulin release: fasting induced adaptation of key glycolytic enzymes in isolated islets. *J Biol Chem* 251:1731–1737, 1976.
75. Trus M, Warner H, Matschinsky F M: Effects of glucose on insulin release and on intermediary metabolism of isolated perifused pancreatic islets from fed and fasted rats. *Diabetes* 29:1–14, 1980.
76. Liang Y, Najafi H, Smith RM, Zimmerman EC, Magnuson MA, Tal M, et al.: Concordant glucose induction of glucokinase, glucose usage, and glucose-stimulated insulin release in pancreatic islets maintained in organ culture. *Diabetes* 41:792–806, 1992.
77. Chen C, Bumbalo L, Leahy JL: Raised intrinsic activity of islet glucokinase in euglycemic hyperinsulinemic rats. *Diabetes* 42,Suppl 1:11A (abstract), 1993.
78. Malaisse WJ, Malaisse-Lagae F, Davies DR, Vandercammen A, Van Schaftingen E: Regulation of glucokinase by a fructose-1-phosphate-sensitive protein in pancreatic islets. *Eur J Biochem* 190:539–545, 1990.
79. Tippett PS, Neet KE: Specific inhibition of glucokinase by long chain acyl coenzymes A below the critical micelle concentration. *J Biol Chem* 257:12,839–12,845, 1982.
80. Lynch RM, Fogarty KE, Fay FS: Modulation of hexokinase association with mitochondria analyzed with quantitative three-dimensional confocal microscopy. *J Cell Biol* 112:385–396, 1991.
81. Robertson RP, Seaquist ER, Walseth TF: G-proteins and modulation of insulin secretion. *Diabetes* 40:1–6, 1991.

82. Srere PA: Complexes of sequential metabolic enzymes. *Ann Rev Biochem* 56:89–124, 1987.
83. Tal M, Wu Y-J, Leiser M, Surana M, Lodish H, Fleischer N, et al.: [Val12] HRAS downregulates GLUT2 in β cells of transgenic mice without affecting glucose homeostasis. *Proc Natl Acad Sci USA* 89:5744–5748, 1992.
84. Tal M, Liang Y, Najafi H, Lodish HF, Matschinsky FM: Expression and function of GLUT-1 and GLUT-2 glucose transporter isoforms in cells of cultured rat pancreatic islets. *J Biol Chem* 267:17,241–17,247, 1992.
85. Van Schravendijk CFH, Kiekens R, Pipeleers DG: Pancreatic β-cell heterogeneity in glucose-induced insulin release. *J Biol Chem* 267: 21,344–21,348, 1992.
86. Giordano E, Bosco D, Cirulli V, Meda P: Repeated glucose stimulation reveals distinct and lasting secretion patterns of individual rat pancreatic β-cells. *J Clin Invest* 87:2178–2185, 1991.
87. Lacy PE, Scharp DW: Islet transplantation in treating diabetes. *Ann Rev Med* 37:33–46, 1986.
88 Posselt AM, Barker CF, Tomaszewski JE, Markmann JF, Choti MA, Naji A: Induction of donor-specific unresponsiveness by intrathymic islet transplantation. *Science* 249:1293–1295, 1990.
89. Sullivan SJ, Maki T, Borland KM, Mahoney MD, Solomon BA, Muller TE, et al.: Biohybrid artificial pancreas: Long-term implantation studies in diabetic, pancreatectomized dogs. *Science* 252: 718–721, 1991.
90. Lacy PE, Hegre OD, Gerasimidi-Vazeou A, Gentile FT, Dionne KE: Maintenance of normoglycemia in diabetic mice by subcutaneous xenografts of encapsulated islets. *Science* 254:1782–1785, 1991.
91. Lanza RP, Borland KM, Lodge P, Carretta M, Sullivan SJ, Muller TE, et al.: Treatment of severely diabetic pancreatectomized dogs using a diffusion-based hybrid pancreas. *Diabetes* 41:886–889, 1992.
92. Newgard CB, Quaade C, Johnson JH, Hughes SD: Engineering of glucose-stimulated insulin release in clonal cells: therapeutic implications. *Diabetes, Nutr, Metab* 5,Suppl 1:15–20, 1992.
93. Ferber S, Schnedl W, BeltrandelRio H, Irminger J-C, Halban P, Newgard CB: Molecular strategies for the treatment of diabetes. *Transplantation Proc*, in press, 1994.
94. German MS, Moss LG, Rutter WJ: Regulation of insulin gene expression by glucose and calcium in transfected primary islet cultures. *J Biol Chem* 265:22,063–22,066, 1990.
95. German MS: Glucose sensing in pancreatic islet beta cells: the key role of glucokinase and the glycolytic intermediates. *Proc Natl Acad Sci USA* 90:1781–1785, 1993.
96. Adams TE, Alpert S, Hanahan D: Non-tolerance and autoantibodies to a transgenic self-antigen expressed in pancreatic B-cells. *Nature* 325:223–228, 1987.
97. Epstein PN, Boschero AC, Atwater I, Cai X, Overbeek PA: Expression of yeast hexokinase in pancreatic β-cells of transgenic mice reduces blood

glucose, enhances insulin secretion, and decreases diabetes. *Proc Natl Acad Sci USA* 89:12,038–12,042, 1992.

98. Brubaker PL, Lee YC, Drucker DJ: Alterations in proglucagon processing and inhibition of proglucagon gene expression in transgenic mice which contain a chimeric proglucagon-SV40 T-antigen gene. *J Biol Chem* 267:20,728–20,733, 1992.
99. McGrory J, Bautista D, Graham FL: A simple technique for the rescue of early region I mutation into human adenovirus type 5. *Virology* 163:614–617, 1988.
100. Gomez-Foix AM, Coats WS, Baque S, Alam T, Gerard RD, Newgard CB: Adenovirus-mediated transfer of the muscle glycogen phosphorylase gene into hepatocytes confers altered regulation of glycogen metabolism. *J Biol Chem* 267:25,129–25,134, 1992.
101. Van Doren K, Hanahan D, Gluzman Y: Infection of eucaryotic cells by helper-independent recombinant adenoviruses: Early region I is not obligatory for integration of viral DNA. *J Virology* 50:606–614, 1984.
102. Schwab DA, Wilson JE: Complete amino acid sequence of rat brain hexokinase, deduced from the cloned cDNA, and proposed structure of a mammalian hexokinase. *Proc Natl Acad Sci USA* 86:2563–2567, 1989.
103. Rosenfeld MA, Yoshimura K, Trapnell BC, Yoneyama K, Rosenthal ER, Dalemans W, et al.: *In vivo* transfer of the human cystic fibrosis transmembrane conductance regulator gene to the airway epithelium. *Cell* 68:143–155, 1992.
104. Herz J, Gerard RD: Adenovirus-mediated transfer of low density lipoprotein receptor gene acutely accelerates cholesterol clearance in normal mice. *Proc Natl Acad Sci USA* 90:2812–2816, 1993.
105. Walsh CE, Liu JM, Xiao X, Young NS, Nienhuis AW, Samulski RJ: Regulated high level expression of a human gamma-globin gene introduced into erythroid cells by an adeno-associated virus. *Proc Natl Acad Sci USA* 89:7257–7261, 1992.

Chapter 7

Glucokinase Gene Expression and Regulation

Mark A. Magnuson, Kevin D. Niswender, and Cathleen C. Pettepher

Summary

Diabetes investigators have been interested in the regulation of glucokinase for years because this enzyme catalyzes the initial step in glucose metabolism by the liver and pancreatic β-cell. However, now that mutations in the glucokinase gene have been associated with early-onset noninsulin-dependent diabetes mellitus, there is increased interest in the mechanisms that enable the gene to be differentially regulated in a cell-specific manner. In this chapter, we provide an overview of our current knowledge of the mechanisms by which the glucokinase gene is regulated and how glucokinase gene mutations might cause the hyperglycemia associated with certain types of diabetes.

Introduction

The phosphorylation of glucose is the first step in glycolysis. This reaction is catalyzed in mammals by a hexokinase gene family that consists of four members. Of these, glucokinase, or hexokinase IV, differs both functionally and structurally from hexokinases I–III.

From: *Molecular Biology of Diabetes, Part I*
Edited by: B. Draznin and D. LeRoith

For instance, glucokinase catalysis shows sigmoidal kinetics, lacks endproduct inhibition by physiological concentrations of glucose-6-phosphate, and has a K_m for glucose that is several fold higher than for hexokinases I–III. Moreover, glucokinase is approx half the size of the other three mammalian hexokinases (~50 vs ~100 kDa). However, two particular features, the K_m for glucose of ~5 m*M* and the lack of a significant inhibitory effect of glucose-6-phosphate, may be the most important since they enable glucokinase to play a key role in glucose utilization by the pancreatic β-cell *(1)* and hepatocyte *(2,3)*, the only two cell types identified to date in which this hexokinase is expressed.

To understand the differential regulation of glucokinase in the β-cell and hepatocyte it is first necessary to appreciate the different roles that these cells play in maintaining glucose homeostasis. The β-cell plays an indispensable role by sensing the plasma glucose concentration and secreting insulin when it rises above a threshold level *(4)*. It is now well established that the metabolism of glucose by β-cells is necessary for it to be sensed *(1)*. Glucose sensing is a multistep process involving several key proteins that link metabolic flux to insulin secretion *(5)*. Since glucokinase catalyzes the first step in glucose metabolism, it is ideally situated to determine many specific features of glucose usage by the β-cell. GLUT-2, a high K_m glucose transporter, also plays an important role since glucose must first enter the β-cell. However, it is glucokinase, not GLUT-2, that functions as the so-called "glucose sensor" of the β-cell *(1)* because glucose transport occurs at rates that greatly exceed the capacity of this enzyme to phosphorylate glucose.

Hepatocytes perform a very different role in maintaining glucose homeostasis. The net consumption or production of glucose by the liver is modulated by insulin and other hormones. This is accomplished by regulating the activity of specific enzymes in several different substrate cycles *(6)*. During periods when insulin levels are high relative to those of glucagon, the entry and metabolism of glucose by hepatocytes is favored. The product of the phosphorylation step, glucose-6-phosphate, can be used either for glycogen synthesis or glycolysis, or it can enter the pentose phosphate shunt, which allows glucose to be converted into other useful metabolites or stored as glycogen. In light of their markedly different functions, it is surprising that the β-cell and hepatocyte express the same glucose transporters and hexokinases. However, both cell types make GLUT-2 and glucokinase, although glucokinase gene expression varies in a manner consistent with the different physiologic functions of the β-cell and hepatocyte. These differences will be discussed in this chapter.

Whereas the function, structure, and regulation of glucokinase have been studied by investigators in different fields, our approach has been to focus how glucokinase gene expression is regulated, both at the transcriptional and posttranscriptional levels, using normoglycemic rats as the model system. The knowledge gained from cloning and characterizing rat glucokinase cDNAs and genomic DNAs *(7–10)* was applied directly to characterizing human glucokinase cDNAs and gene *(11–14)* and this information, in turn, led to the identification of a genetic linkage between glucokinase gene mutations and early onset noninsulin-dependent diabetes mellitus (NIDDM) *(15–18)*. The genetic linkage studies, in combination with an understanding of the biochemistry and tissue-specific regulation of glucokinase, have firmly established a key role for this enzyme in the maintenance of blood glucose homeostasis. However, in spite of the remarkable recent progress that established a link between glucokinase gene mutations and diabetes, it is not yet clear how these mutations cause hyperglycemia. A thorough understanding of glucokinase gene regulation will, therefore, be required in order to explain the basis of the hyperglycemia that is the hallmark of individuals with a defect in this enzyme. Toward this end, we will review our efforts and those of others that demonstrate multiple levels of regulation of glucokinase gene expression, as is illustrated in Fig. 1. Glucokinase gene expression, for the purpose of this chapter, is considered to be the process whereby structural information in the glucokinase gene is converted to an active enzyme.

Alternate Promoters

A fundamental feature of glucokinase gene expression is the use of alternate promoters in the liver and islet *(9,19)*. Dual promoters in the single glucokinase gene determine both the cell-specific regulation of glucokinase and explain the production of cell-specific isoforms, as will be discussed later. The upstream glucokinase promoter is active in at least two neuroendocrine cells, the pancreatic β-

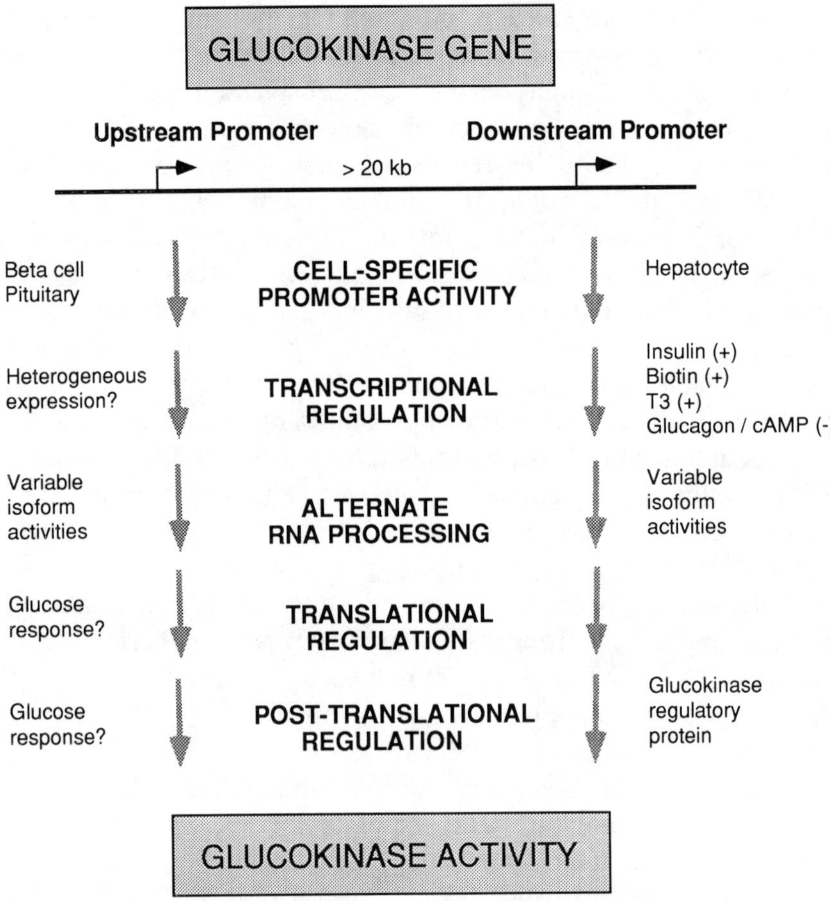

Fig. 1. Regulation of glucokinase gene expression at multiple levels. This diagram illustrates the levels at which glucokinase gene expression and activity can be controlled. Glucokinase gene expression begins with the gene and moves stepwise to the production of an active enzyme. Between these extremes there are a variety of sites of regulation, as indicated.

cell and pituitary corticotrope *(9,20,21)*, whereas the downstream promoter is expressed only in hepatocytes *(9)*. The promoters are separated by at least 20 kb in both the rat and human genomes *(9,12,22)*, although the exact distance remains to be determined. Because the sequences of the two promoters are dissimilar, it has been assumed since their discovery that they are independently regulated. This notion has been supported fully by studies performed since that time.

Downstream Promoter Regulation

Regulation of hepatic glucokinase occurs largely at a transcriptional level and is determined by hormones that are involved in metabolic regulation. However, this regulation is complex and the molecular mechanisms involved have only recently begun to be explored. In addition to the modulation of hepatic glucokinase gene transcription by hormones, the amount of glucokinase varies in different hepatocytes, depending upon their location in the hepatic lobule. More glucokinase is found in perivenous hepatocytes than in periportal hepatocytes. This distribution is consistent with the metabolic zonation of hepatic enzymes where glucokinase, a glycolytic enzyme, is expected to be expressed at higher levels in pericentral hepatocytes *(23)*. Hepatic glucokinase levels are also altered dramatically by dietary intake. Expression of glucokinase is low during fasting and increases with feeding of a carbohydrate-rich diet or with an bolus of glucose *(7,24)*. This rise parallels the situation in diabetic rats where hepatic glucokinase levels are undetectable but increase with insulin treatment *(25,26)*. Insulin and glucagon seem to be the most important acute regulators of the gene *(26,27)* although other hormones and dietary agents have also been shown to modulate glucokinase gene expression in some situations.

Insulin and Glucagon

The effects of insulin and glucagon have been studied using both animal models and cultured primary hepatocytes *(10,26–29)*. In both systems, insulin causes a prompt increase in the rate of gene transcription. Transcription in diabetic rats increases approx 20-fold within 45 min of insulin treatment *(10,26)* whereas in cultured hepatocytes, transcription increases within 30 min after adding the hormone *(30)*. The rapid response to insulin suggests that new protein synthesis would not be required for a change in the gene transcription rate to occur. However, it has now been observed by two groups that protein synthesis inhibitors abolish the insulin-dependent accumulation of glucokinase mRNA in hepatocytes *(30,31)* suggesting instead that one or more short-lived proteins may be involved. The stimulatory effect of insulin on hepatic glucokinase gene transcription is opposed by glucagon, acting via cAMP, which inhibits gene transcription in a dominant manner *(29)*. The effects of glucagon are most evident in cultured hepatocytes where glucokinase gene transcription is inhibited when glucagon and insulin are both used at maximum stimulatory concentrations *(27)*.

The *cis*-regulatory elements mediating the effects of insulin and glucagon on hepatic gene transcription have not been identified, nor have the signal transduction pathways. Fusion gene constructs containing up to 5500 base pairs of DNA upstream of the hepatic first exon do not respond to insulin in primary hepatocytes *(32)*. However, the reporter gene signal observed from these constructs was small, so it is possible that some or all of the elements necessary for liver-specific gene expression were missing in the constructs tested. Nevertheless, it is reasonable to assume that the means by which insulin modulates hepatic glucokinase gene transcription is via the phosphorylation or dephosphorylation of one or more transcription factors that alters either their function or DNA binding. Recent studies using okadaic acid, an inhibitor of the serine/threonine protein phosphatases PP1 and PP2A, support this notion since they appear to abolish the transcriptional response of the downstream promoter to insulin *(30)*.

Thyroid Hormone and Biotin

Glucokinase gene expression in the liver is also regulated by thyroid hormones, but the effects are both diet- and age-dependent. In primary cultures of neonatal rat hepatocytes, a dose-dependent increase of glucokinase mRNA, similar in magnitude to that observed with insulin, was observed after the addition of triiodothyronine (T3) *(33)*. However, in adult rats, hepatic glucokinase mRNA increases in response to T3 administration only during refeeding but not during starvation *(34)*. These experiments can be interpreted as supporting a dominant inhibitory effect of glucagon over that of T3 in regulating hepatic glucokinase gene transcription. In any case, the response of hepatic glucokinase to T3 suggests a role in the regulation of lipogenesis, in addition to the more clearly defined role in glucose utilization, since the phosphorylation of glucose is a prerequisite for the conversion of glucose into fatty acids *(34)*.

Finally, biotin, a water soluble vitamin, affects glucokinase activity in liver *(35,36)*. Glucokinase activity increases within 24 hours of administration to starved rats *(37)* as a result of increased glucokinase gene transcription *(35)*. Like the response to other hormones, the intracellular signaling mechanism, *cis*-regulatory element, and *trans*-regulatory factor mediating the biotin response of the hepatic glucokinase gene remain to be identified.

Developmental Regulation

Hepatic glucokinase activity and mRNA is first detected around postnatal d 14 in the developing rat, after which the levels rise to adult concentrations between d 21–31 *(7)*. The expression of glucokinase in the developing liver is associated with a dietary shift from maternal milk that is high in fat to a carbohydrate-rich chow diet *(38)* and with a rise in insulin levels. Suckling rats treated with insulin show a rise in hepatic glucokinase mRNA, indicating that the gene is transcriptionally competent but simply not induced prior to weaning *(39)*. In addition to insulin, glucocorticoids and thyroid hormones may also be necessary for the correct developmental expression of liver glucokinase *(29,33,40,41)*.

Upstream Promoter Regulation

Transcription initiating from the upstream glucokinase promoter has been identified in two different neuroendocrine tissues, the pancreatic islet and pituitary. However, within the various cell types of these two tissues, glucokinase activity has only been detected in β-cells of the pancreas. Transcription of the glucokinase gene from the upstream promoter in pituitary is unexplained, particularly since an active enzyme is not made. Nevertheless, transcription initiating from the upstream promoter appears to be more constitutive in nature than that initiating from the downstream promoter. For instance, although the amount of hepatic glucokinase mRNA in fasted and refed rats varies, islet glucokinase mRNA remains nearly constant *(42)*. Glucose has been shown to regulate islet glucokinase activity *(43)*, but this effect, as discussed later, does not appear to be mediated at a transcriptional level *(44)*. Moreover, insulin and other hormones do not appear to regulate β-cell glucokinase gene expression, thus arguing against a wide variety of hormone response elements in the upstream glucokinase promoter region. Nevertheless, several interesting aspects of glucokinase gene expression in the β-cell have now been identified and studied.

Heterogeneous Expression of Glucokinase Among β-Cells

Isolated β-cells have variable responses to glucose *(45)*, the basis for which appears to be differences in glucose metabolism. In response to a glucose stimulus, proinsulin biosynthesis and immunoreactivity *(46)*, membrane potential *(47)*, and insulin secretory activity *(48)* have all been observed to vary among individual β-cells. Recent observations suggest that these differences may be attributed to variability in the cellular content of both glucokinase and other hexokinases in β-cells. Heimberg et al. reported that single β-cells, sorted by their metabolic response to glucose, have different amounts of both glucokinase activity and mRNA in pools of low and high responding β-cells *(49)*. Utilizing immunocytochemical techniques, Jetton and Magnuson *(50)* have shown that glucokinase is present only in β-cells, and not in α-, δ-, or PP-cells, of normal rat islets. Glucokinase is located in the cytoplasm and does not appear to be associated with GLUT-2, the high K_m glucose transporter of β-cells. However, glucokinase immunoreactivity varies considerably among different β-cells *(50)*. The heterogeneous distribution of glucokinase appears to be largely random. A transcriptional mechanism is likely to be involved in generating this heterogeneity, but this remains to be proven. Nevertheless, the variable insulin secretory responses of individual β-cells to a glucose stimulus, together with the heterogeneous expression of glucokinase, suggests that differences in the cellular content of this enzyme may be a phenomenon of fundamental physiologic importance.

Multiple *Cis*-Acting Elements in the Upstream Promoter

The upstream glucokinase promoter is transcriptionally active in both corticotrope- and insulinoma-derived cell lines, however studies identifying *cis*-regulatory elements have only been conducted in insulinoma cells. Shelton et al. have performed a fusion gene analysis using different fragments of the upstream glucokinase promoter to identify several DNA sequences that may be involved in the neuroendocrine cell-specific expression of glucokinase *(51)*. A DNA fragment containing 294 bp of promoter DNA (from –280 to +14) is expressed efficiently in HIT M2.2.2 cells, a β-cell-derived line, but not in NIH-3T3 cells, a fibroblastic cell line. Thus, most if not all of the sequences responsible for the cell-specific expression of the upstream glucokinase promoter appear to lie in this short DNA fragment. Analysis of a series of block transversion mutants that spanned the 280 bp proximal region of the promoter identified two mutants that reduced transcription ten- or more fold, whereas six others reduced transcription between three- and tenfold *(51)*. Three mutationally sensitive regions bind a factor that is expressed preferentially in pancreatic β-cells. The binding sites for this factor have been designated Upstream Promoter Elements (UPEs) and have a consensus sequence of CAT($^{T}/_{C}$)A($^{C}/_{G}$). Laser UV-crosslinking experiments indicate that the UPE binding protein is ~50 kDa in size *(51)*. Interestingly, this may be the same factor that binds to the CT-boxes in the human insulin promoter *(52,53)*. While the function of the UPEs in regulating glucokinase gene transcription in the β-cell is presently unclear, the UPE-binding activity does not appear to be present in AtT-20 cells, a corticotrope cell line that expresses the upstream glucokinase promoter *(51)*. Thus this protein, although it binds to upstream glucokinase promoter elements, is not a good candidate to explain glucokinase gene expression in both the pituitary and islet.

Another pair of elements with the sequence TGGTCACCA were identified by Shelton et al. in the upstream glucokinase promoter *(51)*. These elements, termed Pal-1 and Pal-2 because of their near palindromic nature, may be better candidates to account for transcription of the upstream glucokinase promoter in both islet and pituitary-derived cell lines. Block mutations of Pal-1 and Pal-2 sequences diminish glucokinase promoter activity in insulinoma cells to ~30% and ~10%, respectively, of wild-type transcriptional activity *(51)*. To date, cell-specific factors that bind to the Pal elements in the upstream promoter have not been identified. Several different proteins have been found to bind to the Pal elements in mobility shift assays, but the ratios of these proteins differ in cells that either express or do not express this gene *(54)*. In any case, because the Pal elements are so mutationally sensitive and since they are conserved in both the human and rat glucokinase promoters *(55)*, they remain good candidates for further exploration of the mechanisms involved in determining the cell-specific expression of the upstream promoter.

Alternate RNA Processing

Alternate processing of glucokinase gene transcripts is a second major mechanism for regulating glucokinase expression. This mechanism leads to the production of cell-specific glucokinase isoforms and appears to determine whether active or inactive glucokinase isoforms are produced. Moreover, the alternate RNA processing associated with the use of two promoters in the glucokinase gene result in different glucokinase mRNAs in the liver, islet, and pituitary. The islet/pituitary exon 1 in rat (termed 1a in humans) is approx 200 bases longer than the hepatic exon 1 (termed 1b in humans) and explains why the glucokinase mRNA is longer in islets than in liver *(9)*. However, another consequence of the two different first exons is that cell-specific glucokinase isoforms are made. Different nucleic acid sequences in the alternate first exons lead to differences in the 15 amino-terminal residues of glucokinase. Despite the sequence variation, the kinetic properties of the enzyme are not affected when assayed by expression either in bacteria or in NIH-3T3 cells *(21)*. This may explain why different glucokinase isoforms were not suspected prior to the cloning of the gene *(3)*.

Alternate Splicing Between Exons 2 and 4

Alternate splicing events, other than those associated with the use of cell-specific first exons, have also been observed. Variant glucokinase mRNAs that contain disrupted reading frames for the enzyme have been identified in liver, pancreas, and anterior pituitary. The changes in the reading frame encoded by these variant mRNAs have a profound influence on glucokinase activity. The first such alternate splicing event was identified in a rat insulinoma glucokinase cDNA *(9)*, however, other alternate splice events have subsequently been described in cDNA clones obtained from both rats *(20,21,56)* and humans *(13)*. In most cases, the alternate splicing occurs via different splice donor and acceptor sites in exons 2, 3, and 4 of the gene. We examined the utilization and effect of one such alternate splice acceptor site that results in a 51 bp in-frame deletion of nucleic acid sequence in exon 4 of the gene. The protein produced from this alternately spliced mRNA is missing 17 amino acids and is enzymatically inactive when expressed either in eukaryotic or prokaryotic cells *(21)*. Interestingly, this mRNA variant has been detected in both islets and liver by RNA-PCR amplification but constitutes only a small fraction of the total glucokinase mRNA in either tissue *(21)*.

The minor, cryptically-spliced glucokinase mRNAs that seem to be of little consequence in the liver and islet are of greater consequence in the pituitary. Glucokinase mRNA is transcribed from the upstream promoter in the pituitary, however glucokinase activity cannot be detected, even after partial purification of the extract *(21)*. None of the glucokinase mRNAs that we and others *(20,21)* have amplified from pituitary encode an active glucokinase isoform. This has led us to explain the lack of glucokinase activity in the pituitary by the preferential use of several alternate splice sites that are otherwise used only to a minor extent in the islet and liver *(21)*.

Cassette Exon in Liver

In addition to the use of alternate splice donor and acceptor sites in differential processing of glucokinase pre-mRNA, a cassette exon is utilized in a small fraction of hepatic glucokinase mRNA. Hayzer and Iynedjian *(56)* identified a glucokinase mRNA in liver that contains 151 nucleotides inserted between hepatic exon 1 and 2. This cassette exon, designated 2A, was found to be used in conjunction with an alternate splice donor site in exon 2 that deleted 52 nucleotides. Together, the combined insertion and deletion of nucleic acid sequence encodes a unique protein of 498 amino acids *(56)* that lacks enzyme activity when expressed in bacteria *(57)*. A different situation occurs in human liver where a glucokinase mRNA containing a 124 base cassette exon (designated 1c in humans) has been identified. In this case, a different translation initiation codon is utilized producing a protein that differs at the amino terminal end *(13)*. The glucokinase isoform produced from this variant human liver mRNA is functionally active.

Regulation at Other Levels

Several examples of the regulation of glucokinase gene expression at the posttranscriptional and post-RNA processing level have been identified. These include the regulation by glucose in the β-cell, the regulation of glucokinase activity by the glucokinase regulatory protein, and the inhibitory effect of long chain acyl CoAs.

Glucose in the β-Cell

The pancreatic β-cell has several responses to glucose besides that of insulin secretion. A key response may be the induction of glucokinase activity by glucose. This response has been observed in both whole animals and in primary organ culture *(43,44,58)*. For instance, rats made profoundly hypoglycemic by implantation with insulinomas exhibited reduced islet glucokinase activity at the same time that hepatic glucokinase activity was increased *(58)*. Fasted euglycemic rats also have reduced islet glucokinase activity, but this occurs to a lesser degree than in animals bearing insulinoma tumor tissue *(59)*. Glucose also modulates glucokinase activity in cultured islets. Islets cultured for 7 d in 3 m*M* glucose have a 50% reduction in glucokinase activity compared to freshly isolated islets, whereas islets cultured in 30 m*M* glucose showed over a 200% increase after 7 d *(43)*. Interestingly, the change in glucokinase activity is not paralleled by a increase in the amount of glucokinase mRNA although glucokinase immunoreactivity does rise *(44)*. These observations led to the suggestion that glucose affects glucokinase activity at a posttranscriptional level, perhaps by stabilizing glucokinase mRNA, increasing its translation, or by stabilizing the enzyme itself *(44)*. The alteration in glucokinase enzyme activity in response to glucose almost certainly has major effects on the β-cell since these changes correlate with both glucose usage and with glucose-stimulated insulin secretion by the β-cell *(44)*.

Glucokinase Regulatory Protein

From the initial observation that fructose stimulates glucose phosphorylation in the liver *(60)*, an intriguing posttranslational mechanism for glucokinase regulation has been elucidated. In a series of reports, Van Schaftingen and colleagues identified and described a protein that increases the apparent affinity of glucokinase for glucose in response to certain metabolites of fructose, sorbitol, and D-glyceraldehyde *(61)*. The fructose metabolites, fructose-1-phosphate (F1P) and fructose-6-phosphate (F6P), have either positive or negative effects on glucose phosphorylation by glucokinase. They do not have a direct effect on glucokinase itself, but cause their effects through a 62 kDa monomeric protein termed the glucokinase regulatory protein *(62)*. The F6P-mediated inhibition of glucokinase by the glucokinase regulatory protein may occur through the formation of a heterodimeric complex between the two proteins, thus altering the K_m of the enzyme *(62)*. The regulation of glucokinase by the regulatory protein may allow for the short term physiological control of hepatic glucokinase activity by fructose. It remains to be established whether the regulatory protein plays a role in islet glucose metabolism, although a protein with the same characteristics appears to be present in islets *(63)*.

Other Posttranslational Regulators

Two additional mechanisms have been proposed for the post-translational regulation of glucokinase. One of these is the inhibition of glucokinase by long chain acyl CoAs (e.g., palmitoyl Co-A). This regulation appears to occur by an allosteric mechanism that is not related to the detergent effects of these molecules *(64,65)*. The physiologic relevance of this regulation remains unclear, however, during starvation or in diabetes, when lipids are being metabolized, these products might enable the inhibition of glycolysis by inhibiting glucokinase. The last potential means of regulating glucokinase activity may be phosphorylation by protein kinase A (PKA), which decreases the V_{max} of the enzyme while increasing its K_m for glucose *(66)*. However, these in vitro observations are difficult to reconcile with the absence of PKA phosphorylation sites in the enzyme *(22)* and the lack of evidence modulation of glucokinase activity by PKA in either the liver or β-cell.

Implications for Altered Glucose Homeostasis

It now clear that glucokinase plays an important role in glucose homeostasis and is regulated at multiple levels. Much of the regulation of glucokinase is cell-specific and reflects the different functions of the β-cell and hepatocyte. Moreover, given the variety of means by which glucokinase gene expression is modulated, additional regulatory mechanisms certainly remain to be discovered.

An understanding of glucokinase regulation provides an explanation for hyperglycemia in individuals with glucokinase gene defects, although our knowledge is still far from complete. Some individuals with glucokinase mutations have been shown to have diminished insulin secretion in response to glucose *(67)*. The decrease in insulin secretion in response to a standard glucose load argues that diminished glucokinase activity in the islet increases the glucose set point. Indeed, an increase in the concentration of glucose necessary for maximal insulin secretion was predicted ten years ago by Matschinsky to be a consequence of decreased islet glucokinase activity *(4)*. However, the extent to which decreased insulin secretion accounts for the hyperglycemia is difficult to determine directly in humans. It is clear, however, that most if not all of the mutations described adversely affect either the glucose K_m or V_{max} of the enzyme *(68)*. The mutations found in diabetic pedigrees occur throughout the gene, although there may be some bias for exons 5, 7, and 8 *(68)*. It is interesting to note, however, that none of the mutations described thus far affect either the liver or β-cell isoform of the enzyme specifically. This might indicate a necessity to interfere with glucose utilization in both cell types in order to manifest hyperglycemia. Indeed, the differential regulation of glucokinase in the liver and β-cell, and the two stage feedback loop that has previously been described *(10,58)*, should be considered when offering explanations for the hyperglycemia in people with glucokinase gene mutations (*see* Fig. 2). Given the different and independent roles of glucokinase in the liver and β-cell, mutation of the enzyme in both locations is likely to be more deleterious than a mutation in either location alone.

After years of biochemical, physiological, and molecular biological studies, the central importance of glucokinase to glucose homeostasis was, perhaps, most clearly established by the identification of linkage between mutations in the glucokinase gene on chromosome 7 and early onset NIDDM *(15,16,17,18)*. Although it was a crucially important advance, it is now clear that many other forms of both early and late onset noninsulin-dependent diabetes mellitus are not explained by mutations in the glucokinase gene. Indeed, not all of the pedigrees with early onset NIDDM have glucokinase gene mutations, further illustrating the genetic heterogeneity of the disease *(69)*. For instance, early onset NIDDM in a large pedigree has also been linked to the adenosine deaminase locus on chromosome 20 *(70)*. In pedigrees with early onset NIDDM that are not caused by glucokinase gene defects, it remains possible that either glucokinase, or the glucokinase gene, could be indirectly involved. For instance, defects in the glucokinase regulatory protein, or the transcription factors involved in glucokinase gene expression in the liver or islet, might also be able to cause diabetes. Mutations that affect glucokinase gene expression, either by affecting the transcriptional regulation of the gene, the cell-specific pattern of RNA processing, or the posttranslational regulation of the enzyme, could all potentially diminish glucokinase activity and thus induce or contribute to diabetes. Thus, a

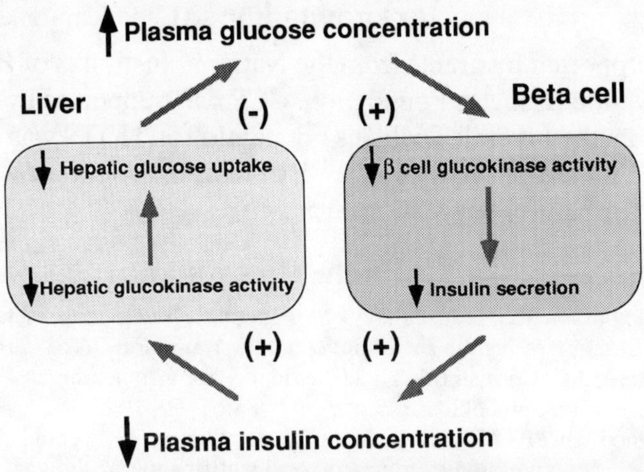

Fig. 2. Deleterious impact of glucokinase mutations on plasma glucose and insulin levels. The role that glucokinase gene mutations may play in causing hyperglycemia is illustrated by the two stage feedback loop shown. Glucokinase mutations reduce the amount of glucokinase activity in the β-cell thus elevating the glucose set point and decreasing the insulin secretory response of the islet to elevated concentrations of glucose. This results in low plasma insulin levels and the diminished uptake of glucose by the liver. In addition, the ability of the liver to utilize glucose is exacerbated by the reduced glucokinase activity in hepatocytes due to glucokinase gene mutations. Hyperglycemia in early onset NIDDM resulting from glucokinase mutations may, therefore, be owing both to diminished insulin secretion by the β-cell and to diminished uptake of glucose by the liver although the relative importance of each remains to be determined.

thorough understanding of the regulation of glucokinase gene expression remains relevant to understanding the pathogenesis of NIDDM.

Last, just as the various mechanisms by which glucokinase is regulated must be considered as potential sites of dysregulation, some of these sites might also be considered potential targets for therapeutic intervention. If a decrease in the amount of glucokinase increases the glucose set point of the β-cell, then increasing the amount of glucokinase should lower the glucose set point. If this could be accomplished by manipulating the amount of glucokinase in the β-cell, a new means to treat diabetes might become available.

Acknowledgment

Supported by grants from the National Institutes of Health and the Juvenile Diabetes Foundation. CCP was supported by a Fellowship from the Juvenile Diabetes Foundation and KDN was supported by the Vanderbilt Medical Scientist Training Program. We thank T. Jetton for helpful suggestions.

References

1. Meglasson MD, Matschinsky FM: Pancreatic islet glucose metabolism and regulation of insulin secretion. *Diabetes Metab Rev* 2:163–214, 1986.
2. Storer AC, Cornish BA: Kinetic evidence for a "mnemonical" mechanism for rat liver glucokinase. *Biochem J* 165:61–69, 1977.
3. Iynedjian PB, Möbius G, Seitz HJ, Wollheim CB, Renold AE: Tissue-specific expression of glucokinase: identification of the gene product in liver and pancreatic islets. *Proc Natl Acad Sci USA* 83:1998–2001, 1986.
4. Meglasson MD, Matschinsky FM: New perspectives on pancreatic islet glucokinase. *Am J Physiol* 13:E1–E13, 1984.
5. Matschinsky FM: Glucokinase as glucose sensor and metabolic signal generator in pancreatic beta-cells and hepatocytes. *Diabetes* 39:647–652, 1990.
6. Granner D, Pilkis S: The genes of hepatic glucose metabolism. *J Biol Chem* 265:10,173–10,176, 1990.
7. Iynedjian PB, Ucla C, Mach B: Molecular cloning of glucokinase cDNA. Developmental and dietary regulation of glucokinase mRNA in rat liver. *J Biol Chem* 262:6032–6038, 1987.
8. Andreone TL, Printz RL, Pilkis SJ, Magnuson MA, Granner DK: The amino acid sequence of rat liver glucokinase deduced from cloned cDNA. *J Biol Chem* 264:363–369, 1989.
9. Magnuson MA, Shelton KD: An alternate promoter in the glucokinase gene is active in the pancreatic beta cell. *J Biol Chem* 264:15,936–15,942, 1989.
10. Magnuson MA, Andreone TL, Printz RL, Koch S, Granner DK: Rat glucokinase gene: structure and regulation by insulin. *Proc Natl Acad Sci USA* 86:4838–4842, 1989.
11. Koranyi LI, Tanizawa Y, Welling CM, Rabin DU, Permutt MA: Human islet glucokinase gene. Isolation and sequence analysis of full-length cDNA. *Diabetes* 41:807–811, 1992.
12. Tanizawa Y, Matsutani A, Chiu KC, Permutt MA: Human glucokinase gene: isolation, structural characterization, and identification of a microsatellite repeat polymorphism. *Mol Endocrinol* 6:1070–1081, 1992.
13. Tanizawa Y, Koranyi LI, Welling CM, Permutt MA: Human liver glucokinase gene: cloning and sequence determination of two alternatively spliced cDNAs. *Proc Natl Acad Sci USA* 88:7294–7297, 1991.
14. Nishi S, Stoffel M, Xiang K, Shows TB, Bell GI, Takeda J: Human pancreatic beta-cell glucokinase: cDNA sequence and localization of the polymorphic gene to chromosome 7, band p 13. *Diabetologia* 35:743–747, 1992.

15. Froguel P, Vaxillaire M, Sun F, Velho G, Zouali H, Butel MO, et al.: Close linkage of glucokinase locus on chromosome 7p to early-onset noninsulin-dependent diabetes mellitus. *Nature* 356:162–164, 1992.
16. Vionnet N, Stoffel M, Takeda J, Yasuda K, Bell GI, Zouali H, et al.: Nonsense mutation in the glucokinase gene causes early-onset noninsulin-dependent diabetes mellitus. *Nature* 356:721,722, 1992.
17. Stoffel M, Froguel P, Takeda J, Zouali H, Vionnet N, Nishi S, et al.: Human glucokinase gene: isolation, characterization, and identification of two missense mutations linked to early-onset noninsulin-dependent (type 2) diabetes mellitus. *Proc Natl Acad Sci USA* 89:7698–7702, 1992.
18. Hattersley AT, Turner RC, Permutt MA, Patel P, Tanizawa Y, Chiu KC, et al.: Linkage of type 2 diabetes to the glucokinase gene. *Lancet* 339:1307–1310, 1992.
19. Magnuson MA: Glucokinase gene structure. Functional implications of molecular genetic studies. *Diabetes* 39:523–527, 1990.
20. Hughes SD, Quaade C, Milburn JL, Cassidy L, Newgard CB: Expression of normal and novel glucokinase mRNAs in anterior pituitary and islet cells. *J Biol Chem* 266:4521–4530, 1991.
21. Liang Y, Jetton TL, Zimmerman EC, Najafi H, Matschinsky FM, Magnuson MA: Effects of alternate RNA splicing on glucokinase isoform activities in the pancreatic islet, liver, and pituitary. *J Biol Chem* 266:6999–7007, 1991.
22. Iynedjian PB: Mammalian glucokinase and its gene. *Biochem J* 293:1–13, 1993.
23. Eilers F, Bartels H, Jungermann K: Zonal expression of the glucokinase gene in rat liver. Dynamics during the daily feeding rhythm and starvation-refeeding cycle demonstrated by *in situ* hybridization. *Histochemistry* 99:133–140, 1993.
24. Sharma C, Manjeshwar R, Weinhouse S: Effects of diet and insulin on glucose-adenosine triphosphate phosphotransferases of rat liver. *J Biol Chem* 238:3840–3845, 1963.
25. Weinhouse S: Regulation of glucokinase in liver. *Curr Top Cell Regul* 11:1–50, 1976.
26. Iynedjian PB, Gjinovci A, Renold AE: Stimulation by insulin of glucokinase gene transcription in liver of diabetic rats. *J Biol Chem* 263:740–744, 1988.
27. Iynedjian PB, Jotterand D, Nouspikel T, Asfari M, Pilot PR: Transcriptional induction of glucokinase gene by insulin in cultured liver cells and its repression by the glucagon-cAMP system. *J Biol Chem* 264:21,824–21,829, 1989.
28. Sibrowski W, Seitz HJ: Rapid action of insulin and cyclic AMP in the regulation of functional messenger RNA coding for glucokinase in rat liver. *J Biol Chem* 259:343–346, 1984.
29. Spence JT, Pitot HC: Hormonal regulation of glucokinase in primary cultures of adult rat hepatocytes. *J Biol Chem* 254:12,331–12,336, 1979.
30. Nouspikel T, Iynedjian PB: Insulin signalling and regulation of glucokinase gene expression in cultured heptocytes. *Eur J Biochem* 210:365–373, 1992.

31. Matsuda T, Noguchi T, Yamada K, Takenaka M, Tanaka T: Regulation of the gene expression of glucokinase and L-type pyruvate kinase in primary cultures of rat heptocytes by hormones and carbohydrates. *J Biochem (Tokyo)* 108:778–784, 1990.
32. Noguchi T, Takenaka M, Yamada K, Matsuda T, Hashimoto M, Tanaka T: Characterization of the 5' flanking region of rat glucokinase gene. *Biochem Biophys Res Commun* 164:1247–1252, 1989.
33. Narkewicz MR, Iynedjian PB, Ferre P, Girard J: Insulin and tri-iodothyronine induce glucokinase mRNA in primary cultures of neonatal rat hepatocytes. *Biochem J* 271:585–589, 1990.
34. Höppner W, Seitz HJ: Role of thyroid hormones in the regulation of hepatic glucokinase and phosphoenolpyruvate-carboxykinase gene expression during the starvation–refeeding transition. *Biochem Soc Trans* 18:845–847, 1990.
35. Chauhan J, Dakshinamurti K: Transcriptional regulation of the glucokinase gene by biotin in starved rats. *J Biol Chem* 266:10,035–10,038, 1991.
36. Li Hsieh YT, Mistry SP: Effect of biotin on the regulation of glucokinase in the intact rat. *Nutr Res* 12:787–799, 1992.
37. Dakshinamurti K, Cheah TC: Liver glucokinase of the biotin deficient rat. *Can J Biochem* 46:75–80, 1968.
38. Walker DG, Eaton SW: Regulation of development of hepatic glucokinase in the neonatal rat by the diet. *Biochem J* 105:771–777, 1967.
39. Haney PM, Estrin CR, Caliendo A, Patel MS: Precocious induction of hepatic glucokinase and malic enzyme in artificially reared rat pups fed a high-carbohydrate diet. *Arch Biochem Biophys* 244:787–794, 1986.
40. Girard J, Decaux JF, Bossard P: Regulation of the initial expression of hepatic phosphoenolpyruvate carboxykinase and glucokinase genes during development. *Diabete Metab* 18:74–80, 1992.
41. Walker DG, Holland G: The development of hepatic glucokinase in the neonatal rat. *Biochem J* 97:845–854, 1965.
42. Iynedjian PB, Pilot PR, Nouspikel T, Milburn JL, Quaade C, Hughes S, et al.: Differential expression and regulation of the glucokinase gene in liver and islets of Langerhans. *Proc Natl Acad Sci USA* 86:7838–7842, 1989.
43. Liang Y, Najafi H, Matschinsky FM: Glucose regulates glucokinase activity in cultured islets from rat pancreas. *J Biol Chem* 265:16,863–16,866, 1990.
44. Liang Y, Najafi H, Smith RM, Zimmerman EC, Magnuson MA, Tal M, et al.: Concordant glucose induction of glucokinase, glucose usage, and glucose–stimulated insulin release in pancreatic islets maintained in organ culture. *Diabetes* 41:792–806, 1992.
45. Pipeleers DG: Heterogeneity in pancreatic beta-cell population. *Diabetes* 41:777–781, 1992.
46. Schuit FC, In't Veld PA, Pipeleers DG: Glucose stimulates proinsulin biosynthesis by a dose-dependent recruitment of pancreatic beta cell. *Proc Natl Acad Sci USA* 85:3865–3869, 1988.
47. Dean PM, Matthews EK: Glucose-induced electrical activity in pancreatic islet cells. *J Physiol* 210:255–264, 1970.

48. Orci L: The insulin cell: its cellular environment and how it processes proinsulin. *Diabetes Metab Rev* 2:71–106, 1986.
49. Heimberg H, De Vos A, Van Schaftingen E, Pipeleers D, Schuit F: Heterogeneity in glucose sensitivity among pancreatic B-cells is correlated to differences in glucose phosphorylation rather than glucose transport. *EMBO J* 12:2873–2879, 1993.
50. Jetton TL, Magnuson MA: Heterogeneous expression of glucokinase among pancreatic beta cells. *Proc Natl Acad Sci USA* 89:2619–2623, 1992.
51. Shelton KD, Franklin A, Khoor A, Beechem J, Magnuson MA: Multiple elements in the upstream glucokinase promoter are necessary for transcription in insulinoma cells. *Mol Cell Biol* 12:4578–4589, 1992.
52. Boam DSW, Docherty K: A tissue-specific nuclear factor binds to multiple sites in the human insulin-gene enhancer. *Biochem J* 264:233–239, 1989.
53. Boam DSW, Clark AR, Docherty K: Positive and negative regulation of the human insulin gene by multiple trans-acting factors. *J Biol Chem* 265:8285–8296, 1990.
54. Moates J, Shelton K, Magnuson M: The palindromic repeat elements in the upstream glucokinase promoter are determinants of neuroendocrine cell-specific transcription. *75th Annual Meeting of the Endocrine Society*, Las Vegas, NV, Abstract # 1298, 1993.
55. Magnuson MA, Jetton TL: Evolutionary conservation of elements in the upstream glucokinase promoter. *Biochem Soc Trans* 21:160–163, 1993.
56. Hayzer DJ, Iynedjian PB: Alternative splicing of glucokinase mRNA in rat liver. *Biochem J* 270:261–263, 1990.
57. Quaade C, Hughes SD, Coates WS, Sestak AL, Iynedjian PB, Newgard CB: Analysis of the protein products encoded by variant glucokinase transcripts via expression in bacteria. *FEBS Lett* 280:47–52, 1991.
58. Bedoya FJ, Matschinsky FM, Shimizu T, O'Neil JJ, Appel MC: Differential regulation of glucokinase activity in pancreatic islets and liver of the rat. *J Biol Chem* 261:10,760–10,764, 1986.
59. Tiedge M, Lenzen S: Regulation of glucokinase and GLUT–2 glucose-transporter gene expression in pancreatic B-cells. *Biochem J* 279:899–901, 1991.
60. Clark DG, Filsell OH, Topping DL: Effects of fructose concentration on carbohydrate metabolism, heat production and substrate cycling in isolated rat hepatocytes. *Biochem J* 184:501–507, 1979.
61. Van Schaftingen E, Vandercammen A, Detheux M, Davies DR: The regulatory protein of liver glucokinase. *Adv Enzyme Regul* 32:133–148, 1992.
62. Vandercammen A, Van Schaftingen E: The mechanism by which rat liver glucokinase is inhibited by the regulatory protein. *Eur J Biochem* 191:483–489, 1990.
63. Malaisse WJ, Malaisse LF, Davies DR, Vandercammen A, Van Schaftingen E: Regulation of glucokinase by a fructose-1-phosphate-sensitive protein in pancreatic islets. *Eur J Biochem* 190:539–545, 1990.
64. Tippett PS, Neet KE: An allosteric model for the inhibition of glucokinase by long chain acyl coenzyme A. *J Biol Chem* 257:12,846–12,852, 1982.

65. Tippett PS, Neet KE: Specific inhibition of glucokinase by long chain acyl coenzymes A below the critical micelle concentration. *J Biol Chem* 257:12,839–12,845, 1982.
66. Ekman P, Nilsson E: Phosphorylation of glucokinase from rat liver *in vitro* by protein kinase A with a concomitant decrease of its activity. *Arch Biochem Biophys* 261:275–282, 1988.
67. Velho G, Froguel P, Clement K, Pueyo ME, Rakotoambinina B, Zouali H, et al.: Primary pancreatic beta-cell secretory defect caused by mutations in glucokinase gene in kindreds of maturity onset diabetes of the young. *Lancet* 340:444–448, 1992.
68. Gidh–Jain M, Takeda J, Xu LZ, Lange AJ, Vionnet N, Stoffel M, et al.: Glucokinase mutations associated with noninsulin-dependent (type 2) diabetes mellitus have decreased enzymatic activity: implications for structure/function relationships. *Proc Natl Acad Sci USA* 90:1932–1936, 1993.
69. Froguel P, Zouali H, Vionnet N, Velho G, Vaxillaire M, Sun F, et al.: Familial hyperglycemia due to mutations in glucokinase. Definition of a subtype of diabetes mellitus. *N Engl J Med* 328:697–702, 1993.
70. Bell GI, Xiang KS, Newman MV, Wu SH, Wright LG, Fajans SS, et al.: Gene for noninsulin-dependent diabetes mellitus (maturity-onset diabetes of the young subtype) is linked to DNA polymorphism on human chromosome 20q. *Proc Natl Acad Sci USA* 88:1484–1488, 1991.

Chapter 8

Fundamentals of Fuel Sensing and Intermediary Metabolism in Pancreatic A- and B-Cells

Guizhu Li, Prabakaran Kesavan, Habiba Najafi, Lijun Wang, Peter Ronner, Donna Berner, Yin Liang, and Franz M. Matschinsky

Introduction

The endocrine cells of the pancreatic islet organ respond very effectively to the blood's small nutrient molecules: Glucose and the mixture of 20 standard amino acids are potent stimulants at physiological concentrations, and fatty acids and ketone bodies also appear to be effective. The high efficacy of these molecules contrasts with the inertness of major metabolites, as for instance pyruvate, lactate, glycerol, uric acid, urea, and ammonia, which have no influence on these cells at physiological concentrations. The examination of this issue is naturally greatly influenced by the prevailing views about the biochemical nature of fuel sensing, in particular the essential role that intermediary metabolism plays in this process *(1)* as contrasting to concepts of fuel sensing mechanisms that might be based on direct fuel interactions with membrane receptors and ion channels *(2)*, cir-

From: *Molecular Biology of Diabetes, Part I*
Edited by: B. Draznin and D. LeRoith

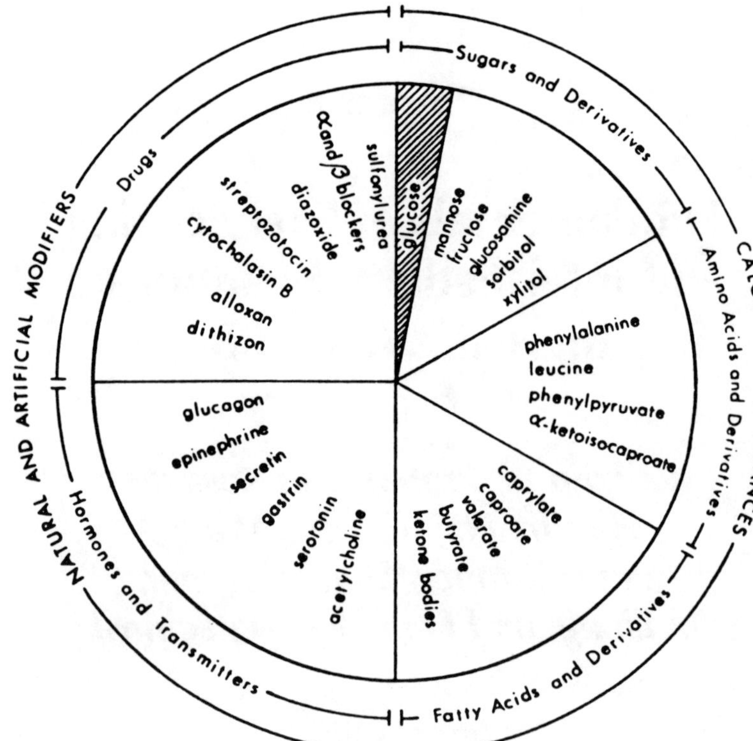

Fig. 1. The chemosensitivity of pancreatic islet B-cells (from Matschinsky et al. *[2]*).

cumventing catabolism of the agonists. It is currently widely accepted that the effect of most nutrient agonists on pancreatic endocrine cells is a result of their catabolism *(3)*. It is the purpose of this brief review to provide a perspective on this topic.

Overview of the Broad Fuel Sensing Capabilities of Pancreatic Islet Cells

In this overview, fuel sensing is equated with stimulation or inhibition by various nutrient agonists of hormone secretion from islet A- or B- cells. (Note that nutrient modification of D- and PP- cell and of islet neuronal tissue function is not discussed here.) A certain perspective of the topic can be gained by glancing at Fig. 1, which provides an impression of the wide spectrum of chemosensitivity of pancreatic B-cells, for which cell type the knowledge is most comprehensive. Pancreatic B-cells respond to two major classes of agonists: a great variety of small nutrient molecules and a similarly great range of natural and artificial noncalorigenic modifier substances. Here, we are primarily concerned with the former, but realize that the latter might influence islet cell function by modifying intermediary metabolism in addition to other mechanisms of action.

D-glucose is the only nutrient molecule independently effective in causing insulin release at physiological concentrations *(3)*. This somewhat categorical statement is based on results with the isolated perfused rat pancreas considered to be the most physiological preparation currently in use. The glucose threshold for the B-cells, of animal and humans in the fed state, is about 5 m*M* and levels for half-maximal and maximal effects are about 10 and 25 m*M*, respectively. The α-anomer is more potent than the β-anomer. Many other sugars, sugar derivatives, and sugar alcohols are stimulators or inhibitors at pharmacological concentrations and are not infrequently stimulators in a glucose-dependent manner. Fructose, for example requires the presence of permissive levels of glucose to be effective. There is considerable animal species specificity as to the potency of these sugars and sugar derivatives. For example, humans, and dogs are responding to the polyols sorbitol and xylisol but rats do not *(2)*. Amino acids and their derivatives are potent B-cell secretagogues. For example, the mixture of 20 standard amino acids at physiological concentrations is effective, but only in the presence of glucose *(4)* (Table 1). It cannot be overemphasized that at physiological concentrations no single standard amino acid is capable of causing insulin release even in the presence of glucose. However, given the presence of at least 2.5 m*M* glucose, the B-cells are very sensitive to the physiological mixture of 20 amino acids, with a threshold of 0.5–1.0 m*M*, and levels for half-maximal and maximal effectiveness at about 5 and 15 m*M*, respectively. L-leucine is unique in its capability of causing insulin release from B-cells at extreme pharmacological levels provided certain other requirements are met *(2)*. Several amino acid metabolites (α-ketoisocaproate, α-ketocaproate, phenylpyruvate) are stimulators of B-cells even in the absence of glucose, but only at pharmacological concentrations *(2,5,6)*. Fatty acids are usually inert at physiological concentrations, when glucose is absent, but elicit

Table 1
The Permissive Action of Glucose and Release Patterns
of Insulin Release Owing to Various Natural and Model Nutrient Molecules
as Studied with the Isolated Perfused Rat Pancreas

Agent	Effect in the absence of glucose	Effect in the presence of glucose	Releasing profile in the presence of glucose
Sugars			
fructose	Ø	+	C
Amino acids			
alanine	Ø	+	A
a-aminobutyrate	Ø	+	A
norvaline	Ø	+	A
valine	Ø	Ø	—
norleucine	Ø	+	A
leucine	+	+	I
isoleucine	Ø	+	B
BCH	Ø	+	I
phenylalanine	Ø	+	I
arginine	Ø	+	B or D
20 standard amino acids	Ø	+	B and C
Fatty acids			
propionate	Ø	Ø	—
butyrate	Ø	+	H
valerate	Ø	+	H
isovalerate	Ø	+	J
caproate	(+)	+	H
β,β-dimethylacrylate	Ø	+	H
phenylacetate	Ø	+	H
Ketone bodies			
acetoacetate	Ø	+	C
β-hydroxybutyrate	Ø	+	C
α-Ketomonocarboxylic acids			
pyruvate	Ø	(+)	—
α-O-butyrate	Ø	+	A–B
α-O-valerate	Ø	+	C
α-O-isovalerate	Ø	+	C
α-O-caproate	+	+	C
α-O-isocaproate	+	+	C
α-O-β-methylvalerate	Ø	+	C
α-O-octanoate	+	+	G
α-O-nonanoate	+	+	H
phenylpyruvate	+	+	C

(continued)

Table 1 (*continued*)

α-Hydroxymonocarboxylic acids			
α-OH-isovalerate	Ø	+	A
α-OH-caproate	Ø	(+)	—
α-OH-isocaproate	Ø	(+)	—
α-OH-β-methylvalerate	Ø	Ø	—
phenyllactate	Ø	(+)	—

The concentration of the stimulus was usually 5 m*M* and glucose was 5 m*M*. The explanation for the capital letters representing different releasing profiles are found in Fig. 3 (from Matschinsky et al. *[2]*).

insulin release in the presence of 5 m*M* glucose and when present at pharmacological levels *(2,5,6)*. The effectiveness of ketone bodies acetoacetate or β-hydroxybutyrate depends similarly on the permissive action of glucose. It is worth noting that many important metabolites are inert at physiological levels (e.g., lactate, pyruvate, glycerol, succinate, malate, urea, uric acid, ammonia).

The chemosensitivity of A-cells differs strikingly from that of B-cells. D-glucose is an inhibitor of stimulated glucagon release *(4)*. Even as little as 1 m*M* glucose reduces L-amino acid induced glucagon release. (There is debate whether this effect is direct or indirect *[7,8)]*.) Amino acids—in particular physiological levels of the natural mixture of the 20 amino acids—are powerful stimulators of glucagon release *(4)*. Ketone bodies appear to be inert and information on the effect of fatty acids is limited. Common metabolites (e.g., lactate, pyruvate, succinate, malate, glycerol, ammonia, urea, uric acid) seem to be inert at physiological levels.

A highly informative way of characterizing the chemosensitivity of pancreatic islet A- and B-cells is to study isolated perifused islets that had been maintained in organ culture under well defined conditions and expose them to a linear ramp of increasing fuel concentrations such that the threshold for release, the dose dependency characteristics, and the maximal responsiveness can be assessed in a single experiment (Fig. 2). This is strikingly illustrated with results that were obtained with a standard amino acid mixture in the absence or presence of 4 m*M* glucose. Prior to the test islets were cultured for 7 d in 1, 10, or 30 m*M* glucose. The experiment demonstrates the marked difference in responsiveness of A- and B-cells to glucose and

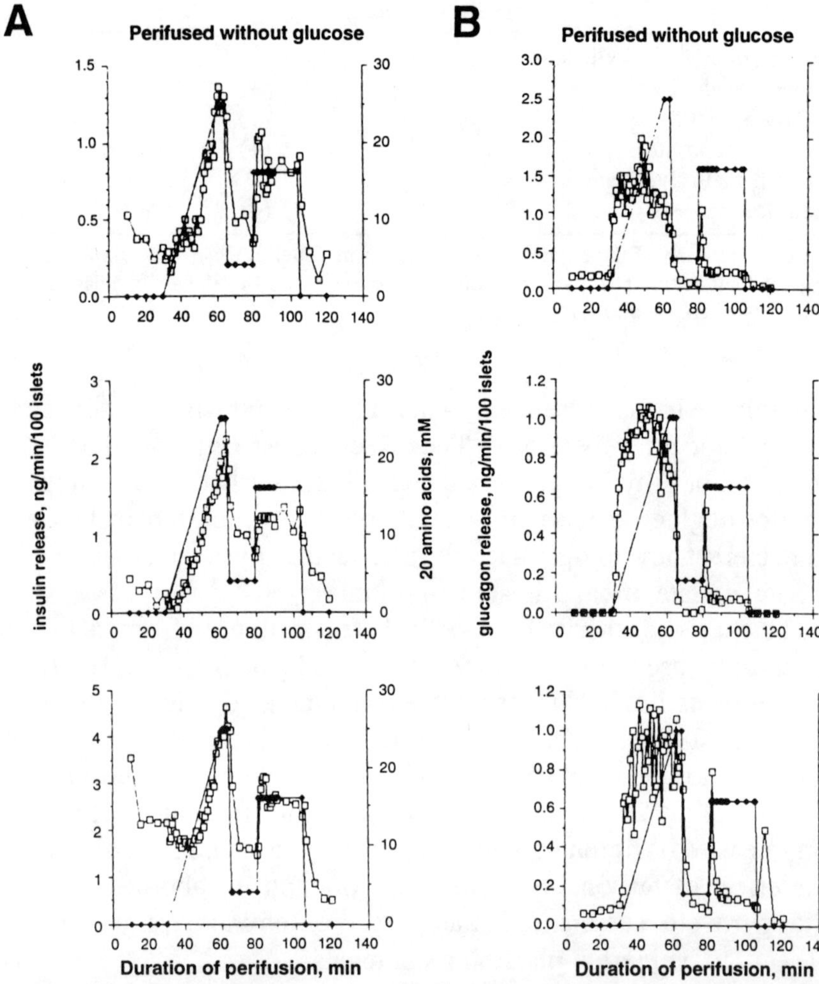

Fig. 2. Fuel sensitivity of pancreatic A- and B-cells. Rat islets were cultured for 7 d in 1, 10, or 30 m*M* glucose (presented from top to bottom in each panel) and were then stimulated with amino acids in the absence (**A,B**) or presence (**C,D**) of 4 m*M* glucose. From 30–60 min a physiological mixture of the 20 standard amino acids was infused in a ramp-like fashion such that the levels rose from 0–25 m*M* in 30 min followed by stepwise reduction of the stimulus to 4 m*M* and restimulation with a 25 min square wave of 16 m*M*. Perifusate samples were obtained at 1 min intervals after switches and less frequently during steady states and the two hormones insulin and glucagon were determined. Results of single perfusion experiments are shown.

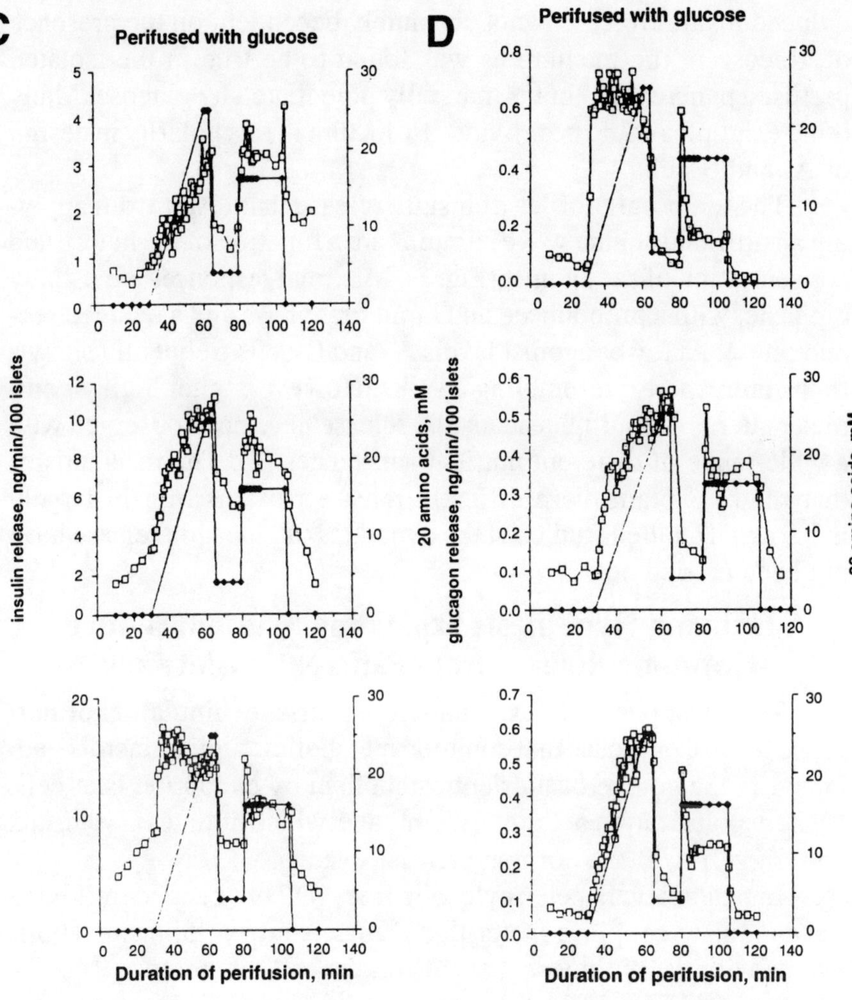

Fig. 2 *(continued).*

amino acids. A-cells cultured in low glucose are exquisitely sensitive to amino acids and are inhibited even by low glucose in the perfusate, whereas B-cells cultured under the same conditions exhibit a greatly diminished responsiveness to these fuels. Culturing islets in 30 m*M* glucose greatly alters this situation such that the B-cells are now extremely sensitive to both fuels and that the responsiveness of A-cells is reduced. It is noteworthy that in cultured islets amino acid induced insulin release is not absolutely dependent on the presence of glucose in the medium as was found to be true in the isolated perfused pancreas *(4)* but is markedly potentiated by glucose. Many other examples could be provided to document this polarity in design of A- and B-cells.

The temporal profiles of insulin release that result from applying an artificial square wave stimulus are a function of the nature and concentration of the agonist (Fig. 3). Maximal responses are usually biphasic, with a pronounced and rapid first phase and a delayed second phase. At lower agonist levels A- and B-cells frequently show a transient response resembling a spike. However, other highly complex patterns of multiphasic insulin release have been observed with a wide range of different nutrient substances *(2)*. The mechanisms that might explain these different release patterns remain largely unknown. Detailed studies of the dynamics of glucagon release have not been carried out.

A Unifying Hypothesis Explaining Nutrient Induced Hormone Release from Pancreatic Islet Cells

The most plausible explanation of nutrient stimulation of hormone release proposes that common metabolic coupling factors generated in the course of nutrient catabolism by endocrine islet cells cause depolarization of the cell membrane, which initiates Ca^{2+} influx and triggering of the hormone release event.

In pancreatic B-cells, cytosolic free ADP has been identified as the candidate coupling factor that connects intracellular metabolic events with the biophysical events on the cell membrane *(9)*. ADP activates adenine nucleotide sensitive K^+ channels that are physiologically inhibited by ATP. This leads to depolarization of the cell. Such nucleotide sensitive K^+ channels have been found in A-cells as well and may play a similar role there (*see below* and *[10]*). Much effort is being devoted to assess whether nutrients that are effective as secretagogs do indeed cause the postulated decrease of free ADP levels to explain their effects. Only very recently has it been possible to determine the islet tissue levels of free ADP reliably *(11)*. By measuring the levels of ATP, P-creatine, and creatine, and using the equilibrium constant of the creatine kinase reaction it was possible to calculate the levels of free cytosolic ADP. It remains to be seen

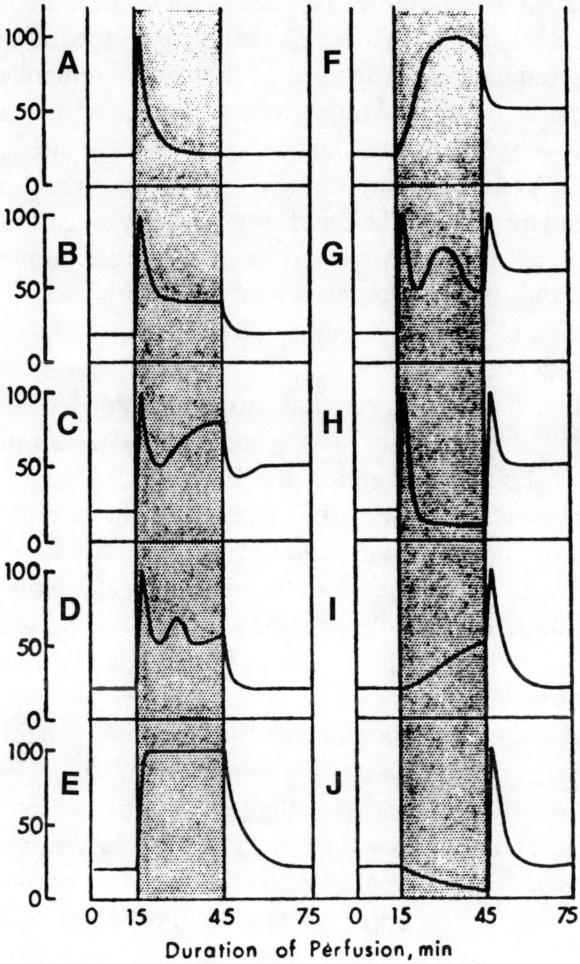

Fig. 3. Patterns of multiphasic insulin release from the isolated perfused pancreas. Typical secretion profiles are presented. The patterns are schematic drawings. Relative rates are plotted. The figure also contains the keys for the last column of Table 1 (from Matschinsky et al. *[2]*).

whether this explanation applies to the stimulation of B-cells by amino acids, fatty acids, and ketone bodies (all in the presence of permissive levels of glucose) and whether it applies to A-cells stimulated by amino acids, as predicted here. Other metabolic coupling factors, in addition to free ADP, have been proposed for B-cells.

Most provocative is the concept of lipid related coupling factors, e.g., Malonyl-CoA and Acyl-CoA *(12–15)*. The following sequence of events is considered for the case of their involvement in glucose-induced insulin release. High glucose enhances the synthesis of malonyl-CoA by increasing the tissue levels of citrate that activates of acetyl-CoA carboxylase; Malonyl-CoA then curbs the mitochondrial catabolism of acyl-CoA and consequently causes the cytosolic acyl-CoA levels to rise; Acyl-CoA activates protein kinase C either directly or indirectly through enhanced diacylglycerol provision; Protein kinase C enhances insulin release by mechanisms to be elucidated. Evidence in favor of the physiological relevance of this proposed sequence of events remains circumstantial.

It is reemphasized that these concepts of metabolic coupling appear to suffice in explaining the fuel stimulation of B-cells. It remains to be seen whether similar mechanisms are operative in the A-cells. In support of this view, it was found that A-cells are endowed with adenine nucleotide sensitive K-channels *(10)*. However such a view is difficult to reconcile with the paradoxical opposite effects of the two major nutrient stimuli of amino acids and of glucose because amino acids serve as agonists and glucose as antagonists of A-cells. One plausible explanation might be that only amino acids are effective fuels for A-cells, whereas glucose metabolism of A-cells might be very slow because of intrinsically low rates of transport and phosphorylation. The inhibitory action of glucose on A-cells might occur indirectly through release of insulin or gamma-amino-butyrate from B-cells followed by receptor mediated inhibition of A-cells.

Characteristic Design Features of Glucose Metabolism of Islet Cells

The preceding discussion automatically draws attention to the crucial involvement of islet cell intermediary metabolism in nutrient sensing and hormone release. An outline of the characteristic design features of intermediary metabolism in these cells promises to provide the biochemical basis for much of the physiological and biophysical observation that have been discussed so far. The glycolytic and oxidative pathways of glucose catabolism constitute the centerpiece of B-cell intermediary metabolism, consistent with the observation that under optimal physiological experimental conditions glucose appears to be the only low molecular physiological nutrient molecule that stimulates insulin release *per se*. All other physiologically relevant nutrients require the presence of glucose to be effective in this regard. (This distinction between glucose and nonglucose nutrient stimuli is somewhat blurred in studies with cultured islet, as discussed earlier.) The pathways of glucose catabolism of islet tissue have been worked out *(1–3)*. Glucose enters the B-cell primarily via the glucose transporter GLUT-2. The capacity of this transporter is at least 100-fold in excess of actual glycolysis. Glucose phosphorylation by hexokinase I might be quantitatively significant when glucose levels are lower than 1 m*M* but hexokinase IV or glucokinase plays an increasingly important role quantitatively as glucose levels rise to postprandial levels of 7–8 m*M*. Glucokinase is thus the predominant enzyme, particularly postprandially. However, the relative contribution of these two enzymes to glucose phosphorylation at different glucose levels has not been worked out in detail. Islets have glucose-6-phosphatase that may lead to glucose cycling, albeit of small magnitude *(16,17)*. The glycogen apparatus is, however, of very limited quantitative importance in the physiological setting *(18)*. Isomerization of glucose-6-P to fructose-6-P and phosphorylation of the latter to fructose-1,6-P_2 is achieved with enzyme capacities exceeding by far the capacities of glucose phosphorylation *(3)*. The pentose-P shunt operates at a rate of less than 10% of the glycolytic rate. The regulation of the metabolic processes that control the level of the nodal metabolite glucose-6-P is naturally complex considering the involvement of multiple enzymes and pathways and has not been fully established. However, the activities of the six enzymes directly involved in glucose-6-P metabolism appear to be tuned and throttled precisely to guarantee that metabolic flux through the main pathway of glycolysis is determined primarily by the substrate affinity, sigmoidicity, and capacity of glucokinase and that it is proportional to the level of blood glucose.

There are two other outstanding design features of B-cell glucose metabolism: the capacity to oxidize NADH by hydrogen shuttles that transfer reducing equivalents from the cytosol to the mitochondria and several ways to metabolize pyruvate *(19)*. The α-glycerol-P shuttle appears to be uniquely important in B-cells. The capacity of this shuttle is substantial and its unidirectionality contributes to its efficacy. Pyruvate metabolism is accomplished by at least four enzymes; i.e., lactic dehydrogenase, pyruvate dehydrogenase, malic enzyme, and pyruvate carboxylase. The combination of effective oxidation of cytosolic NADH and of pyruvate metabolism assures that glucose remains the principal determinant of flux through glycolysis and mitochondrial oxidative processes. Glucose increases oxygen consumption suggesting that oxidative processes (i.e., the citric acid cycle and electron transport) are primarily regulated by substrate availability through mass action. However, as glucose levels rise pyruvate oxidation becomes more predominant owing to regulatory mechanisms that are poorly understood *(20)*. It is extrapolated that ATP production increases *pari passu* with enhanced respiration and that ADP levels fall. Glucose metabolism of the B-cell thus appears to be under little feedback control and seems to be governed by "push" rather than by "pull" mechanisms, which contrasts with the regulation of glucose metabolism in most tissues. This is teleologically plausible. ATP serves as an inhibitor and ADP as an activator of the adenine nucleotide sensitive K^+ channels of B-cells *(9)*. Free ADP qualifies as the preeminent metabolic coupling factor of pancreatic B-cells since ATP levels are virtually constant and free ADP levels fluctuate as a function of substrate availability under physiological circumstances. It needs to be appreciated that it is the level of free ADP that is important here. Levels of free ADP have been estimated and were found to be about 50 μM and appeared to fall when islets were exposed to physiological glucose changes *(11)*.

Because of the technical obstacles of scarcity, microscopic size and cellular heterogeneity of islets of Langerhans it is not surprising that our knowledge of intermediary metabolism of pancreatic A-cells is extremely fragmentary. It has been known for some time that glucose transport into A-cells is fundamentally different from that into B-cells and that their energy metabolism is less dependent on glucose availability *(22,23)*. Not surprisingly, normal A-cells seem to lack the B-cell glucose sensor glucokinase *(24)*.

This sketch of pancreatic islet glucose metabolism is probably correct in its general terms. However, many important qualitative and quantitative details need to be worked out to arrive at a totally reliable and comprehensive picture. The greatest difficulty arises from the cellular heterogeneity of the islet of Langerhans. Practically all studies with islet tissue are compromised by the fact that about 25% of the islet tissue is of other than B-cell origin. It remains a formidable task to correct for this cellular heterogeneity in enzyme and metabolite determinations of intact islets. Quantitative histochemical methods have provided some information on islet tissue almost exclusively composed of A-cells or B-cells, which supports many results obtained with intact composite islets *(11,21–23)*. Additional approaches need to be found to overcome this difficulty. The application of cell sorting methods followed by the generation of pure B-cell and A-cell islets that should be suitable for biochemical and physiological studies promises to offer one solution to this intractable problem that has plagued islet cell research for decades.

Other Design Features of Intermediary Metabolism of Pancreatic Islet Cells

The knowledge about the metabolic pathways that are involved in the catabolism of B-cell nutrient secretagogs other than glucose remains very limited. From the fact that amino acids, fatty acids, and the ketone bodies acetoacetate and β-hydroxybutyrate stimulate insulin release (provided permissive levels 2.5–4.0 m*M* of glucose are present) it can be surmised that the membrane transporters and enzymes allowing metabolism of these fuels are present in B-cells *(5,6,25–27)* (Fig. 4). The metabolism of certain individual amino acids has been studied: e.g., branched chain amino acids *(25)*. Unphysiologically high levels were usually employed in these investigations. These studies have discovered that certain α-keto monocarboxylic acids, metabolites of these amino acids, are powerful glucose independent secretagogues and that all of them potentiate glucose *(5,6,25)*. Since many of these α-keto monocarboxylic are suitable substrates for metabolism, the results fit into the general concept that secretagogues have to be degraded to be effective *(25)*. It is, however, not clear whether α-keto-octanoate and α-keto-nonanoate *(2,5,6)*, both very potent in the presence of glucose, are indeed fuels or whether they may work through other mechanisms. Fatty acids and their metabolites acetoacetate and β-hydroxybutyrate appear to be suitable substrates for B-cell metabolism *(26,27)*. However, the enzymes involved in the catabolism of these nutrients have not been investigated in detail. The question of regulation of metabo-

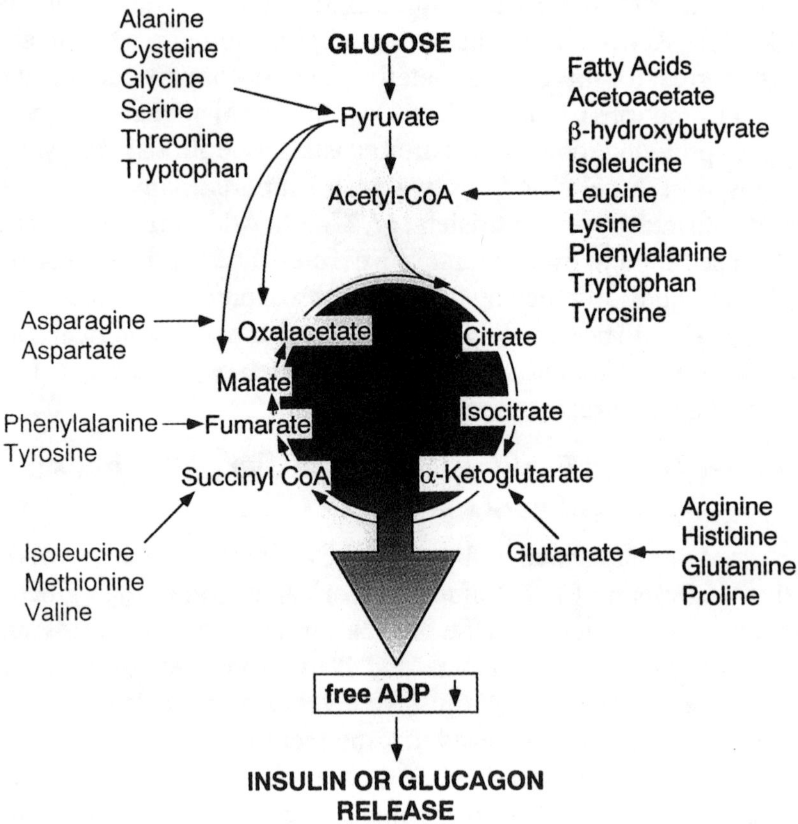

Fig. 4. The central role of the citric acid cycle in the metabolism of physiological nutrients that impact on pancreatic A- and B-cells.

lism of long chain fatty acids, and ketone bodies is of primary importance for the understanding of the results. It appears that in B-cells the catabolism of amino acids, fatty acids, and ketone bodies is under strong negative feedback control such that high substrate pressure alone is not sufficient to force their rapid metabolism, which contrasts with the biochemical design of glucose metabolism. Biosynthesis of complex lipids and protein biosynthesis may be enhanced by high levels of fatty acids or amino acids, respectively, which contrasts with the inability of B-cells to synthesize glycogen effectively when glucose is high. It also needs to be appreciated that islets have a very low capacity for fatty acid synthesis from malonyl-CoA and acetyl-CoA, even though malonyl-CoA is readily produced when islets are exposed to high glucose *(13,14)*. The ability of high glucose to augment the level of malonyl-CoA in pancreatic islets could have physiological significance *(12)*. There are several ways by which malonyl-CoA could influence islet cell intermediary metabolism and the intracellular signaling processes. Malonyl-CoA might be a coupling factor *per se* directly affecting membrane channels or transporters that are involved in stimulus secretion coupling or it might redirect fatty acids from catabolism to anabolic lipid synthesis, such that energy metabolism is primarily a function of glucose concentration when the level of this substrate is high. One possible corollary of this effect could be an elevation of cytosolic acyl-CoA esters, which are known to modify protein kinase C and other enzymes. Therefore acyl-CoA might function as a metabolic coupling and signaling factor. In isolated perifused islets acyl-CoA esters rise slowly after high glucose, much slower than the rise of malonyl-CoA, which seems to argue against involvement in first phase insulin release *(14)*. This additional acyl-CoA that slowly accumulates during prolonged glucose stimulation probably resides in the cytosol because the palmityl-carnitine transferase that is involved in shuttling fatty acids into the mitochondria is likely inhibited by malonyl-CoA. The desensitization to fatty acids and ketone bodies in starvation may be in part the result of the reduced permissive effect of glucose, owing to increased adrenergic input and finally might be caused by extended fatty acid metabolism itself *(see below)*.

Adaptation of Islet Cell Intermediary Metabolism to Fuel Deprivation or Overload

Extended nutrient deprivation or overload, in particular of glucose, influence profoundly the intermediary metabolism and secretory function of pancreatic islet cells. High glucose in the culture media induces glucokinase, the rate limiting step of glycolysis, increases glucose usage and enhances insulin release *(28)* (Fig. 5). The biochemical basis of glucose induction of glucokinase remains to be elucidated fully. Glucose appears to act translationally or posttranslationally. It is our working hypothesis that glucose stabilizes the enzyme and decreases its turnover and thus elevates the

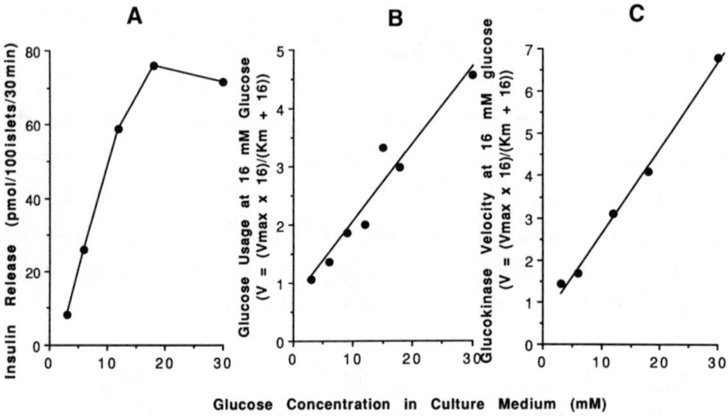

Fig. 5. Glucose induction of glucose stimulated insulin release (**A**), glucose usage (**B**), and glucokinase (**C**) in islets cultured for 7 d at various glucose concentrations (from Liang et al. *[28]*).

tissue level of glucokinase. Other enzymes of intermediary metabolism are also induced by high glucose *(19)*. The molecular basis of this general enzyme induction remains to be clarified. It also remains to be established whether exposure to excessive levels of amino acids and fatty acids influences the intermediary metabolism and function of pancreatic islet cells. It will be important to assess whether the glucose-fatty acid cycle as proposed by Randle operates also in pancreatic islet cells, particularly in B-cells *(29)*. Glucokinase, pyruvate dehydrogenase, and P-fructokinase are usually implicated as sites where elevated acyl-CoA, acetyl-CoA and citrate, respectively, might mediate the inhibition of glucose metabolism by increased fatty acid oxidation. Excessive fat intake or poorly suppressible free fatty acid levels in obesity owing to insulin resistance might be involved in the development of impaired glucose responsiveness of pancreatic B-cells. In support of this possibility elevated citrate levels were found in islet tissue of ob/ob, C57 black/6J mice *(30)*. Recent work of Sako and Grill also supports the proposal that the glucose fatty acid operates in pancreatic B-cells *(31)*. These investigators showed that 48 h lipid infusion in the rat inhibited glucose induced insulin secretion in the isolated perfused pancreas and glucose oxidation of isolated islets through a process that appeared to be coupled to fatty acid oxidation. A vicious cycle could develop whereby excessive fat intake or

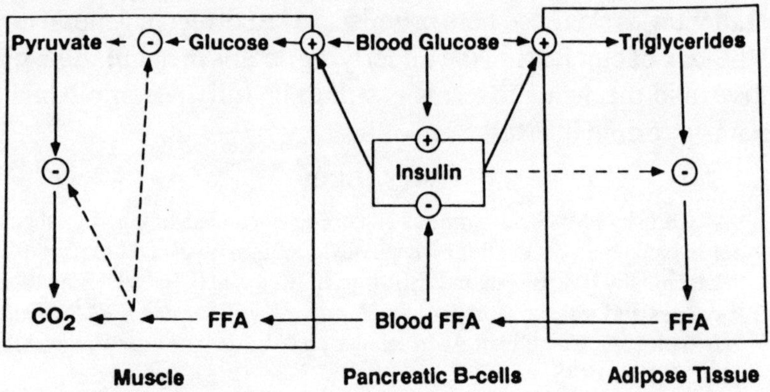

Fig. 6. The glucose fatty acid cycle might affect pancreatic B-cells and aggravate impairment of glucose tolerance.

insulin resistance would result in abnormally high serum free fatty acid levels that could interfere with glucose mediated insulin release and could further aggravate the impairment of glucose homeostasis (Fig. 6). It remains to be fully investigated whether, and if so, how A- and B-cells might be influenced by chronic overexposure to free fatty acids.

Summary

The biochemical design of pancreatic islet B-cells appears to be such that intermediary metabolism of the physiological nutrient molecules is the predominant determinant of hormone release from these cells, with glucose metabolism of central importance. In A-cells the metabolism of amino acids seems to play the predominant role with glucose of little importance. The linkage between metabolism and releasing function of A- and B-cells appears to be mediated by several metabolic coupling factors. Free ADP appears to be the most important one among these and acyl-CoA has been proposed as another candidate. Chronically high glucose induces glucokinase in B-cells and increases glycolysis, glucose oxidation, and insulin release, whereas chronic overexposure to free fatty acid is proposed to impair glucose responsiveness through inhibition of B-cell glucose metabolism. Neurotransmitters, enteric hormones, and drugs affect hormone release from pancreatic islet cells directly through their respective receptors, but they may influence A- and B-cell function also indirectly by modifying intermediary metabolism. The overall view as sketched here promises to be correct in general terms, but the task of elucidating the underlying details in qualitative, quantitative, and mechanistic terms is still to be fully accomplished and remains a formidable task.

References

1. Matschinsky FM: Glucokinase as glucose sensor and metabolic signal generator in pancreatic beta-cells and hepatocytes. *Diabetes* 39:647–652, 1990.
2. Matschinsky FM, Ellerman J, Stillings S, Raybaud F, Pace C, Zawalich W: Hexoses and insulin secretion. In *Handbook of Experimental Pharmacology*, vol. 23/2, Hasselblatt A, Bruchhausen FV, eds. Springer Verlag, Berlin, pp. 79–109, 1975.
3. Meglasson MD, Matschinsky FM: Pancreatic islet glucose metabolism and regulation of insulin secretion. *Diabetes Metab Rev* 2:163–214, 1986.
4. Pagliara AS, Stillings SN, Hover B, Martin DM, Matschinsky FM: Glucose modulation of amino acid-induced glucagon and insulin release in the isolated perfused rat pancreas. *J Clin Invest* 54:819–832, 1974.
5. Fertel R, Kotler-Brajtburg J, Holowach-Thurston J, Matschinsky FM: Insulin secretion due to alpha-keto monocarboxylic acids (alpha-KMCAs). *Diabetes* Suppl I 359:1972.
6. Fertel RH: Thesis: Part I, The effect of α-carbon substituted short chain monocarboxylic acids on insulin release; Part II, The penetration of hexoses into the islets of Langerhans, Washington University, St. Louis, MO, 1972.
7. Pipeleers DG, Shmit FM, Van Schravendijke CFH, Van De Winkel M: Interplay of nutrients and hormones in the regulation of glucagon release. *Endocrinology* 117:817–823, 1985.
8. Unger, RH: Glucagon physiology and pathophysiology in the light of new advances. *Diabetologia* 28:574–578, 1985.
9. Hopkins WF, Fatherazi S, Peter-Reisch B, Corkey BE, Cook DL: Two sites for adenine neucleotide regulation of ATP sensitive potassium channels in mouse pancreatic β-cells and HIT cells. *J Membr Biol* 129:287–295, 1992.
10. Ronner P, Matschinsky FM, Hang TL, Epstein AJ, Buettger C: Sulfonylurea binding sites and ATP sensitive K-channels in alpha-TC glucagonoma and beta-TC insulinoma cells. *Diabetes*, in press, 1993.
11. Ghosh A, Ronner P, Cheong E, Khalid P, Matschinsky FM: The role of ATP and free ADP in metabolic coupling during fuel-stimulated insulin release from islet B-cells in the isolated perfused rat pancreas. *J Biol Chem* 266:22,887–22,892, 1991
12. Prentki M, Matschinsky FM: Ca^{2+}, cAMP, and phospholipid-derived messengers in coupling mechanisms of insulin secretion. *Physiol Rev* 67:1185–1248, 1987.
13. Corkey BE, Glennon MC, Chen KS, Deeney JT, Matschinsky FM, Prentki M: A role for malonyl-CoA in glucose-stimulated insulin secretion from clonal pancreatic beta-cells. J Biol Chem 264:21,608–21,612, 1989.
14. Liang Y, Matschinsky FM: Content of CoA-esters in perifused rat islets stimulated by glucose and other fuels. Diabetes 40:327–333, 1991.

15. Louis NA, Witters LA: Glucose regulatin of Acetyl-CoA carboxylase in hepatoma and islet cells. *J Biol Chem* 267:2287–2293, 1992.
16 . Waddell ID, Burchell A: The microsomal glucose-6-phosphatase enzyme of pancreatic islets. *Biochem J* 255:471–476, 1988.
17. Khan A, Chandramouli V, Ostenson CG, Ahren B, Schumann WC, Low H, et al.: Evidence of the presence of glucose cycling in pancreatic islets of ob/ob mouse. *J Biol Chem* 264:9732–9733, 1989.
18. Matschinsky FM, Ellerman JE: Metabolism of glucose in the islets of Langerhans. *J Biol Chem* 243:2730–2736, 1968.
19. MacDonald MJ: Elusive proximal signals of β-cells for insulin secretion. *Diabetes* 39:1461–1466, 1990.
20. Malaisse WJ: Regulation of insulin secretion nutrients: The fuel concept, in *Nutrient Regulation of Insulin Secretion*, Flatt PR, ed, Portland Press, London, pp. 83–100, 1992.
21. Matschinsky FM, Ghosh AK, Meglasson MD, Prentki M, June V, von Allman, D: Metabolic concomitants in pure, panceratic beta cells during glucose-stimulated insulin secretion. *J Biol Chem* 261:14,057–14,061, 1986.
22. Matschinsky FM, Pagliara AS, Stillings SN, Hover BA: Glucose and ATP levels in pancreatic islet tissue of normal and diabetic rats. *J Clin Invest* 58:1193–1200, 1976.
23. Matschinsky FM, Pagliara AS, Hover BA, Pace CS, Ferrendelli JA, Williams A: Hormone secretion and glucose metabolism in islets of Langerhans of the isolated perfused pancreas from normal and streptozotocin diabetic rats. *J Biol Chem* 251:6053–6061, 1976.
24. Jetton T, Magnuson MA: Heterogeneous distribution of glucokinase in B-cells of pancreatic islet. *Proc Natl Acad Sci USA* 89:2619–2624, 1992.
25. Hutton JC, Sener A, Malaisse WJ: Interactions of brandished chain amino acids and ketoacids upon pancreatic islet metabolism and insulin secretion. *J Biol Chem* 255:7340–7346, 1980.
26. Berne C: Fatty acid and ketone body oxidation in pancreatic islets. *Biochem J* 152:661–666, 1975.
27. Malaisse WJ, Best L, Kawazu S, Malaisse-Lague F, Sener A: Fuel metabolism in islets. *Arch Biochem Biophys* 224:102–110, 1983.
28. Liang Y, Najafi H, Smith RM, Zimmerman E, Magnuson M, Tal M, et al.: Concordant glucose induction of glucokinase, glucose usage and glucose stimulated insulin release in pancreatic islets maintained in organ culture. *Diabetes* 41:792–806, 1992.
29. Randle PJ, Garland PB, Hales CN, Newsholme EA: The glucose fatty acid cycle. Its role in insulin sensitivity and the metabolic disturbances of diabetes mellitus. *Lancet* i:785–789, 1963.
30. Matschinsky FM, Rutherford CR, Ellerman JE: Accumulation of citrate in pancreatic islets of obese hyperglycemic mice. *Biochem Biophys Res Commun* 33:855–862, 1968.
31. Sako Y, Grill WA: 48-hour lipid infusion in the rat time-dependently inhibits glucose induced insulin secretion and B-cell oxidation through a process likely coupled to fatty acid oxidation. *Endocrinology* 127:1580–1589, 1990.

Chapter 9

Glucose Toxicity and the Insulin Gene

R. Paul Robertson, L. Karl Olson, J. Bruce Redmon, Hui-Jian Zhang, and Howard C. Towle

Introduction

Glucose is the primary regulator of insulin exocytosis from the pancreatic islet β-cell. More recently, glucose has been appreciated as an important physiological regulator at several other points in the pathway leading from insulin gene transcription through the formation of insulin mRNA and the eventual processing of insulin precursors and insulin itself *(1–7)*. Consequently, glucose can be considered to be a fundamentally important regulator of the entire sequence of events initiated in the earliest stages of insulin gene expression leading to the eventual release of the hormone from islet β-cells into the general circulation for distribution to a wide array of target tissues.

Although glucose is normally a physiologic regulator, concern has been raised that excessively high concentrations of this fuel might be potentially deleterious for β-cell function. Exposure of the β-cell to chronically elevated glucose levels in vivo may eventually lead to dysfunctional states described variously as "glucose desensitization,"

From: *Molecular Biology of Diabetes, Part I*
Edited by: B. Draznin and D. LeRoith

"glucose toxicity," or "β-cell exhaustion." Although experimental data *(8–25)* have been published that support these concepts, little is available that provides insights into the mechanisms of these phenomena.

The information provided in this chapter emanates from studies designed to assess potential mechanisms whereby glucose in excessive concentrations may adversely affect insulin gene expression and thereby interrupt the normal flow of events that begin with insulin gene transcription and lead to the formation, storage, and exocytosis of insulin. Although ideally such studies would be conducted using pure β-cells, the technology involved in isolating β-cells is quite labor-intensive and results in relatively low cellular yields. Consequently, we have used a clonal line of pancreatic islet β-cells, the HIT-T15 cell, for our experiments.

The HIT-T15 Cell Line

In 1981 Santerre et al. described a novel cell line, designated HIT-T15, derived from Simian virus 40-transfection of Syrian hamster pancreatic islets *(26)*. This cell line was shown by both light and electron microscopy to be morphologically similar to native β-cells of the pancreatic islet. HIT cells were shown to contain and release insulin. This cell line was one of the earliest demonstrated to have insulin secretory responsiveness to increases in glucose concentration (Fig. 1). Furthermore, HIT cells placed in a perifusion chamber were shown to demonstrate biphasic insulin release when exposed to a maximally stimulatory concentration of glucose (Fig. 2). The phasic pattern of insulin release from HIT cells is virtually identical to the pattern observed from islets isolated from Syrian hamsters. Thus, the HIT cell reproduces the insulin secretory dynamics one would expect from islet β-cells both under static and perifusion conditions. However, the EC_{50} for glucose-induced insulin secretion is left-shifted (Fig. 1).

An intriguing aspect of the HIT cell is that its insulin response to glucose eventually disappears as the cell line is chronically passaged *(26–28)*. By passage 85, the HIT cell has markedly decreased insulin secretion when exposed to stimulating concentrations of glucose (Fig. 3). This deterioration of insulin secretion can also be seen when agonists such as arginine and potassium are used (Figs. 4 and 5). The decrease in insulin secretion is accompanied by parallel

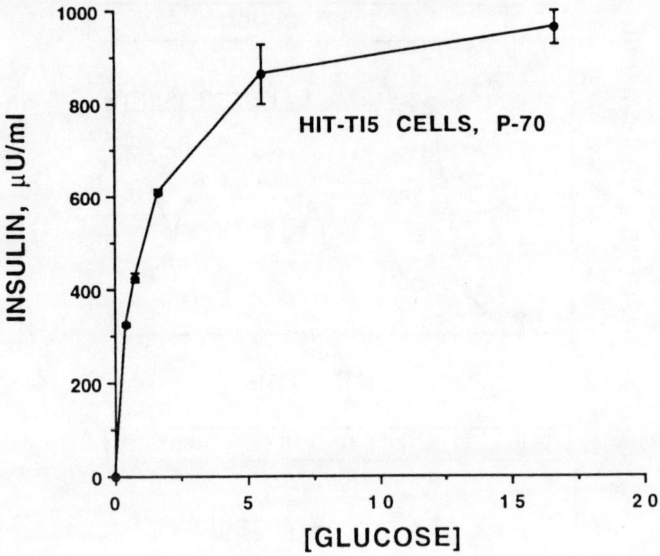

Fig. 1. Glucose dose-insulin response curve in an early passage 70 of HIT cells grown in RPMI-1640 media containing 11.1 m*M* glucose.

decreases in cellular insulin content (Fig. 6) and levels of insulin mRNA (Fig. 7). In the process of trying to understand these passage-related changes in insulin secretion, insulin content, and insulin mRNA *(29)*, we considered whether chronic exposure to the relatively high glucose concentrations in the media conventionally used for culturing HIT cells might paradoxically have an adverse effect on insulin gene expression and insulin secretion, i.e., glucose toxicity.

Influence of Chronic Exposure to High Glucose Concentrations on HIT Cell mRNA Levels and Insulin Secretion

HIT cells are conventionally cultured in RPMI 1640 media that contain 11.1 m*M* glucose. As can be appreciated from Fig. 1, this glucose concentration is maximally stimulatory for insulin secretion from HIT cells. We designed experiments to determine whether chronic exposure to this maximally stimulating concentration of glucose might have deleterious effects on insulin gene expression and insulin secretion *(29)*. In these studies we compared insulin mRNA levels, insulin content, and insulin secretion from passage 70 (the

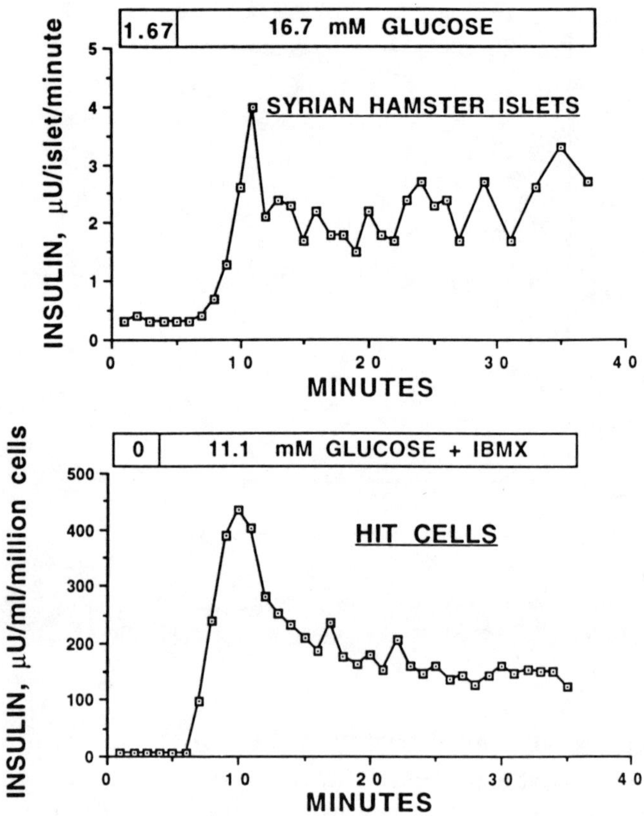

Fig. 2. Comparison of phasic insulin secretion from isolated Syrian hamster islets and HIT cells in response to maximal stimulatory concentrations of glucose.

youngest passage available to us) through passage 96 HIT cells that had been cultured in RPMI 1640 containing either 0.8 or 11.1 m*M* glucose. The reason these two concentrations were selected is that a glucose concentration of 0.8 m*M* is minimally stimulatory, whereas a glucose concentration of 11.1 m*M* is maximally stimulatory for insulin secretion. In this manner we tested the hypothesis that chronic exposure to maximally stimulatory concentrations of glucose might play a role in the passage-related decline in insulin mRNA levels, insulin content, and insulin secretion.

Throughout these experiments, it was essential to consider whether culturing the cells in media containing these two differing

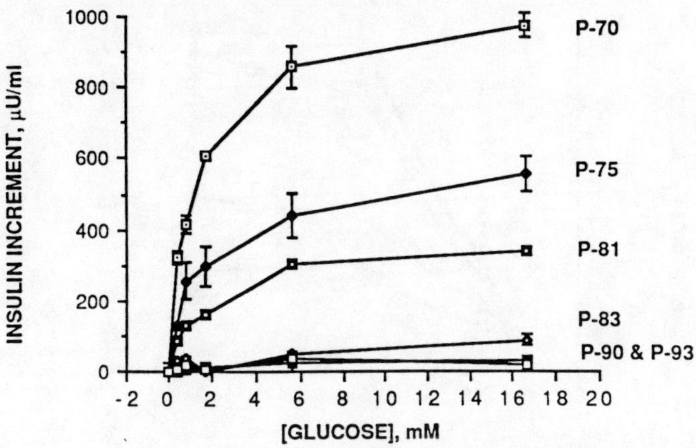

Fig. 3. Passage-dependent loss of glucose-induced insulin secretion from HIT cells serially grown from passage 70 through passage 93. Reprinted with permission from ref. *(28)*.

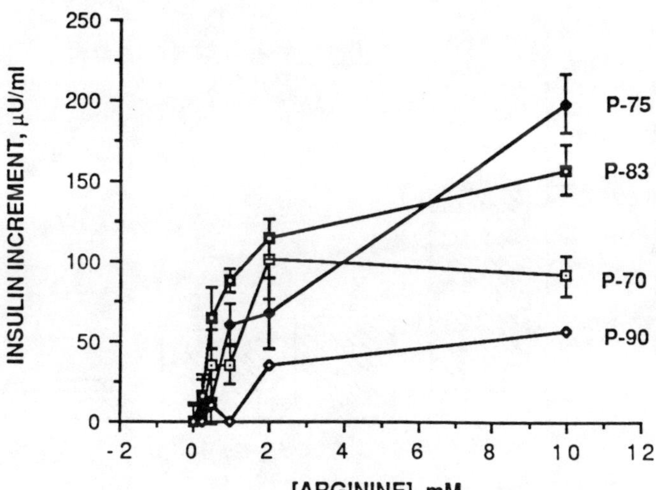

Fig. 4. Passage-dependent loss of arginine-induced insulin secretion from HIT cells grown serially from passage 75 through passage 90. Reprinted with permission from ref. *(28)*.

glucose concentrations might lead to differences in the rate of cell replication and, thus, the rate of cell aging. If so, this might be expected to alter insulin secretion. It was ascertained by daily total cell counts for seven consecutive days for passages 75, 85, and 95

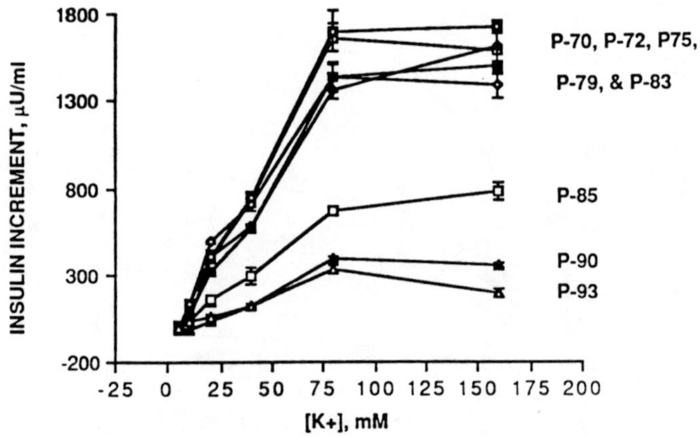

Fig. 5. Passage-dependent loss of potassium-induced insulin secretion from HIT cells grown serially from passage 70 through passage 93. Reprinted with permission from ref. *(28)*.

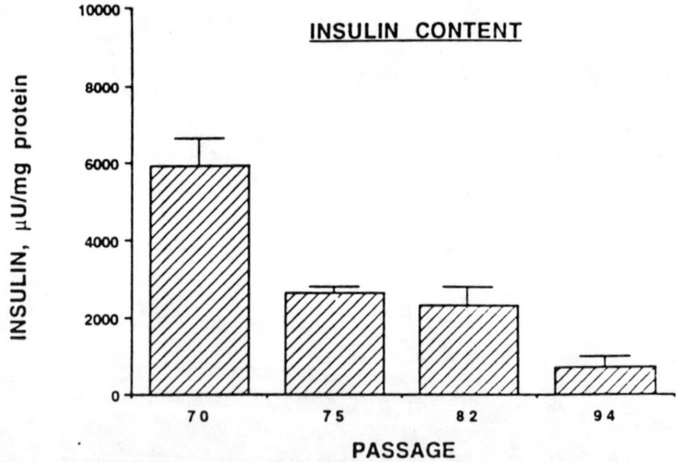

Fig. 6. Passage-dependent decrements in insulin content of HIT cells grown serially from passage 70 through passage 94. Reprinted with permission from ref. *(28)*.

that the population doubling times and cumulative doubling times were not significantly different (Fig. 8). Thus, it did not appear as though culturing the cells in media containing a low glucose concentration slowed the replication process of HIT cells.

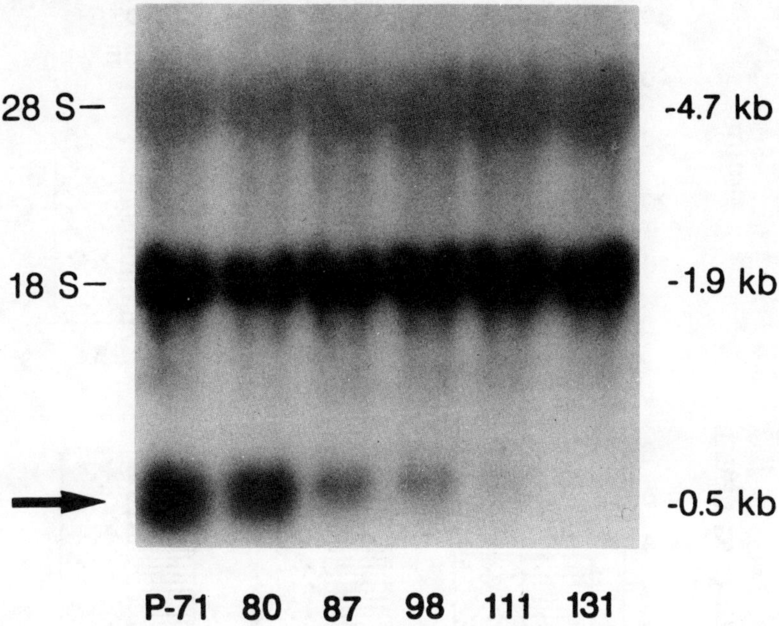

Fig. 7. Passage-dependent decrements in insulin mRNA levels in HIT cells cultured serially from passage 71 through 131. Arrow designates insulin mRNA. Reprinted with permission from ref. *(29)*.

Northern analysis of insulin mRNA levels in HIT cells cultured under conditions of either low or high glucose concentrations revealed strikingly different results (Fig. 9). Exposure of HIT cells to 11.1 m*M* glucose in the culture media caused the anticipated decline in insulin mRNA levels when cells were progressively passed from passage 70 to 96. However, when culture media containing 0.8 m*M* glucose was used instead, insulin mRNA levels were preserved such that the level of insulin message in passage 96 was virtually indistinguishable from the level in passage 75. Subcultures of HIT cells from late passages grown in media containing either low or high glucose concentrations provided correspondingly dissimilar results when glucose concentration-insulin response experiments using static incubations were performed (Fig. 10). As expected, late passages of cells grown in media containing high glucose concentration failed to release insulin when exposed to stimulatory concentrations of glu-

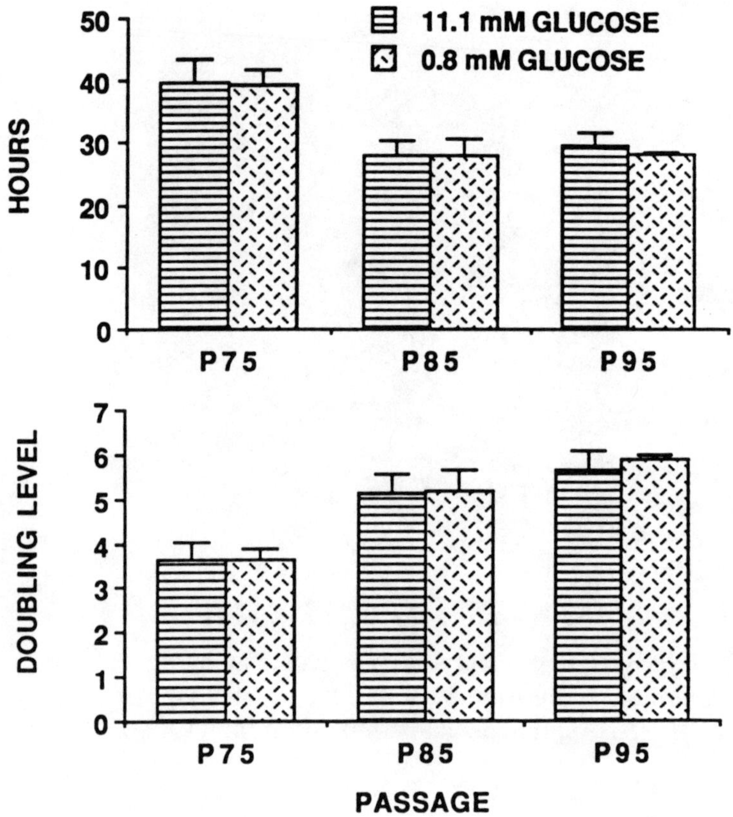

Fig. 8. Comparison of HIT cell population doubling times and cumulative doubling levels in passages 75, 85, and 95. Cells were serially cultured either in 11.1 m*M* or 0.8 m*M* glucose. Reprinted with permission from ref. *(29)*.

cose. In marked contrast, late passages of cells grown in media containing low glucose concentrations had preserved insulin secretory responses. The magnitude of these preserved responses was similar to that observed in HIT cells from passages in the early 70s cultured in media containing 11.1 m*M* glucose. Moreover, perifusion of late passages of HIT cells grown in media containing low glucose concentrations revealed preserved first and second phase glucose-induced insulin secretion whereas HIT cells grown conventionally in media containing 11.1 m*M* glucose failed to demonstrate insulin release during perifusion (Fig. 11).

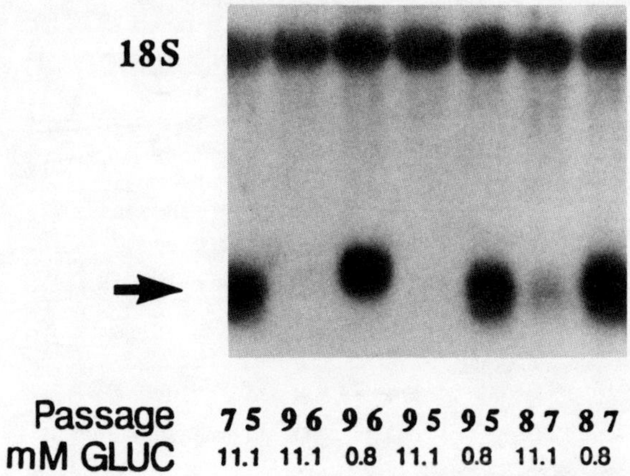

Fig. 9. Decrements in HIT cell insulin mRNA in passages 87, 95, and 96 when cultured in 11.1 m*M* glucose. These decrements are prevented by culturing cells in 0.8 m*M* glucose. Reprinted with permission from ref. *(29)*.

Mechanism of the Paradoxical Effect of a High Glucose Concentration to Decrease Insulin mRNA and Insulin Secretion

To understand the adverse effects of culturing HIT cells in media containing a high glucose concentration, we first turned to studies of insulin gene transcription *(30)*. A chloramphenicol acetyl transferase (CAT) gene linked to the human insulin gene enhancer-promoter sequence was constructed and termed INSCAT. HIT cells were transiently transfected with INSCAT using a liposome-mediated (Lipofectin) method. Thirty hours after transfection cells were harvested and CAT activity was assayed. Control transfections were carried out using RSVCAT, a CAT gene linked to the Rous sarcoma virus promoter region. The data were analyzed as relative INSCAT to RSVCAT expression to control for variability in transfection efficiency observed between cells cultured in media containing either low or high glucose concentrations. HIT cells from passages 73 to 76 cultured in 11.1 m*M* glucose readily expressed CAT activity, whereas the expression of CAT activity in late passages of HIT cells cultured in 11.1 m*M* glucose was markedly decreased (Fig. 12). The decrease in relative CAT activity observed in late passages of HIT cells cul-

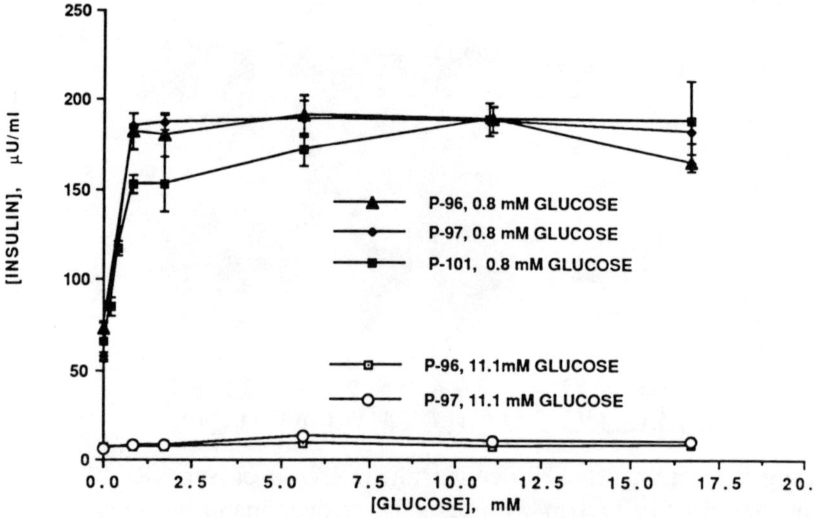

Fig. 10. Preservation of insulin responses to increasing concentrations of glucose in late passages of HIT cells cultured in 0.8 m*M* glucose rather than 11.1 m*M* glucose. Reprinted with permission from ref. *(29)*.

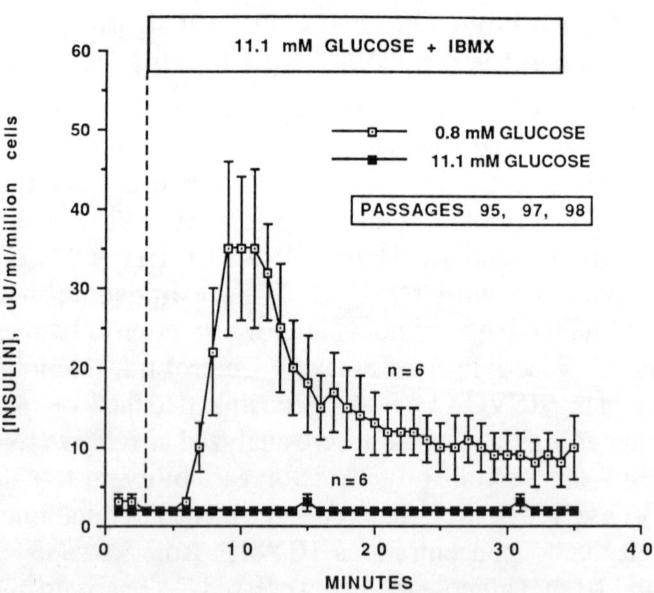

Fig. 11. Preservation of phasic insulin secretion in late passages of HIT cells cultured in 0.8 m*M* glucose rather than 11.1 m*M* glucose. Reprinted with permission from ref. *(29)*.

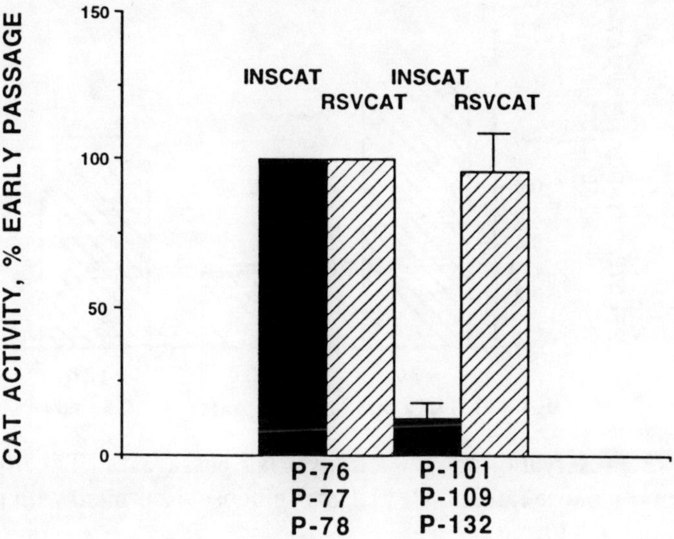

Fig. 12. Comparison in early and late passages of CAT (chloramphenicol acetyl transferase) activity in cells transfected with the CAT gene driven by the human insulin enhancer-promoter region. Controlled transfections were done with RSVCAT. Reprinted with permission from ref. *(30)*.

tured in the higher glucose concentration was specific for INSCAT, since RSVCAT expression was the same for both early and late passages of HIT cells. Compared to late passages of HIT cells chronically cultured in 11.1 mM glucose, cells chronically cultured in 0.8 m*M* glucose had a markedly higher degree of CAT activity when transfected with INSCAT (Fig. 13). In these studies, insulin promoter activity from late passages of HIT cells serially passaged in 0.8 m*M* glucose was approx 70% compared to earlier passages of HIT cells, whereas activity was roughly 30% for late passages of HIT cells cultured in 11.1 m*M* glucose. These data indicate that late passages of HIT cells chronically cultured in media containing the lower glucose concentration had preserved insulin promoter activity. This was consistent with the hypothesis that the mechanism through which the lower glucose concentration preserved both insulin mRNA and insulin content involved preserving insulin gene transcription.

In searching for possible mechanisms to explain the adverse effects on insulin gene transcription caused by culturing HIT cells chronically in high glucose concentrations, we examined the possi-

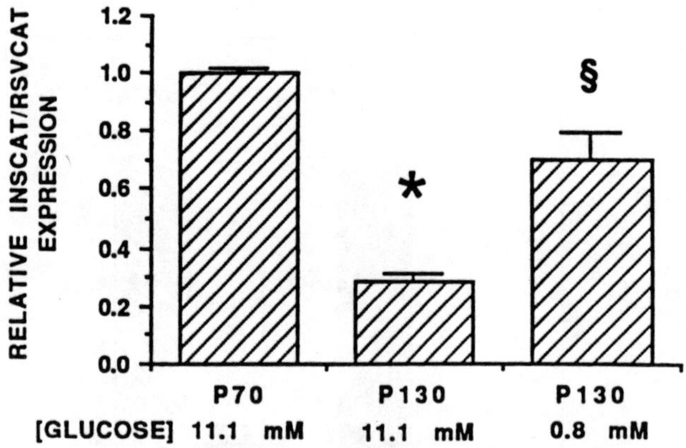

Fig. 13. Preservation of CAT activity in late passages of HIT cells grown in 0.8 m*M* glucose rather than 11.1 m*M* glucose. Reprinted with permission from ref. *(30)*.

bility that there may be alterations in the binding activity of transcription factors that interact and regulate the enhancer-promoter of the human insulin gene *(30)*. We focused our studies on the CT motifs of the human insulin gene characterized and shown to bind a β-cell specific transcription factor, IUF-1, by Docherty and his colleagues *(31)*. To study the binding to the CT motifs, electrophoretic mobility shift assays were performed using [^{32}P]-oligodeoxynucleotide corresponding to the DNA sequences of human insulin gene which contained the CT2 motif and nuclear extracts from various passages of HIT cells. The specificity of the DNA-protein complex formed with the nuclear extracts was determined by use of an excess of unlabeled oligodeoxynucleotide corresponding to the same DNA sequences. The results demonstrated that nuclear extracts made from earlier passages of HIT cells cultured in media containing 11.1 m*M* glucose formed a specific DNA–protein complex to sequences containing the CT2 motif of the human insulin gene (Fig. 14). These could be successfully competed for by an excess of unlabeled oligodeoxynucleotide. If we mutated six base pairs corresponding to the CT motif within this unlabeled oligodeoxynucleotide, it no longer competed for the labeled probe, suggesting that this DNA binding factor binds directly to the CT motif on the enhancer of the human insulin gene. Nuclear extracts made from late passages of HIT cells chroni-

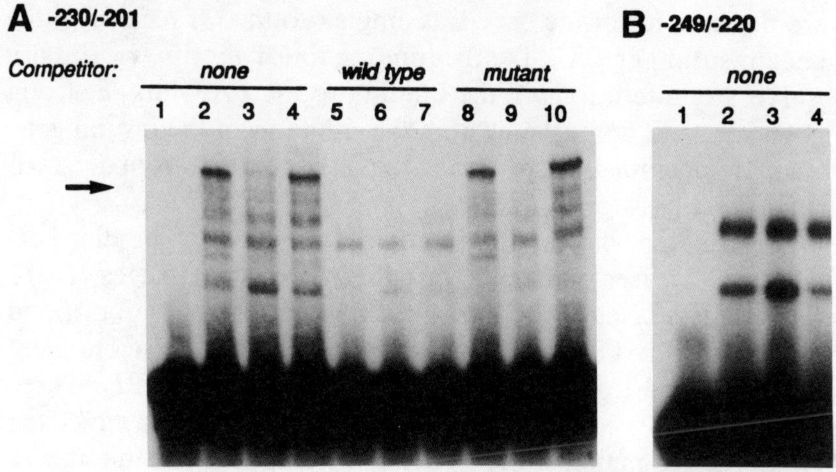

Fig. 14. Analysis of protein binding to the insulin promoter sequences from –230 to –201 and –249 to –220 using nuclear extracts from early passage and late passage of HIT cells serially passaged in either 11.1 m*M* or 0.8 m*M* glucose. (**A**) EMSA using [^{32}P]-labeled insulin promoter sequence –230 to –201. Lane 1, free probe; lanes 2,5,8, nuclear extract from HIT cell passage 74; lanes 3,6,9, nuclear extract from HIT cell passage 133 serially passaged in 11.1 m*M* glucose; lanes 4,7,10, nuclear extracts from HIT cells passage 133 serially passaged in 0.8 m*M* glucose. 100-fold molar excess of unlabeled wild type sequence –230 to –201 added, lanes 5–7; 100-fold molar excess of unlabeled mutated sequence –230 to –201 added lanes 8–10. Arrow indicates DNA-protein complex present in early passages of HIT cells and late passages of HIT cells cultured in 0.8 m*M* glucose, but not in late passages of HIT cells cultured in 11.1 m*M* glucose. (**B**) EMSA using [^{32}P]-labeled insulin promoter sequence –249 to –220. Lane 1, free probe; lanes 2–4, nuclear extracts from HIT cell passage 74 and passage 133 serially passaged in 11.1 m*M* glucose and 0.8 m*M* glucose, respectively. Reprinted with permission from ref. *(30)*.

cally cultured under conditions of this high glucose concentration failed to form this specific DNA-protein complex. In contrast, nuclear extracts from late passages of HIT cells chronically cultured under 0.8 m*M* glucose concentrations had preserved the ability to form this DNA-protein complex. As observed with the CT2 motif, nuclear extracts from late passages of HIT cells cultured in high glucose were not able to form a specific complex to the CT1 motif of the human insulin gene. Unlike the binding to CT motifs, we did not observe any alterations in the binding to the FAR box, a strong regulatory motif conserved within the enhancer of the insulin gene from many mammalian species, with nuclear extract from our various HIT cell passages.

To examine whether the loss of this protein–DNA binding correlated to decreased expression of INSCAT in late passages of HIT cells serially passed in high glucose concentrations, site-directed mutations of the CT binding sites within INSCAT vectors were constructed and tested in various HIT cell passages *(31)*. Three mutant INSCAT vectors were constructed; mCT2CAT in which the CT2 motif was mutated, mCT1CAT in which the CT1 motif was mutated, and mCT1CT2CAT in which both the CT1 and CT2 motifs were mutated. The expression of the vector in which both of the binding sites were mutated was markedly decreased in both early and late passages of HIT cells regardless of the glucose concentrations used in the culture media (Fig. 15). These data confirmed that the protein-DNA binding sites present within the CT motifs of the human insulin gene play a functional role in the regulation of insulin gene transcription and that the loss of corresponding protein–DNA binding will lead to decreased insulin gene transcription. Since these experiments utilized the CT regions of the human insulin gene enhancer-promoter region described by Docherty and colleagues, we interpret these data to indicate that the protein loss in the nuclear extracts of HIT cells grown in media containing high glucose concentrations may be the protein designated by Boam and Docherty as IUF-1 *(31)*.

Summary and Conclusion

The experiments described in this chapter were performed to understand the loss of insulin secretion in a cell line of pancreatic islet β-cells, the HIT-T15 cell, grown chronically in media containing a glucose concentration that maximally stimulates insulin secretion. This high glucose concentration has also been associated with decreased levels of insulin mRNA and insulin content. Our experiments indicate that chronic exposure to a high glucose concentration

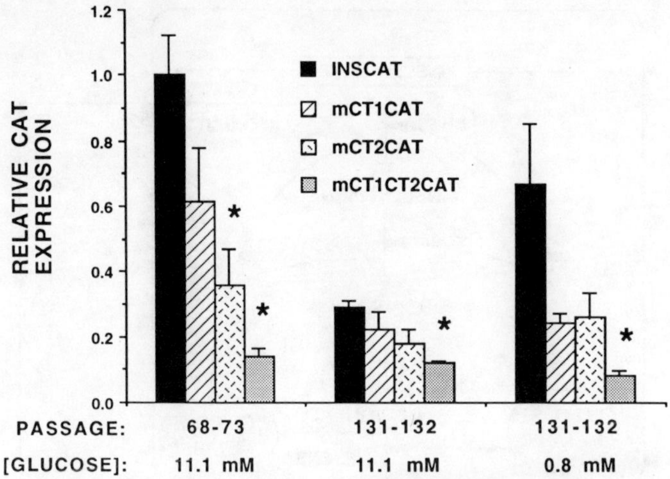

Fig. 15. Functional analysis of the CT motifs contained within the human insulin gene promoter. Early and late passages of HIT cells serially passaged in 11.1 m*M* and 0.8 m*M* glucose were transiently transfected with INSCAT with either the CT1 (mCT1CAT), CT2 (mCT2CAT), or both the CT1 and CT2 (mCT1CT2CAT) motifs mutated. Reprinted with permission from ref. *(30)*.

is associated with a marked decrease in insulin gene transcription. This appears to be related to alteration and/or loss of a nuclear protein–DNA complex involving the CT_1 and CT_2 motifs of the human insulin gene enhancer-promoter. This suggests that chronic exposure to a high glucose concentration results in defective production of this insulin gene transcription factor and/or inactivation of the transcription factor. In this sense, our data provide a potential mechanism for glucose toxicity at the level of the insulin gene. We believe that an important distinction may exist between glucose toxicity and the phenomena termed as glucose desensitization (Fig. 16). In this context, we view glucose toxicity as an irreversible, adverse effect on the formation of insulin because of interference with insulin gene transcription, presumably by interruption of the formation or activation of nuclear factors that enhance insulin gene transcription. Insulin desensitization is considered to be a reversible phenomenon that may take place at the level of insulin exocytosis.

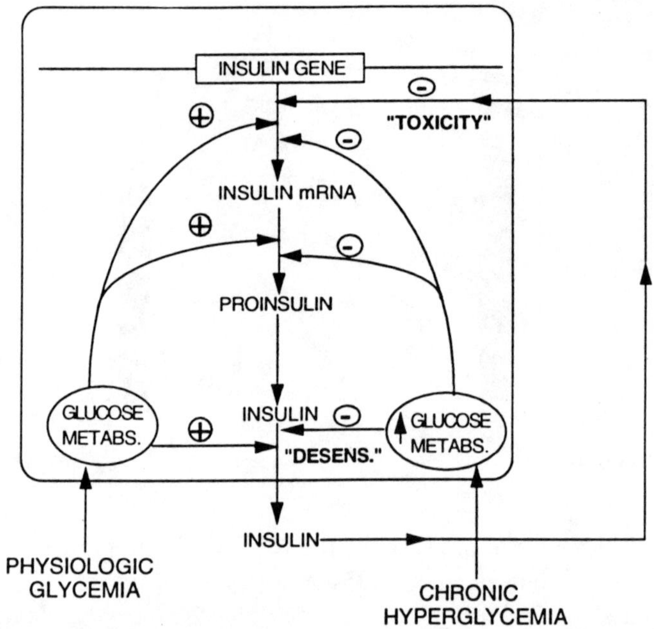

Fig. 16. Hypothetical differentiation of "glucose desensitization" from "glucose toxicity." Glucose desensitization is viewed as a short-term, reversible effect expressed primarily at the level of insulin exocytosis. Glucose toxicity is viewed as an irreversible consequence of more prolonged exposure to deleterious levels of glucose. This toxic effect is expressed at the level of insulin gene transcription and paradoxically prevents normal increases in insulin gene expression in response to high concentrations of glucose.

Acknowledgments

This work was supported by NIH R01 DK-38325 (RPR), NIH F32 DK-08742 (LKO), NIH KO8 DK-02134 (JBR), and NIH R01 DK-26919 (HCT). This chapter is largely a review of refs. *(28–30)* written by the authors. As such, most of the same figures and similar text has been used.

References

1. Hammonds P, Schofield PN, Ashcroft SJH: Glucose regulates preproinsulin messenger RNA levels in a clonal cell line of simian virus 40-transformed β cells. *FEBS Lett* 213(1):149–154, 1987.
2. Giddings SJ, Chirgwin J, Permutt MA: Effects of glucose on proinsulin messenger RNA in rats in vivo. *Diabetes* 31:624–629, 1982.

3. Brunstedt J, Chan SJ: Direct effect of glucose on the preproinsulin mRNA level in isolated pancreatic islets. *Biochem Biophys Res Comm* 106(4):1383–1389, 1982.
4. Hammonds P, Schofield PN, Ashcroft SJH, Sutton R, Gray DWR: Regulation and specificity of glucose-stimulated insulin gene expression in human islets of Langerhans. *FEBS Lett* 223(1):131–137, 1987.
5. Welsh M, Nielsen DA, MacKrell AJ, Steiner DF: Control of insulin gene expression in pancreatic β-cells and in an insulin-producing cell line, RIN-5F cells. *J Biol Chem* 260(25):13,590–13,594, 1985.
6. German MS, Moss LG, Rutter WJ: Regulation of insulin gene expression by glucose and calcium in transfected primary islet cultures. *J Biol Chem* 265(36):22,063–22,066, 1990.
7. Efrat S, Surana M, Fleischer N: Glucose induces insulin gene transcription in a murine pancreatic β-cell line. *J Biol Chem* 266(17):11,141–11,143, 1991.
8. Turner RC, McCarthy ST, Holman RR, Harris E: β-cell function improved by supplementing basal insulin secretion in mild diabetes. *Br Med J* 1:1252–1254, 1976.
9. Schmeltz R, Wendorff HJ, Field JB: Effect of control of blood glucose on plasma insulin responses to various stimuli in secondary failures to oral hypoglycemic agents and in newly diagnosed, maturity onset, ketosis-resistant diabetics. *J Clin Endocrinol Metab* 46:519–527, 1978.
10. Kosaka K, Kuzuya T, Akanuma Y, Hagura R: Increase in insulin response after treatment of overt maturity-onset diabetes is independent of the mode of treatment. *Diabetologia* 18:23–28, 1980.
11. Hidaka H, Nagulesparan M, Klimes I, Clark R, Sasaki H, Aronoff SL, et al.: Improvement of insulin secretion but not insulin resistance after short term control of plasma glucose in obese type II diabetics. *J Clin Endocrinol Metab* 54:217–222, 1982.
12. Vague P, Moulin JP: The defective glucose sensitivity of the B cell in non insulin dependent diabetes. Improvement after twenty hours of normoglycaemia. *Metab Clin Exp* 31:139–142, 1982.
13. Bonner-Weir S, Trent DF, Weir GC: Partial pancreatectomy in the rat and subsequent defect in glucose-induced insulin release. *J Clin Invest* 71:1544–1553, 1983.
14. Unger RH, Grundy S: Hyperglycaemia as an inducer as well as a consequence of impaired islet cell function and insulin resistance: implications for the management of diabetes. *Diabetologia* 28:119–121, 1985.
15. Giugliano D, Di Pinto P, Ceriello A, Paolisso G, Saccomanno F, Torella R, et al.: Glycemic control with an artificial pancreas improves insulin responses to both oral and I.V. glucose in non-obese noninsulin-dependent diabetic subjects. *Acta Diabetol Lat* 22:203–213, 1985.
16. Glaser B, Leibovich G, Nesher R, Hartling S, Binder C, Cerasi E: Improved beta-cell function after intensive insulin treatment in severe non-insulin-dependent diabetes. *Endocrinologica* 118:365–373, 1988.

17. Rossetti L, Shulman GI, Zawalich W, DeFronzo RA: Effect of chronic hyperglycemia on *in vivo* insulin secretion in partially pancreatectomized rats. *J Clin Invest* 80:1037–1044, 1987.
18. Imamura T, Koffler M, Helderman JH, Prince D, Thirlby R, Inman L, et al.: Severe diabetes induced in subtotally depancreatized dogs by sustained hyperglycemia. *Diabetes* 37:600–609, 1988.
19. Leahy JL, Bonner-Weir S, Weir GC: Minimal chronic hyperglycemia is a critical determinant of impaired insulin secretion after an incomplete pancreatectomy. *J Clin Invest* 81:1407–1414, 1988.
20. Giroix M-H, Serradas P, Portha B: The desensitization of normal B-cells to glucose *in vitro* is transient and not related to high glucose levels. *Endocrinology* 125:1999–2007, 1989.
21. Grodsky GM: A new phase of insulin secretion. How will it contribute to our understanding of β-cell function? *Diabetes* 38:673–678, 1989.
22. Robertson RP: Type II diabetes, glucose "non-sense," and islet desensitization. *Diabetes* 38:1501–1505, 1989.
23. Rossetti L, Giaccari A, DeFronzo RA: Glucose toxicity. *Diabetes Care* 13:610–630, 1990.
24. Korsgren O, Jansson L, Sandler S, Andersson A: Hyperglycemia-induced B cell toxicity. The fate of pancreatic islets transplanted into diabetic mice is dependent on their genetic background. *J Clin Invest* 86:2161–2168, 1990.
25. Sako Y, Grill VE: Coupling of β-cell desensitization by hyperglycemia to excessive stimulation and circulating insulin in glucose-infused rats. *Diabetes* 39:1580–1583, 1990.
26. Santerre RF, Cook RA, Crisel RMD, Sharp JD, Schmidt RJ, Williams DC, et al.: Insulin synthesis in a clonal cell line of simian virus 40-transformed hamster pancreatic β-cells. *Proc Natl Acad Sci USA* 78:4339–4343, 1981.
27. Ashcroft SJH, Hammonds P, Harrison DE: Insulin secretory responses of a clonal cell line of simian virus 40-transformed B cells. *Diabetologia* 29: 727–733, 1986.
28. Zhang H-J, Walseth TF, Robertson RP: Insulin secretion and cAMP metabolism in HIT cells. Reciprocal and serial passage-dependent relationships. *Diabetes* 38:44–48, 1989.
29. Robertson RP, Zhang H-J, Pyzdrowski KL, Walseth TF: Preservation of insulin mRNA levels and insulin secretion in HIT cells by avoidance of chronic exposure to high glucose concentrations. *J Clin Invest* 90:320–325, 1992.
30. Olson LK, Redmon JB, Towle HC, Robertson RP: Chronic exposure of HIT cells to high glucose concentrations paradoxically decreases insulin gene transcription and alters binding of insulin gene regulatory protein. *J Clin Invest* 92:514–519, 1993.
31. Boam DSW, Docherty K: A tissue-specific nuclear factor binds to multiple sites in the human insulin-gene enhancer. *Biochem J* 264:233–239, 1989.

Chapter 10

Proinsulin-Processing Endopeptidases

Deborah L. Bennett and John C. Hutton

Introduction

Knowledge of the gene structure of secreted proteins and analysis of their biosynthesis has revealed that many are initially produced as larger biologically inactive precursors that are subjected to limited proteolysis at sites marked by clusters of basic amino acids in characteristic linear sequences. Peptide hormones and neurotransmitters that are secreted via the regulated secretory pathway in neuroendocrine tissues are generally processed at pairs of basic amino acids, typically Lys Arg and Arg Arg and much less frequently at Lys Lys or Arg Lys sites. Growth factors and receptor molecules that follow the constitutive pathway are processed at sites marked by a more complex array of basic amino acids, typically a pair of basic amino acids with a further basic amino acid in the P4 position (for review, *see* ref. *1*). In the majority of cases where the most C-terminal amino acid in the cluster is an arginine residue, cleavage of the amide bond occurs on the C-terminal side of this arginine. When it is a lysine residue, cleavage often occurs on the N-terminal side and probably involves a different enzymatic process in many cases. Basic amino acids exposed at the C-termini after endoproteolytic cleavage are removed by carboxypeptidase H (E) (CPH) within the regulated pathway of secretion. Whether a similar activity is present in the constitutive pathway is not clear.

From: *Molecular Biology of Diabetes, Part I*
Edited by: B. Draznin and D. LeRoith

Such posttranslational proteolysis is ancient in evolutionary terms and appears to serve a similar physiological role in all eukaryotes in the activation of biological function of proteins. It also probably fulfils other molecular, cellular, and physiological functions, including folding, intracellular movement and sorting, and regulation of the physicochemical properties of the product. The mere presence of paired basic amino acids, however, is no guarantee that a proprotein will be processed at that site. Cell to cell variation in the processing machinery moreover can mean that different products with unrelated biological activities can be produced from the same proprotein molecule. Such differential processing may also occur within the same cell in response to physiological stimuli or developmental cues.

Emphasis will be given in this chapter to the endopeptidases responsible for the maturation of insulin from proinsulin. These enzymes are of special interest since they are usually rate-limiting in posttranslational maturation in the regulated pathway and thus of regulatory importance. How defects in these enzymes or in the processing machinery of β-cells might result in abnormal maturation of insulin in diabetes and islet cell neoplasia is then discussed.

Structural Motifs in Proinsulin as Sites for Cleavage

Human proinsulin consists of a B-chain (30 amino acids) linked to the connecting C-peptide (31 amino acids) by Arg^{31} Arg^{32}, which in turn connects to the insulin A-chain (21 amino acids) by the Lys^{64} Arg^{65} sequence. The A and B chains in proinsulin are connected by two interchain disulfide bonds (A7-B7 and A20-B19), with an intrachain bond between amino acid residues A6 and A11 (Fig. 1). Processing of proinsulin into insulin and C-peptide occurs at the pairs of basic amino acids at the B-chain/C-peptide and A-chain/C-peptide junctions. Proinsulin, like insulin in most animal species, binds Zn^{2+} ions and forms hexamers and higher order complexes. It has a higher solubility and lesser propensity to form crystals than does insulin, features that are likely to be of physiological importance in that they ensure that proinsulin can traverse the secretory pathway from the endoplasmic reticulum to the secretory granule in a soluble form, but once converted, form a condensed proteolytically resistant product.

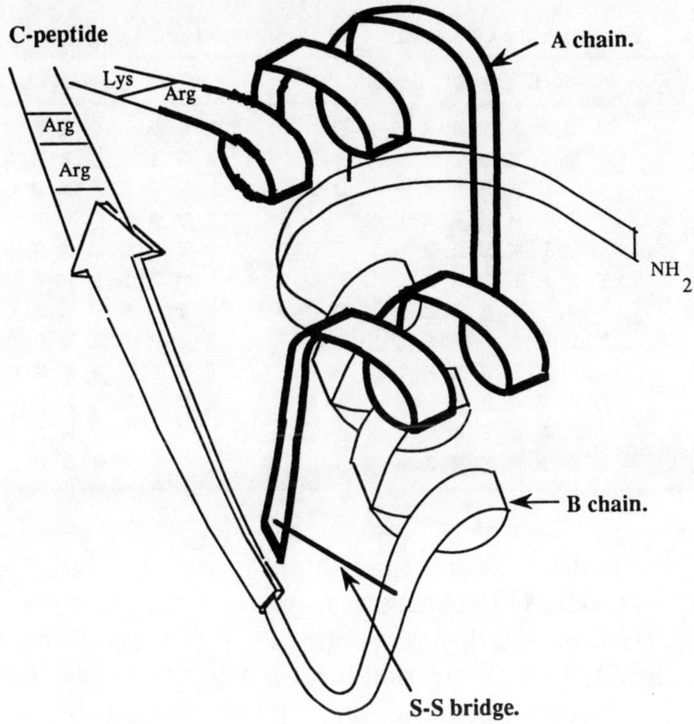

Fig. 1. A model of proinsulin structure. The carbon backbone of insulin based on the crystal structure is shown to illustrate the probable relative positions of the sites of cleavage of proinsulin and their relative proximity. The C-peptide whose structure is ill-defined and not included constitutes about a third of the molecular mass of the molecule. A β-strand toward the COOH terminus of the B-chain is depicted by the extended arrow.

Among the known sequences of vertebrate proinsulins, the dibasic site separating the C-peptide and A-chain is invariably a Lys Arg sequence (Table 1). The dibasic site separating the B-chain and C-peptide is Lys Arg in fish and amphibians but Arg Arg in higher vertebrates. Additional basic amino acids appear in the P4 position in the case of the B-C and C-A junction of a number of species. This arrangement is reminiscent of the processing sites of constitutively secreted proteins and it seems likely that the P4 position contributes to their ability to act as substrates to the converting enzymes.

Table 1
Evolutionary Conservation of Proinsulin Processing Sites

Species	B-chain/C-peptide	C-peptide/A-chain
Human	Y T P **K** T **R R** E A E D L	E G S L Q **K R** G I V E Q
Bovine	Y T P **K** A **R R** E V E G P	E G P P Q **K R** G I V E Q
Rat I	Y T P **K** S **R R** E V E D P	E V A **R** Q **K R** G I V D Q
Rat II	Y T P M S **R R** E V E D P	E V A **R** Q **K R** G I V D Q
Hamster	Y T P **K** S **R R** G V E D P	E V A Q Q **K R** G I V D Q
Guinea pig	Y I P **K** D **R R** E L E D P	E M A L Q **K R** G I V D Q
Chicken	Y S P **K** A **R R** D V E Q P	E Y A **K** V **K R** G I V E Q
Xenopus	Y Y P **K** I **K R** D I E Q A	E Y Q **K** M **K R** G I V E Q
Salmon	F F Y T P **K R** D V D P L	T E M M V **K R** G I V E Q
Hagfish	D P T **K** M **K R** D T G A L	E V L **K** S **K R** G I V E Q
Mullosc IRP	Q P A M V **K R** N A E T D	L T Y L T **K R** Q G T T N
Locust IRP	Y N T M F **K K** A S Q D V	G A V F **R R R** T **R** G V F

The length of the C-peptide in higher vertebrates varies between 26 and 38 residues *(2)* and shows a greater sequence variation than insulin. The sequence of the C-peptide flanking the processing site at the B-chain/C-peptide junction is more highly conserved than the remaining C-peptide sequence and typically consists of two acidic amino acids separated by a hydrophobic amino acid or an amino acid with a short neutral side chain. As no biological function is attributable to the C-peptide and it does not appear to be essential for sorting of the prohormone *(3)*, such conservation suggests that the flanking residues may have a role in the recognition of the dibasic sequence by processing enzymes *(2)*.

The secondary structure around the proinsulin processing sites may provide an additional recognition feature as many proprotein cleavage sites have been predicted to occur in β-turns adjacent to regions of high helical content or propensity to form a β-sheet. An alternative model envisions the dibasic site within an omega loop structure (for review, *see* ref. *1*). Accordingly, proinsulin residues 19–31 and 53–66 are predicted to form β-turns, and residues 46–54 and 69–76 to form omega loops. The three dimensional structure of proinsulin is not documented at the present time though NMR data points to a close conformational relationship of the A and B chains in proinsulin to that in insulin. Subtle differences nevertheless are evident, for example a stable local structure at the C-peptide/A-chain junction termed the CA knuckle *(4)*, which is postulated to form a specific recognition structure for the proinsulin processing endopeptidase that cleaves at this site. In the absence of more specific information it is assumed that the Arg Arg site follows a β-strand and the Lys Arg site precedes an alpha helical structure. The C-peptide is presumed to be flexible and the large number of charged residues not to form salt bridges to basic residues within insulin. Within this model it is notable that the two processing sites lie in close proximity to one another.

Intracellular Site of Proinsulin Conversion

Newly synthesized preproinsulin is directed to the endoplasmic reticulum (ER) by the binding of its signal peptide to the signal recognition particle (Fig. 2). After translocation into the ER lumen, the signal peptide is rapidly removed and folding of nascent proinsulin and formation of the three disulfide bonds occurs. Unlike many secreted proteins, insulin does not appear to undergo posttranslational glycosylation, phosphorylation, or sulfation. Proinsulin travels from the ER through the *cis*, *medial*, and *trans* Golgi by a vesicular transport mechanism, probably by bulk flow. In the *trans* Golgi network (TGN) the prohormone appears to condense into electron-dense aggregates, which become enveloped in membrane-bearing partial clathrin coats. The enveloped material then pinches off to form immature secretory granules (condensing vacuoles). Further maturation of the granule is characterized by the loss of clathrin coating, condensation of the electron-dense core, and the appearance in some granules of rhomboid crystals typical of insulin (Fig. 2). Arvan and colleagues have postulated that membrane remodeling accompanies the removal of the clathrin coat and that resultant vesicles might traffic back to the TGN and can undergo constitutive exocytosis (Fig. 3). Other models envisage the fusion of immature granules to form larger structures with concomitant shedding of membrane. The evidence for either model, however, is indirect and further elucidation may depend on the generation of suitable markers for the granule membrane, which at present are not available.

Subcellular fractionation, immunoelectron microscopy, and pulse chase radiolabeling studies all point to the secretory granule as being the major site of proinsulin conversion into insulin. A minor

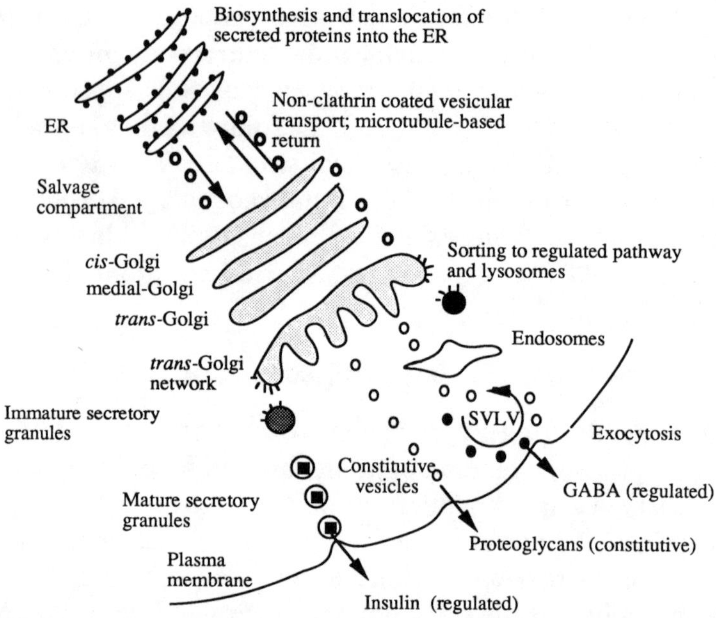

Fig. 2. The secretory pathway in the pancreatic b-cell. Preproinsulin is translocated into the lumen of the endoplasmic reticulum and the presequence removed. Sorting of proinsulin into the regulated pathway of secretion occurs at the level of the trans Golgi network (TGN) in regions of the membrane bearing a partial clathrin coat. The granules are typically large (250–300 nm), have an electron-dense core, and are a prominent feature in the cell since they remain in the cytoplasm for extended periods. Proteins which do not aggregate or interact with specific receptors in the TGN may exit in small vesicles (50–100 nm) to endosomal structures or go directly to the plasma membrane. The latter pathway may represent a default route that is responsible for constitutive secretion. The former may give rise to synaptic vesicle-like vesicles found in neuroendocrine cells that are responsible for the regulated exocytosis of GABA or other biogenic amines.

portion of proinsulin may be converted in pregranule compartments, though this is unlikely to exceed 10–15% of the total conversion and be confined to cleavage at only one of the pairs of basic amino acids to yield a molecule that would still be sorted into the granule. Key factors in the sorting of proinsulin and other secretory granule proteins into the regulated pathway may be the pH and free Ca^{2+} concen-

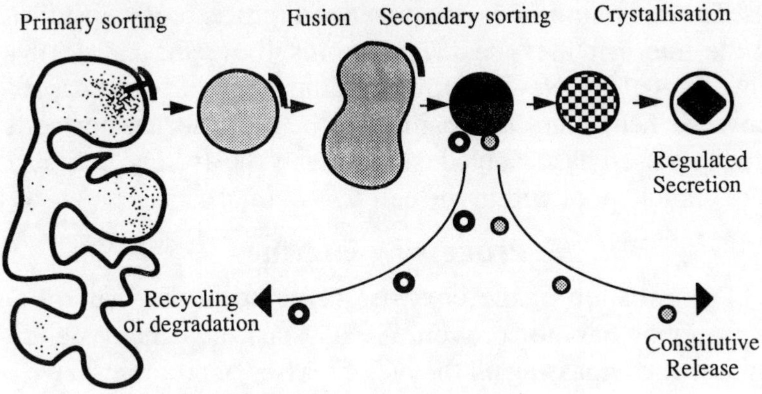

Fig. 3. A model of granule maturation. The nascent secretory granule bears a partial clathrin coat and has a protein core of an amorphous nature. Maturation is characterized by uncoating of the membrane, and condensation and crystallization of the matrix. These changes might simply reflect dissociation of the clathrin coat from the outside and proteolytic conversion of proinsulin to insulin inside. Indirect evidence, however, suggests that immature granules can fuse with one another, and that granule membrane and key catalytic components within it may be removed by vesicle budding from either the nascent granule or fused nascent granules. Such budded vesicles may be recycled to the Golgi, delivered to lysosomes, or undergo exocytosis. Their fluid phase is likely to contain more soluble granule core components and thus constitute a secondary sorting process.

tration in the TGN that induce aggregation of the proteins. A gradient of decreasing pH and increasing Ca^{2+} appears to exist between the various compartments of the Golgi stack to the mature granule. Apart from the involvement of the vacuolar proton translocase and other ion conductance pathways little is known about how such gradients are established and maintained. pH and Ca^{2+} are also of primary importance in the regulation of the enzymes involved in conversion as discussed below.

In normal rodent islets, more than 95% of newly synthesized proinsulin is sorted into the regulated pathway, which it reaches approx 30 min after its synthesis. Proteolytic processing then proceeds with a $t_{1/2}$ of around 45 min and eventually reaches about 95% completion as indicated from the hormone content of radiolabeled cells. The remaining 5% is comprised of unprocessed proinsulin (2%) and the intermediates, des-31,32-proinsulin (2%), and des-64,65-proinsulin (<1%). Newly-formed granules appear to be capable of exocytosis hence the composition of the radiolabeled hormone secreted in pulse-chase labeled islets reflects the average composition of the granule pool within the cell *(see below).*

Processing Enzymes

The isolation of the enzymes involved in the maturation of prohormones has not proven an easy task and many candidate enzymes encompassing all the major classes of proteases have been proposed at one time or another. Much attention is focused at the moment on a family of serine proteases related to bacterial subtilisins whose members include enzymes capable of cleaving prohormones at Lys Arg and Arg Arg sequences and others which cleave constitutively-secreted proteins at sites marked by the sequence Arg X X Arg. The following review summarizes the molecular cloning of candidate genes and the evidence for the involvement of these enzymes based upon enzymological and cell transfection studies. It is well to remember however that cleavage of Lys Lys or Arg Lys motifs in prohormones are not always easily explained by involvement of members of this family.

The Type 1 and Type 2 Proinsulin Endopeptidases

Ion-exchange chromatography of insulin secretory granule proteins has revealed the presence of two soluble, Ca^{2+}-dependent, acidic endopeptidase activities capable of correctly processing human proinsulin in vitro to give insulin *(5).* The activity designated type 1 cleaves exclusively on the C-terminal side of the Arg^{31} Arg^{32} sequence of proinsulin, whereas the type 2 activity cleaves predominantly on the C-terminal side of the Lys^{64} Arg^{65} sequence. The exposed basic residues are then removed by the action of carboxy peptidase H to produce insulin *(6)* (Fig. 4).

Classification of the type 1 and type 2 endopeptidase activities by inhibitor studies has been inconclusive. Phenylmethylsulphonylfluoride (PMSF) and diisopropylfluorophosphate (DFP) are not inhibitory, neither is pepstatin A. Both activities display some thiol character in that they are inhibited by low concentrations of Hg^{2+} and organomercurials but not by alkylating agents (*N*-ethylmaleimide,

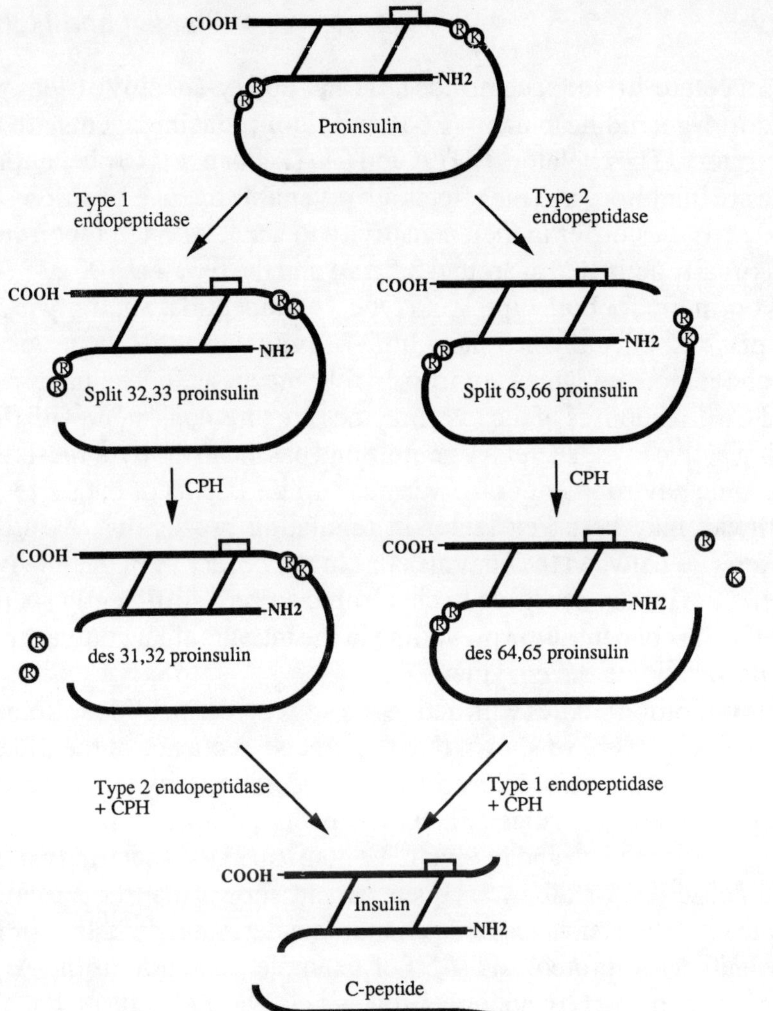

Fig. 4. Reaction pathway for proinsulin conversion. After initial cleavage of the paired basic sequences, the COOH-terminal amino acids are very rapidly removed by carboxypeptidase activity. A second round of endopeptidase and carboxypeptidase action produces insulin, C-peptide, and free amino acids. The right hand branch of the pathway may be favored in compartments such as the Golgi where type 1 activity is limited by low ambient Ca^{2+}. The left hand branch may be favored in secretory granules as a kinetic advantage is produced by the preference of the type 2 enzyme for des 31,32 proinsulin over proinsulin. The relative amounts of the intermediates des 31,32 proinsulin and des 64,65 proinsulin found in the cell may be a complex function of the relative activities of type 1 and type 2 enzymes, their kinetic properties, and the sequence in which the enzymes are activated or inactivated in the cell.

iodoacetate or iodoacetamide). Trans-epoxy-succinyl-l-leucylamido-(4-guanidino)butane (E64) and thiol reducing agents are not inhibitory. The chelators EDTA and CDTA but not 1,10 phenanthroline are inhibitory and the effects are reversible by Ca^{2+} addition. The two activities differ in their sensitivity to Ca^{2+}, with the type 1 half-maximally activated at around 2.5 m*M* and the type 2 at 100 μ*M*. The pH optimum for both type 1 and type 2 endopeptidase activity is 5.5. At pH 7.4 both enzymes show little activity and at pH values of 8.0 or above both enzymes are irreversibly inactivated. The pH profile and Ca^{2+} responses of the two enzymes are thus consistent with their being active in the secretory granule and has led to the hypothesis that the ionic environment of the various compartments of the secretory pathway may be a key factor in regulating processing. A further difference between the enzymes lies in the observation that the type 2 enzyme is very sensitive to chaotropic anions, sufficiently so, that the Cl^- ion concentration prevailing in the intragranular compartment could inactivate the enzyme *(12)*.

Inhibition studies with active-site-directed tripeptide sulfonium salt derivatives have shown that the precise sequence at the dibasic site is an important determinant of the specificity of these two endopeptidase activities *(7)*. Experiments performed with mutant proinsulins in vitro and in vivo have confirmed the specificity of the two activities for dibasic sequences and shown that the structural context of the cleavage site is crucial in determining whether or not it is subject to proteolysis *(8)*. For example, mutation of the Arg^{31} Arg^{32} site to Arg Gly not only prevents cleavage at that site but also reduces the susceptibility of the Lys^{64} Arg^{65} site to proteolytic attack. Since these sites are probably in close spatial proximity (Fig. 1), it is conceivable that the Arg^{32} to Gly mutation could affect the accessibility of the type 2 endopeptidase to the Lys^{64} Arg^{65} site or that the induced conformation is no longer suitable for cleavage *(4)*.

The idea that conformational changes in the peptide backbone around the dibasic sites affect the susceptibility to proteolytic attack is further borne out by the finding that the type 2 activity preferentially cleaves the intermediate des-31,32-proinsulin over intact proinsulin, whereas the type 1 activity recognizes the des-64,65-proinsulin intermediate and proinsulin to a similar extent *(9)*. A consequence of this may be that, of the two processing pathways available (Fig. 4), conversion via the des-31,32-proinsulin intermediate is more favored (Fig. 4). It has been argued *(9)* that this is consistent with the detection of higher levels of des-31,32-proinsulin compared to des-64,65-proinsulin in the pancreas and in the circulation of humans *(10)*, however further kinetic data and cell biological studies are needed to establish this point.

The activities of the proinsulin type 1 and 2 endopeptidases are not confined to proinsulin. The insulin granule also contains chromogranin A, a secretory protein whose function may be related to autocrine or paracrine regulation within the islet *(11)*. In the β-cell it is processed at Lys Arg sites and its products cosecreted with insulin *(12)*. The pH, Ca^{2+}-dependence and inhibitor profile of the processing in vitro by granule lysates suggest the involvement of the type 2 endopeptidase activity. The type 2 endopeptidase also processes POMC to a series of products similar to those produced in the neurointermediate lobe of the pituitary *(13)*. POMC transfected into pancreatic β-cells is processed in a similar manner *(14)*. The type 1 activity is capable of converting liver proalbumin to albumin by cleavage at an Arg Arg site *(15)*. A naturally occurring proalbumin mutant in which the Arg Arg site is replaced by Arg Gln is not processed by either the type 1 or type 2 endopeptidase *(15)*. The type 1 and 2 enzymes thus both recognize pairs of basic amino acids as sites for cleavage in proproteins and have a broad substrate specificity. There are differences in their relative abilities to cleave at particular dibasic sites, some of which may relate to the sequence of amino acids at the point of cleavage, and some relating to regulation by pH and Ca^{2+}.

Molecular Cloning of Proprotein Endopeptidases

Kex2

The key to the molecular cloning of the enzymes responsible for the endoproteolytic conversion of proinsulin was provided by genetic studies in conjugation-deficient yeast strains and the subsequent discovery of mammalian homologs of the defective gene *KEX2*.

In the yeast *Saccharomyces cerevisiae*, maturation of α-mating factor and prokiller toxin requires cleavage at both Lys Arg and Arg Arg residues ref. *16* and references therein). The endoprotease involved in this processing has been mapped to the *KEX2* locus by gene complementation studies of conjugation-defective strains that fail to process precursor forms of α-mating factor and killer toxin. The 4118 bp *KEX2* gene encodes a 814 amino acid protein which possesses a hydrophobic signal sequence, a catalytic domain, a P domain, a serine/threonine-rich domain and a transmembrane domain followed by a region rich in acidic amino acids (Fig. 5). Sequence analysis of *KEX2* indicates that the catalytic domain shows striking identity (30%) to the subtilisin family of serine proteases particularly around the active site Asp, His, and Ser residues that correspond to the charge relay system in subtilisin, and the catalytically important Asn residue that stabilizes an intermediate state during catalysis.

Studies on the partially purified enzyme *(17)* have shown that *KEX2* is a Golgi-localized, membrane-associated endopeptidase with a pH optimum of 7.0–7.5 that efficiently hydrolyses synthetic substrates containing Arg Arg and Lys Arg but not Lys Lys or a single Arg residue. The activity is not inhibited by tosyl-lysyl-chloromethylketone (TLCK) or tosyl-phenyl-alanine-chloromethylketone (TPCK), whereas Tyr Ala Lys Arg-chloromethylketone (YAKRCK) is inhibitory at micromolar concentrations. It is resistant to inhibition by PMSF whereas DFP is effective at relatively high concentrations ($K_{1/2}$ = 10 m*M*). The enzyme contains important free thiol groups as indicated by its sensitivity to *p*-chloromercuribenzoate and dithiothreitol (DTT). However unlike classic cysteinyl proteases it is unaffected by mercaptoethanol and epoxide inhibitors such as E64 and is marginally affected by iodoacetic acid and iodoacetamide. The activity is inhibited by Zn^{2+} and other heavy metals including Cu^{2+} and Cd^{2+}. Activity is dependent on Ca^{2+} in the micromolar range and is abolished reversibly by chelators such as EDTA and EGTA but not by 1,10 phenanthroline, an inhibitor of zinc-containing metalloproteases.

The *KEX2* enzyme has been shown to cleave a wide variety of both regulated- and constitutively secreted proproteins at Lys Arg and Arg Arg sites in cell transfection studies. This includes proinsulin *(18)*, proalbumin *(19)*, and POMC *(20)*. The *KEX2* activity also mimics the predicted properties of the proalbumin convertase of hepatocyte microsomes in that it rapidly cleaves the propeptide Arg Gly Val Phe Arg Arg from the N-terminal end of proalbumin but does not cleave physiologically unprocessed human proalbumin variants *(21)*. Antitrypsin Pittsburgh, an inhibitor of in vivo proalbumin cleavage also inhibits *KEX2* in a reversible manner *(21)*.

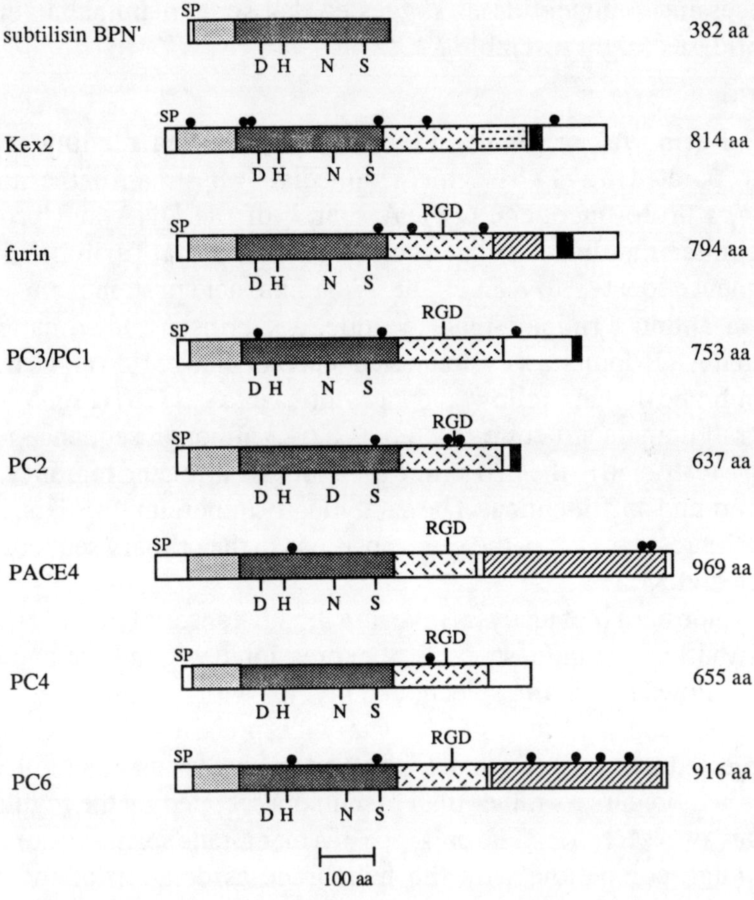

Fig. 5. Structures of subtilisin and subtilisin-related proprotein convertases. The various subregions are designated as follows: signal peptide (SP); proregion (▨); catalytic domain (■); P domain (◪); cysteine-rich region (▨), serine/threonine-rich region (⬚); transmembrane domain (■) and amphiphatic region (■). The catalytic Asp, His, Asn (Asp), and Ser residues are indicated by their single letter code. Putative sites of glycosylation (●) and the ArgGlyAsp sequence implicated in the recognition of fibronectin by its receptor are also shown.

The striking similarity between the processing of mammalian prohormones and the yeast propheromones, the ability of *KEX2* to process mammalian prohormones in cell transfection studies, and the similar inhibitor profiles of *KEX2* and the proinsulin and proalbumin processing endopeptidases suggested that some mammalian endopeptidases might resemble *KEX2*.

Furin

Furin was originally identified as an open reading frame incorporated in a 21 kb fragment immediately upstream of the human *fes/fps* proto-oncogene *(22)*. A search of the DNA and protein sequence databases subsequently revealed that furin had high sequence identity to *KEX2*. The 794 amino acid protein is made up of an amino terminal signal peptide, a subtilisin-related catalytic domain, a P domain, a cysteine rich receptor-like region and a transmembrane domain followed by a cytoplasmic tail *(23)* (Fig. 5). The overall domain structure resembles *KEX2* although sequence identity is restricted to the 270 amino acid subtilisin-related region where it is around 45% identical. The catalytically important Asp, His, Asn, and Ser residues are in the same positions in the primary sequence of furin and *KEX2*.

Northern blot analysis reveals a 4.5 kb transcript of wide tissue distribution, the highest levels of expression being in liver and kidney followed by brain, spleen, and thymus with low levels in heart, muscle, lung, and testes *(24)*. The widespread tissue distribution suggested that furin might be involved in processing constitutively secreted precursors rather than precursors secreted by the regulated pathway of secretion. The presence of a membrane spanning domain, although compatible with the membrane association of the proalbumin convertase, was inconsistent with the solubility of the insulin granule endopeptidases.

The protein encoded by furin mRNA is a Golgi-localized, Ca^{2+}-dependent ($K_{1/2}$ = 200 μ*M*) serine endoprotease with a pH optimum of 6.0–8.5 *(25)*. Activity is reversibly inhibited by EDTA and EGTA, and also inhibited by Zn^{2+}, Hg^{2+}, and the reducing agent DTT. It is not sensitive to the thiol protease inhibitor E64, nor to moderate concentrations of the thiol reagent iodoacetamide. The serine protease inhibitors PMSF and DFP suppress activity but only at high concentrations (10–30 m*M*). The enzyme is able to cleave the fluorogenic peptide Boc-Arg Val Arg Arg-MCA efficiently, but not simple dibasic substrates such as Boc-Leu Lys Arg or Boc-Leu Gly Arg-MCA *(25)*.

Table 2
Substrate Specificity of Furin, PC2, and PC3[a]

Substrate	Enzyme	Cleaved	Partially cleaved	Not cleaved
mPOMC	Furin	PLEFKR ED*		
	PC3	PREGKR ST*	PPKDKR YG*	KNAHKK GQ*
		PLEFKR ED*		PLEFKK ED
	PC2	PREGKR ST*		PLEFKK ED
		PLEFKR ED*		PLEFRK ED
hProrenin	Furin	SQRMKR ST	SQRMKR LT	SQPMKR LT*
				SQPMKR ST
	PC3	SQPMKR LT*		SQPMAR LT
	PC2			SQPMKR LT*
m*Ren2*	Furin	DVRTKR SS	DVRTORSS	DVFTKR SS*
Prorenin	PC3	DVFTKR SS*		DVFTOR SS
		DVRXXR SS		
	PC2			DVFTKR SS*
rProrenin	PC3			GEFIKK SS
hProalbumin	Furin	RGVFRR DA		
hpro-C3	Furin	AARRRR SV		
hPro-β-nerve growth factor	Furin	THRSKR SS		
hPro-von Willebrand factor	Furin	SHRSKR SL*	SHRSKK SL	SHRSKG SL
			SHKSKR SL	SHRSED SL
				SHKSDR SL
pro-factor IX	Furin	LNRPKR YN*		LNRPKT YN
rPlasma prekallikrein	PC3			TKINAR IV
	PC2			
hProrelaxin	PC3	STWSKR SL*		
		HSRKKR QL		
hProgastrin	PC3	ADPSKR QG		ADPSRK QG
	PC2	ADPSRR QG		ADPSRK QG
		ADPSKK QG*		

[a]Cleavage recognition sites are underlined. Where more than one cleavage site is shown, the native sequence(s) are indicated by an asterisk (*).

Cell transfection studies have shown that when furin is coexpressed with precursors having the consensus motif Arg X Lys/Arg Arg in endocrine and nonendocrine cells their cleavage is enhanced (Table 2). For example, processing of human pro-von Willebrand factor

(26), mouse pro-β-nerve growth factor *(27)* and complement pro-C3 and proalbumin *(28)* have been demonstrated in this way. Prorenin containing a simple dibasic cleavage site (Lys Arg) is not processed by cotransfected furin in growth hormone secreting GH_4C_1 cells *(29)* or nonendocrine kidney COS-1 cells *(30)*. Inclusion of an Arg residue in the P4 position, however, permits processing to occur. The minimal motif is probably Arg X X Arg, an hypothesis supported by the finding that replacement of the P2 Arg or P3 Lys of the tetrabasic cleavage site (Arg Lys Arg Arg) of the human insulin receptor with alanine has no effect on processing in unregulated CHO cells, whereas replacing either the P1 or P4 Arg significantly inhibits processing. The Golgi localization and wide tissue distribution of furin mRNA, its processing-site specificity, and proprotein substrate specificity indicate a role in the processing of proprotein precursors as they pass through the *trans*-Golgi, rather than in the conversion of prohormones and other peptides secreted by the regulated pathway.

The human proinsulin B-chain/C-peptide junction (Lys Thr Arg Arg) but not the C-peptide/A-chain junction (Leu Gln Lys Arg) is a substrate for recombinant human furin as assayed in vitro (Bailyes, Thomas, and Hutton; personal communication). It is conceivable that furin acting in the Golgi could also account for the small amount of des 64,65 proinsulin II observed at early time points in pulse-chase studies of rat islets *(5)* since the C-A junction of rat proinsulin II also bears a consensus sequence for this enzyme (Arg X Lys Arg; Table 1). This raises the question of whether the actual levels of furin activity in the pancreatic β-cell are sufficient to contribute to insulin processing and whether its localization overlaps with the compartment involved in sorting of the prohormone. Cell transfection studies, useful though they have been in broadly identifying the substrate specificities of enzymes of the family, have not been particularly informative in this regard since the substrate and enzyme are usually expressed at equimolar concentrations, often under conditions where major perturbations in the integrity of the processing and sorting compartments are occurring.

PC2 and PC3 (PC1)

Soon after the identification of furin as a *KEX2* homolog, two cDNA sequences designated PC2 and PC3 (also termed PC1) were cloned from human and mouse insulinoma and pituitary cDNA libraries. The approach in each case depended on application of the polymerase chain reaction (PCR) with primers corresponding to sequences surrounding the active site residues of *KEX2* and furin (*see* ref. *31* and references therein). PC2 and PC3 encode 638 and 753 amino acid proteins, respectively, consisting of a signal peptide and a subtilisin-related catalytic domain similar to furin and *KEX2* (Fig. 5). There is no apparent transmembrane domain and the C-terminal domain is similar to that of furin and *KEX2* only in as much as it is rich in acidic amino acids. However, both sequences contain a potential C-terminal amphiphilic helical segment similar to the putative membrane anchor of carboxypeptidase H *(32)*. The subtilisin-related domains of PC2 and PC3 exhibit 45–65% amino acid identity with other members of the subtilisin-related family and the Asp-His-Ser catalytic triad is placed in an equivalent position. In PC2, however, the catalytically important Asn residue is replaced by an Asp residue.

Northern blot analysis of PC2 reveals mRNA transcripts of 2.8 and 5 kb in insulinoma, pituitary, hypothalamus and brain with low levels present in adrenal, kidney, liver, and exocrine pancreas *(33)*. The principal forms of PC3 mRNA are 3 and 5 kb forms that are abundant in pituitary, hypothalamus and adrenal, present to a lesser extent in insulinoma and low in whole brain, kidney, liver and exocrine pancreas *(33)*. The association of PC2 and PC3 mRNAs with neuroendocrine tissues suggests they are more likely candidates for endopeptidases associated with the regulated pathway of secretion. *In situ* hybridization studies have demonstrated a distinct localization of the PC2 and PC3 transcripts in pituitary and brain. Thus, whereas both PC2 and PC3 are found in the intermediate lobe of the pituitary, albeit at different levels, only PC3 is easily detected in the anterior lobe. In extrahypothalamic regions of the brain, including cortex, hippocampus, thalamus, and spinal cord, PC2 transcripts predominate over PC3 although many regional variations are detected *(34)*. The specific combinations of putative convertase expression suggest that specific enzymatic pathways are involved in precursor processing and that these combinations are responsible for region-specific differences of posttranslational processing.

Cell transfection studies have shown that both PC cDNAs can code for functional enzymes (Table 2). PC2 and PC3 can process

POMC at dibasic amino acid sites in cell lines that secrete the proprotein either in a regulated or constitutive manner *(35)*. POMC is processed into ACTH and β-LPH along with small amounts of β-endorphin by PC3, the same set of peptides known to be produced in the anterior pituitary in vivo. Coexpression of POMC, PC2, and PC3 results in the intermediate pituitary pattern of cleavages. Further evidence for the essential role of PC2 and PC3 in processing POMC has been provided by experiments with antisense constructs of PC3, which reduce its expression in AtT20 cells and lead to suppression of POMC processing *(36)*. PC3, but not PC2, is capable of processing human type 2 prorelaxin on the C-terminal side of Lys Arg and Arg Lys Lys Arg sequences, when expressed in human kidney cells *(37)*. Mouse prorenin is cleaved efficiently by PC3 at its Lys Arg activation site in regulated GH_4C_1 cells *(38)*. The prorenin cleavage site mutant Arg Arg is cleaved but not the cleavage site mutants, Lys Lys, Arg Lys, Gln Arg, Arg Gln, or Lys Arg Pro *(38)*. PC3 is also capable of cleaving mutant mouse prorenins in GH_4C_1 cells at the monobasic Arg X X Arg site *(39)*.

PC2 expressed in *Xenopus* oocytes can hydrolyze the fluorogenic substrates, Boc-Gln Arg Arg-amidomethyl coumarin and Boc-Gly Lys Arg-amidomethyl coumarin but not Boc-Gln Gly Arg- amidomethyl coumarin, with the activity directed against the Lys Arg substrate three times that detected with the Arg Arg substrate *(40)*. The activity is activated by millimolar concentrations of Ca^{2+} ions, has a pH optimum of 5.5 with no activity below pH 4.0 or above pH 7.0. Its inhibitor profile is similar to that reported for *KEX2 (40)*. Studies performed with proinsulin as substrate show a very similar profile and one that resembles the activity of the type 2 endopeptidase. Likewise, PC3 expressed in *Xenopus* oocytes has been shown to have the same specificity, inhibitor profile, pH optimum, and Ca^{2+}-dependency as the type 1 endopeptidase activity when assayed against human proinsulin *(41)*.

Antibodies raised to the catalytic domain of rat PC2 have shown that PC2 immunoreactivity is localized to insulin secretory granules and coincides with type 2 activity on ion-exchange chromatography of insulinoma secretory granule proteins *(42)*. The identity of PC2 with the type 2 activity is further supported by the ability of PC2 antisera to immunoprecipitate type 2 but not type 1 activity from extracts of insulinoma secretory granules *(43)*.

In cell transfection studies, PC2 selectively cleaves rat proinsulin I at the C-peptide/A-chain (Lys Arg) junction, whereas PC3 generates mature insulin but cleaves preferentially at the B-chain/C-peptide (Arg Arg) junction *(43)*. This is consistent with them being identical to the type 2 and type 1 proinsulin endopeptidases, respectively. The ability of PC3/type 1 to cleave at the C-peptide/A-chain junction in this study may be owing to the presence of an Arg residue at the P4 position relative to the cleavage site (Arg Gln Lys Arg) in the rat proinsulin sequence compared to the human cleavage site (Leu Gln Lys Arg) (Table 1).

Present evidence thus strongly support the idea that the type 1 proinsulin endopeptidase is PC3 (PC1) and the type 2 enzyme is PC2. Their molecular characteristics, tissue distribution, and intracellular localization are entirely consistent with their role as proteases of the regulated pathway of secretion responsible for cleavage of substrates at sites marked by Lys Arg and Arg Arg sequences. The original inference that type 1 activity recognizes only Arg Arg sequences and that type 2 prefers Lys Arg sites is borne out only in so far as it relates to the specific substrate human proinsulin. With other substrates, both Arg Arg and Lys Arg sequences are recognized by both enzymes, with activity further enhanced by the presence of basic amino acids upstream from the dibasic pair. What the basis is for the preference of one enzyme or the other for a particular substrate is unclear, nevertheless it appears to be of primary importance in determining what products are generated from precursors that incorporate multiple processing sites and alternative processing pathways.

PACE4, PC4, PC5, and PC6

Other members of the subtilisin-related protease family that have been identified include PACE4 *(31)*, PC4 *(44,45)*, PC5 *(46)* and PC6 *(47)*. PACE4 was isolated from human osteosarcoma tissue and encodes a 969 amino acid protein that contains similar domains to other subtilisin-related serine proteases (Fig. 5). Unique features are an extended signal peptide, a relatively large C-terminal cysteine rich region, and no obvious transmembrane domain or C-terminal amphiphatic α-helix. It has a widespread tissue distribution, with the highest levels found in liver.

PC4 was isolated from rat and mouse testis cDNA and encodes a 654 (rat) or 655 (mouse) amino acid protein. Northern blot analysis has shown that PC4 mRNA expression is restricted to the germ cells of the testis where it is developmentally regulated *(44,45)*. The nature of its native substrate or cleavage specificity remains elusive. PC4 is not able to cleave prorenin at its Lys Arg processing site or a prorenin mutant with an Arg X Lys Arg sequence in cell transfection studies *(45)*.

Northern blot analysis of rPC5 demonstrates a ubiquitous pattern of tissue distribution similar to that of furin mRNA *(46)*. The highest levels are found in the adrenal cortex and gut with lower levels in many other peripheral tissues and tissues of the central nervous system. No sequence information on PC5 has been reported at the time of preparation of this review (June, 1993).

PC6 was isolated from mouse intestinal cDNA and encodes a 915 amino acid protein. It shows the greatest sequence similarity to PACE4 and contains similar domains such as the C-terminal cysteine-rich region (Fig. 5). Northern blot analysis indicates that PC6 transcripts are most abundant in the intestine but are also present in many other tissues and cell lines. Coexpression of PC6 and native or mutant prorenin in GH_4C_1 cells results in conversion of native prorenin (X X Lys Arg) to mature renin and enhances the cleavage of a prorenin mutant (Arg X Lys Arg). The prorenin mutant, Arg X X Arg, is cleaved with a very low efficiency and X X Gln Arg not at all. The cleavage profile of PC6 is therefore similar to that of PC3 (Table 2) *(39)*.

Further investigation of these newer family members are clearly warranted and in the absence of information on their catalytic properties, cellular localization, and tissue distribution one cannot discount them having a role, if not in processing of proinsulin, then in other islet prohormones or in the processing of proproteins that are critical to the maintenance of the secretory machinery of the cell.

Biosynthesis and Posttranslational Modification of the Subtilisin-Related Endopeptidases

KEX2 and furin are both synthesized as larger precursors that are subjected to autocatalytic processing at basic amino acid sites to produce the mature protein (Fig. 6). A comparison of the structures of PC2 and PC3 with *KEX2* and furin suggested that they would also be subjected to posttranslational maturation at sites marked by basic

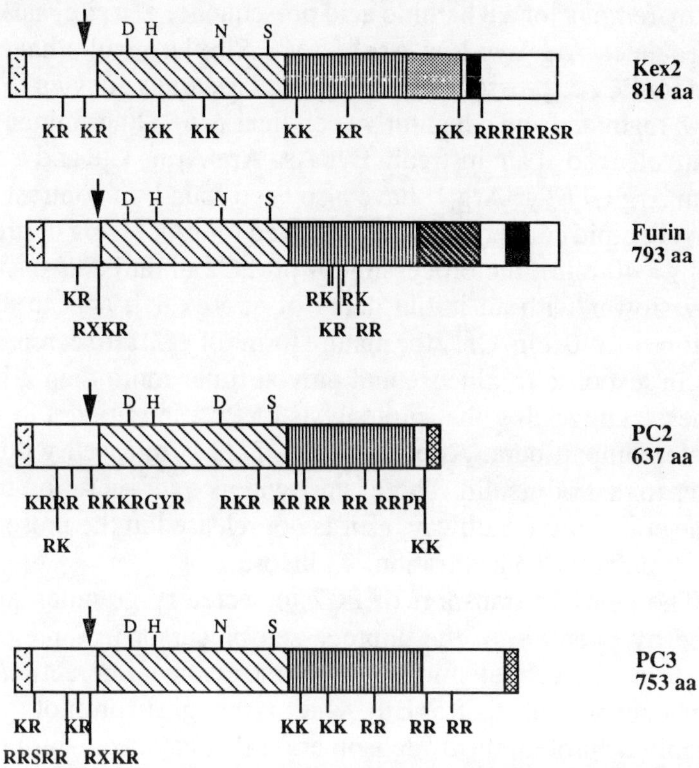

Fig. 6. Schematic representation of KEX-2 and vertebrate furin, PC2 and PC3 proteins showing the positions of basic amino acid sites. The various subregions are designated as follows: signal peptide (□); proregion (□); catalytic domain (▧); P domain (▥), cysteine-rich region (▧), serine/threonine-rich region (▒), transmembrane domain (■) and amphiphatic region (▩). Amino acids are shown by their single letter code. X, variant residues. The positions of N-terminal proteolysis are indicated by arrows.

amino acid residues (Fig. 6). This has been confirmed by N-terminal sequence analysis of mature PC2 and PC3 from bovine adrenal *(48)*, anglerfish islets *(49)* and rat insulinoma *(42)*. Mature PC2 begins at amino acid residue 109 after the Arg Arg Lys Arg site and mature PC3 at residue 111 after the Arg Ser Lys Arg site.

Studies on the biosynthesis of PC2 in isolated rat islets of Langerhans have shown that it is synthesized initially as a 75 kDa precursor that undergoes limited proteolytic processing to a 65 kDa form by removal of a 84 amino acid prosequence at a site marked by the sequence Arg Lys Lys Arg^{108} *(50)*. Similar results have been found for PC2 expressed in microinjected *Xenopus* oocytes *(51)* and in both regulated and constitutive cell lines *(46)*. Other minor forms that are cleaved at an upstream Lys Arg Arg Arg^{81} site and a downstream Arg Gly Tyr Arg^{111} have also been found. In contrast to the relatively rapid conversion rates observed for processing of proinsulin ($t_{1/2}$ = 40 min), the processing of proPC2 in rat islets is significantly slower with an initial delay of approx 1 h and an approx half-time of 140 min. Only the mature forms of PC2 are secreted from islets in response to glucose and only at times more than 2 h after synthesis, suggesting that proteolysis of PC2 is initiated in a pregranule compartment. After this time, PC2 is released with a $t_{1/2}$ similar to that of insulin. There is no evidence for secretion of PC2 via the constitutive pathway, as it is not released in the presence of a substimulatory concentration of glucose.

The delay in transport of PC2 to secretory granules may be caused by retention of the unprocessed precursor in a pregranule compartment. Such retention might be the result of interactions with ER resident proteins such as BiP, which is thought to promote protein assembly or protein disulfide isomerase that catalyzes thiol oxidation and disulfide exchange reactions. Retention in the ER might also result from slow removal of glycosyl residues from N-linked oligosaccharides, which has been shown in the case of some secretory proteins to be necessary for transport to the Golgi complex.

The biosynthesis of PC3 has been studied in both regulated and constitutively secreting cell lines. In contrast to the slow processing of PC2 in rat islets, PC3 is rapidly converted to a 80 kDa protein by removal of the 83 amino acid prosegment presumably at a site marked by the sequence Arg Ser Lys Arg^{110} *(46)*. PC3 also undergoes C-terminal processing *(52)*, possibly at one of several pairs of basic residues that occur in the molecule (Fig. 6). The C-terminally truncated 66 kDa protein produced is the major form found in the islets of Langerhans, although it is not known which of these forms is active.

The nature of the processing events involved in the maturation of PC2 and PC3 are not at present clear. The putative cleavage sites in PC2 and PC3 possess the furin recognition motif and are highly conserved in evolution arguing for activation by such an enzyme in the *trans* Golgi immediately prior to sorting. Mutation of the catalytically important Asp^{167} residue of PC2 to Asn produces an inactive enzyme yet does not affect its processing from the 75 kDa precursor to the mature 68 kDa form in oocytes arguing that activation may occur in trans *(51)*. Furin itself, however, does not appear to be involved since neither a catalytically active recombinant furin incubated with proPC2 in vitro nor cotransfection of PC2 and furin results in changes in the rate of proPC2 conversion (Guest, Bennett, Thomas, and Hutton; unpublished findings).

KEX2 and furin are also subject to posttranslational processing at similar sites by a reaction thought to be autocatalytic and perhaps intramolecular (*see* ref. *31*). Whatever the mechanism in the case of PC2 and PC3, questions remain as to whether the pro-forms, intermediate forms, and truncated forms of the enzymes have intrinsic activity, and if so, whether they differ in kinetic properties from the predominant mature forms found in secretory granules. There is the additional question of where the pro and intermediate forms accumulate in the cell and whether they encounter an environment that is compatible with activity. The answers to such questions are clearly of importance in establishing whether such posttranslational modification of the enzymes play a regulatory role in their activation or sorting to secretory granules.

Translation of insulin mRNA in the β-cell undergoes rapid and marked changes in response to ambient glucose concentrations. PC3 biosynthesis responds in a similar manner, whereas PC2 and carboxypeptidase H change to a much lesser extent *(53,54)*. It follows that the ratio of PC2 to proinsulin in nascent granules will vary with stimulus, an effect that is compounded by the fact that delivery of PC2 to the site of granule assembly in the TGN is delayed relative to that of proinsulin and PC3. Since the V_{max} of the proinsulin endopeptidases appears to be rate limiting, it follows that the initial rate of conversion will depend not only on the magnitude of glucose stimulus but also its duration. This would affect the average composition of the different molecular forms of insulin in the cell for a number of hours after stimulus. This in turn would be reflected in the composition of the insulin peptides secreted since both fully mature and newly formed granules appear competent for exocytosis. Other contributory factors will include again the intensity of stimulus for exocytosis and the overall pool size of stored granules. It is clear from such considerations that variation in the rates of secretion of proinsulin, insulin, and the processing intermediates may be expected under normal circumstances in response to metabolic demands.

Whether such differences in concentration of the intermediates is of physiological significance is not clear. For a start the composition of the secreted forms of insulin is likely to be species-dependent because of the differences in basic amino acid sequence at the P4 position (Table 1). It is thus unlikely to form the basis of an evolutionarily-conserved regulatory mechanism. The whole question of the functional relevance of the secretion of small amounts of proinsulin and processing intermediates remains open in the absence of specific effects attributable to them. These molecules bind the insulin receptor with low affinity and produce insulin-like responses of low potency. However, their half-lives are around tenfold longer than insulin, which means that they can constitute up to a third of the total circulating insulin immunoreactivity in spite of the fact that they account for only 3% of the insulin peptides secreted from the islets.

Prohormone Secretion in Islet Cell Pathology

Proinsulin Gene Mutations

Three mutations have been described that affect the processing of proinsulin to insulin and result in hyperproinsulinaemia. Proinsulin Tokyo results from a point mutation in the codon for residue 65 (CGC to CAC) changing the Lys^{64} Arg^{65} site to Lys^{64} His^{65}. This results in minimal changes in glucose homeostasis and markedly elevated circulating levels of proinsulin-like material *(64)*. Proinsulin Kyoto also results from a point mutation in the codon for residue 65 (CGC to CTC; Arg to Leu) *(65)*. Cleavage at the C-peptide/A-chain junction is prevented resulting in elevation of circulating proinsulin-like materials. A less-readily explained mutant is proinsulin Providence (His^{10} to Asp), resulting from a codon change CAC to GAC *(66)*. This residue is essential for the formation of insulin hexamers and mutation has been reported in one experimental situation to affect the sorting of the nascent proinsulin to secretory granules, thus bypassing normal processing and regulated secretion of the hormone.

All the above mutations may predispose to the development of NIDDM but not all carriers show glucose intolerance, most probably because, as heterozygotes, they produce normal insulin as well as the mutant and have the physiological capacity to compensate. To date only six families with these mutations have been described so it is unlikely that such mutations are frequent causes of diabetes.

Insulin Dependent Diabetes Mellitus

Insulin-dependent diabetes mellitus (IDDM) is the result of the specific loss of insulin-secreting pancreatic β cells probably caused by an autoimmune reaction. Antibodies to a 64 kDa protein, glutamic acid decarboxylase (GAD) *(55)*, insulin, and carboxypeptidase H *(56)* are commonly found in newly diagnosed patients. T-cell proliferative responses to a 38 kDa protein associated with secretory granule membranes are also seen in a large proportion of newly diagnosed type 1 diabetic patients *(57)*. The possibility that proteins associated with the secretory pathway may be prime targets, either involving dense core secretory granules or synaptic vesicle-like vesicles in the islets (GAD) has been advanced and raises the question of whether the type 1/PC3 or type 2/PC2 processing enzymes may be recognized by the humoral or cell-mediated autoimmune response.

Identical twins of patients with IDDM who are discordant for diabetes have elevated circulating levels of proinsulin and the processing intermediates in comparison to a control population. This occurs irrespective of whether the twin subsequently develops diabetes or not and correlates with the presence of islet cell antibodies in these subjects. Autoantibodies directed at the processing enzymes could easily inhibit their activity, however it is difficult to envisage this in a cellular context since the endopeptidases and carboxypeptidase H are released from the cell following exocytosis and not recycled as are other granule membrane proteins. Perhaps a more likely explanation is that such changes occur secondarily to either an active, but limited, autoimmune attack targeted at other β-cell antigens or to a loss in β-cell number or function stemming from a previous attack that was not sufficient to produce clinical diabetes or significant glucose intolerance.

Mild Noninsulin-Dependent Diabetes Mellitus

In mild noninsulin-dependent diabetes mellitus (NIDDM) in which β-cell number, if not function, is largely preserved, the ratio of intact proinsulin and 32,33-split proinsulin to insulin in plasma is elevated in the fasting state *(58)*. The contribution of proinsulin and the intermediates is sufficiently great that it may disguise the fact that the actual level of circulating insulin is depressed even though the total insulin immunoreactivity in the circulation is increased. Disproportionately high levels of pro-forms in the circulation are similarly observed upon glucose tolerance testing in these individuals, suggesting that the origin of the changes lies in the composition of the hormones secreted from the β-cell. Glucose intolerant individuals in the 40–64-yr-old age group show similar changes to the frankly diabetic individuals, which suggests that the changes are not secondary to persistent hyperglycemia and may be an early marker of deteriorating islet function.

The changes in β-cell function which results in elevated secretion of pro-forms of insulin in these circumstances is not clear though a number of testable models can be envisaged (Figs. 7 and 8). It has been suggested that the greater demand for insulin secretion from the β-cell population posed by decreased islet number or insulin resistance results in the release of a proportionately higher number of "immature" granules in which processing was incomplete *(59)*. Given that the granule population is a dynamic one and that nascent granules are as competent in exocytosis as mature granules, then the relative amounts of proinsulin and intermediates released will be a complex function of the rates of exocytosis, *de novo* granule biogenesis, the granule pool size, and rates of conversion in the maturing granule population. Changes in the composition of the secreted protein with diabetes could be viewed as a reflection of a normal physiological response to increased secretory activity or biosynthetic stimulus. Against this model is the experimental evidence that, with partial pancreatectomy, the relative proportions of proinsulin and insulin are unchanged. The increased demand imposed may not be commensurate to that in prediabetic individuals, who may have suffered a far greater loss in β-cell mass and have concomitant insulin resistance. There is the further consideration that in the diseased pancreas, secretion may be occurring from a small subpopulation of healthy islets or from only a subpopulation of β-cells within the islet that are capable of mounting a secretory response to the prevailing levels of glycemia.

The possibility that a defect in the rate or extent of proinsulin processing could account for this phenomenon has been raised and in one instance changes in the activity of the type 1 endopeptidase (PC3 / PC1) has been implicated *(53)*. The proportion of the circulating prohormone relative to total insulin immunoreactivity in the circulation typically changes from approx 10–30% in control subjects to 30–50% in diabetic or glucose-intolerant individuals. Because of differences in circulating half-life this would represent a change in the mean composition of prohormone secreted from the islet from 1–3% to 3–5%, that is a difference, at the most, between 99 and 95% conversion of the prohormone. It is difficult to see that changes in the activity of the processing enzymes *per se*, whether brought about by changes in translation or transcription or competitive inhibition by other granule constituents could result in such a subtle change. The relative amounts of proinsulin, PC2, and PC3 in nascent granules are expected to vary in accordance with the differences in the response of their biosynthesis to stimuli and differences in their rates of delivery to the secretory granule as discussed above. Given this, the question really becomes, why the composition of the secreted peptide changes so little. In this context it is important to recall how little we know of the cellular biology of secretory granule biogenesis, especially with respect to the movement of membrane components in the early stages of granule maturation. It could be that the proinsulin and proinsulin intermediates come not from maturing granules, but in fact from other elements of the secretory pathway that may perform regulated exocytosis. Other models based on the observation that a small number of cells in islets contain proinsulin but not insulin immunoreactivity can be formulated. Whether the proportion of such cells in the islet or the threshold of their secretory response to stimuli is altered in diabetes is unknown.

Islet Cell Neoplasia

Hyperproinsulinaemia is also found in patients with islet cell neoplasias, the levels exceeding those observed in diabetic subjects often by two orders of magnitude. Hyperinsulinaemia is also usually

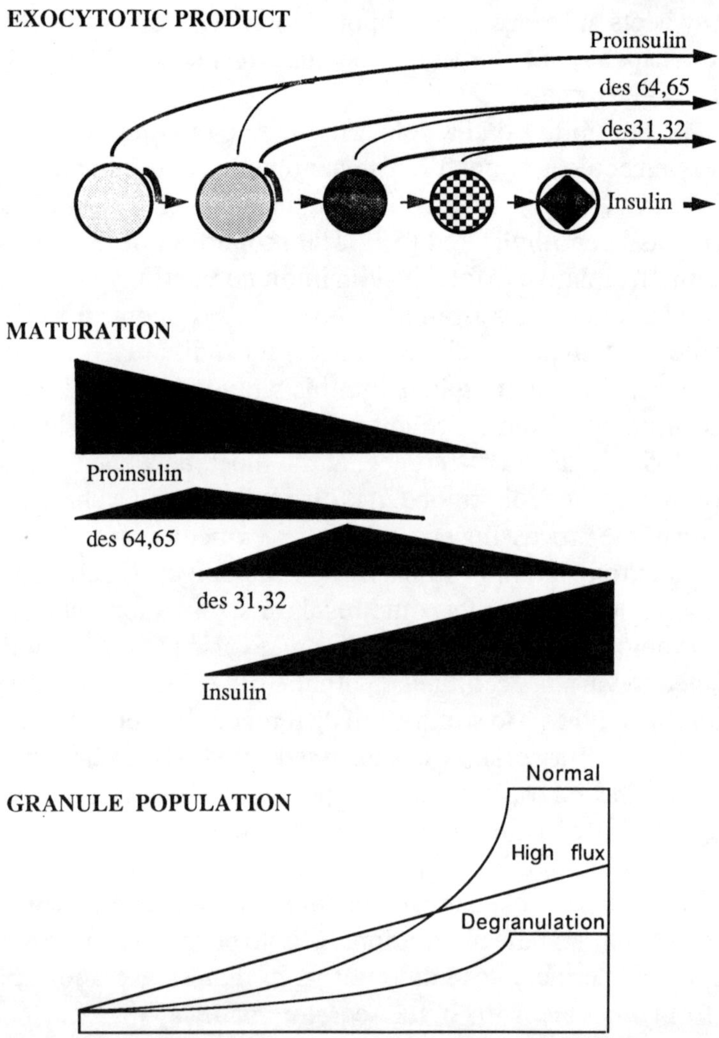

Fig. 7. Mechanism of release of proinsulin and processing intermediates: Conveyor belt model. This model proposes that all secretory granules from the nascent vesicle to the mature granule are competent in exocytosis and that the composition of the released product is a direct function of the time between when it was formed and when it fused with the plasma membrane (upper panel). The relative composition of the precursor, intermediates, and products found in pulse-chase experiments is shown in the centre panel and is a reflection of the order of activation of the type 1 and type 2 endopeptidase and their kinetic properties. The absolute amounts of each component released is a product of the relative composition of granule

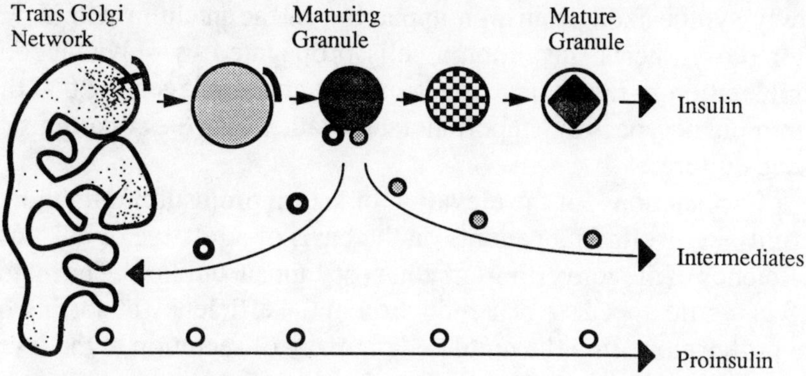

Fig. 8. Mechanism of release of proinsulin, and processing intermediates: Sorting defect model. This model envisages that insulin, proinsulin and intermediates arise from different vesicular compartments. An absolute or relative failure to sort the prohormone into the regulated pathway, such as occurs in the case of insulinomas, results in the constitutive secretion of proinsulin and any processing intermediates that may have formed in the Golgi. Mature granules are envisaged as the source of completely processed material that is released in a regulated manner. The secretion of intermediates is envisaged to occur as a result of regulated exocytosis of vesicles formed by secondary sorting.

present, though to a lesser extent and the circulating proinsulin/insulin ratio can reach very high levels.

Experimental models of islet cell tumors provide some insight into the mechanism involved. βTC3 cells, a β tumor cell line established from insulinomas derived from transgenic mice carrying a hybrid insulin promoter-simian virus-40 large T antigen gene, exhibit a predominantly constitutive release of proinsulin, with up to 80% of

---

form that is undergoing exocytosis and its frequency distribution within the cell (lower panel). Within this model, distortion of the mean composition of the secreted product could arise from changes in the rate of maturation or relative distribution of the various granule forms. Two possible scenarios are depicted that would result in increased secretion of proinsulin and the intermediates. One corresponds to effective degranulation which affects principally the mature granule population. The other depicts a situation where synthesis keeps pace with release but where the mean time of residence of granules in the cell is reduced.

newly synthesized proinsulin appearing in the medium within 1 h after biosynthesis. Insulinoma cells propagated by subcutaneous implantation in rats behave in a similar manner, suggesting that the tumor phenotype is the important factor rather than the conditions of tissue culture.

Explanations for the elevation of serum proinsulin immunoreactivity in insulinoma patients on the basis of a relative or absolute deficiency of the converting enzymes *(60)* appear unlikely. The major defect would appear to be a reduction in the efficiency of sorting of the prohormone into the regulated pathway of secretion at the level of the TGN. Since conversion of proinsulin to insulin occurs principally in the granule compartment, the expectation would be that proinsulin would be released constitutively, that the $t_{1/2}$ of insulin formation would be normal and that insulin itself would be released in a regulated manner. This seems to be the case for the transplantable rat insulinoma and is also supported by the observation that the percentage of serum proinsulin is higher in the fasting state than after stimulation (i.e., after release of stored insulin) and most markedly elevated in cases having poorly granulated tumor cells *(61)*. A second defect appears to relate to the observation that endocrine tumors have decreased granulation and high basal release of polypeptides from dense cored secretory granules. The ensuing high rate of turnover of the granule population as depicted in Fig. 7 would again favor the release of proinsulin and processing intermediates.

A common feature of islets from NIDDM patients and human insulinomas is the presence of amyloid deposits composed of islet amyloid polypeptide (IAPP) *(62)*. The IAPP precursor is a normal constituent of β cell secretory granules where it is copackaged along with proinsulin and processed presumably by the same enzymes involved in the conversion of proinsulin to insulin. Porte *(63)* has hypothesized that a defect in the processing enzymes may result in elevated levels of unprocessed IAPP precursor as well as proinsulin, in a form that is unsuitable for release, which could result in its deposition. A further possibility is that increased levels of the IAPP precursor may compete with proinsulin for the processing enzymes. Against these ideas are the observations that the amyloid deposits appear to contain IAPP that is fully processed, circulating levels of IAPP are not significantly elevated in NIDDM and it is unlikely, given the relatively small amounts of IAPP in islets relative to insulin, that it would be an effective competitive inhibitor of conversion.

Conclusion

The proteolytic conversion of human proinsulin to insulin by the pancreatic β-cell occurs at two sites marked by pairs of basic amino acids and is mediated by two distinct endopeptidases designated type 1 and type 2. Processing occurs principally in the secretory granule compartment by virtue of the fact that the enzymes and substrate are concentrated in that compartment and that the enzymes require a high concentration of Ca^{2+} and an acidic pH for activity. Molecular cloning of the enzymes has been achieved using PCR-based screening for mammalian homologues of the yeast pheromone processing enzyme *KEX2*. The type 1 enzyme corresponds to the PC3 gene product and type 2 to the PC2 gene product, both soluble subtilisin-related enzymes. Studies of the biosynthesis of PC2 and PC3 in islets show that they themselves are subject to proteolytic processing that may be important to their intracellular activation or sorting. These proteins are broadly distributed in neuroendocrine tissues and participate in cell-specific conversion of a number of prohormone precursors with regulation exerted by factors such as the substrate site specificity of the enzymes, the order in which they attack the substrate, their level of expression, and the ionic environment in which they function. The rate of conversion of proinsulin to insulin in the β-cell is slow relative to the speed with which newly-formed secretory granules become competent for exocytosis and small quantities of proinsulin and proinsulin processing intermediates are released normally along with insulin into the circulation. The proportion of unprocessed molecules to insulin increases in diabetes and islet cell neoplasia in humans. In neither case does the defect appear to lie at the level of the processing enzyme and the pathophysiological mechanism may be different in each case.

Acknowledgments

Work from the author's laboratory was supported by the British Diabetic Association, The Wellcome Trust, Medical Research Council and the European Community Bridge Program.

References

1. Hutton JC: Subtilisin-like proteinases involved in the activation of proproteins of the eukaryotic secretory pathway. *Curr Opin Cell Biol* 2:1131–1142, 1990.
2. Gross DJ, Villa-Komaroff L, Kahn CR, Weir GC, Halban PA: Deletion of a highly conserved tetrapeptide sequence of the proinsulin connecting peptide (C-peptide) inhibits proinsulin to insulin conversion by transfected pituitary corticotroph (AtT20) cells. *J Biol Chem* 264: 21,486–21,490, 1989.
3. Powell SK, Orci L, Craik CS, Moore H-PH: Efficient targeting to storage granules of human proinsulins with altered propeptide domain. *J Cell Biol* 106:1843–1851, 1988.
4. Weiss MA, Frank BH, Khait I, Pekar A, Heiney R, Shoelson SE, et al.: NMR and photo-CIDNP studies of human proinsulin and prohormone processing intermediates with application to endopeptidase recognition. *Biochemistry* 29:8389–8401, 1990.
5. Davidson HW, Rhodes CJ, Hutton JC: Intraorganellar calcium and pH control proinsulin cleavage in the pancreatic β-cell via two distinct site-specific endopeptidases. *Nature (London)* 333:93–96, 1988.
6. Davidson HW, Hutton, JC: The insulin-secretory-granule carboxypeptidase H: Purification and demonstration of involvement in proinsulin processing. *Biochem J* 245:575–582, 1987.
7. Rhodes CJ, Zumbrunn A, Bailyes EM, Shaw E, Hutton JC: The inhibition of proinsulin-processing endopeptidase activities by active-site-directed peptides. *Biochem J* 258:305–308, 1989.
8. Taylor NA, Docherty K: Sequence requirements for processing of proinsulin in transfected mouse pituitary AtT20 cells *Biochem J* 286 619–622, 1992.
9. Rhodes CJ, Lincoln B, Shoelson SE: Preferential cleavage of des-31,32-proinsulin over intact proinsulin by the insulin secretory granule type 2 endopeptidase: Implications of a favoured route for prohormone processing. *J Biol Chem* 267:22,719–22,727, 1992.
10. Porte D, Kahn SE: Hyperinsulinaemia and amyloid in NIDDM: Clues to etiology of islet beta cell dysfunction. *Diabetes* 38:1333–1336, 1989.
11. Simon J-P, Aunis D: Biochemistry of the chromogranin A protein family. *Biochem J* 262:1–13, 1989.
12. Hutton JC, Davidson HW, Grimaldi KA, Peshavaria M: Biosynthesis of betagranin in pancreatic β-cells: Identification of a chromogranin A-like precursor and its parallel processing with insulin. *Biochem J* 244:449–456, 1987.
13. Rhodes CJ, Thorne BA, Lincoln B, Nielsen E, Hutton JC, Thomas, G: Processing of proopiomelanocortin by insulin secretory granule proinsulin processing endopeptidases. *J Biol Chem* 268:4267–4275, 1993.
14. Thorne BA, Caton LW, Thomas G: Expression of mouse proopiomelanocortin in an insulinoma cell line: Requirements for β-endorphin processing. *J Biol Chem* 264:3545–3552, 1989.

15. Rhodes CJ, Brennan SO, Hutton JC: Proalbumin to albumin conversion by a proinsulin processing endopeptidase of insulin secretory granules. *J Biol Chem* 264:14,240–14,245, 1989.
16. Bourbonnais Y, Germain D, Latchinian-Sadek L, Boileau G, Thomas DY: Prohormone processing by yeast proteases. *Enzyme* 45:244–256, 1991.
17. Fuller RS, Brake A, Thorner J: Yeast prohormone processing enzyme (KEX-2 gene product) is a Ca^{2+}-dependent serine protease. *Proc Natl Acad Sci USA* 86:1434–1438, 1989.
18. Thim L, Hansen MT, Norris K, Hoegh I, Boel E, Forstrom J, et al.: Secretion and processing of insulin precursors in yeast. *Proc Natl Acad Sci USA* 83:6766–6770, 1986.
19. Sleep D, Belfield GP, Goodey, AR: The secretion of human serum albumin from the yeast *Saccharomyces cerevisiae* using five different leader sequences. *BioTechnology* 8:42–46, 1990.
20. Thomas G, Thorne BA, Thomas L, Allen RG, Hruby DE, Fuller R et al.: Yeast KEX-2 endoprotease correctly cleaves a neuroendocrine prohormone in mammalian cells. *Science* 241:226–230, 1988.
21. Brennan SO, Peach RJ. Bathurst IC: Specificity of yeast KEX-2 protease for variant human proalbumins is identical to the *in vivo* specificity of the hepatic proalbumin convertase. *J Biol Chem* 265:21,494–21,497, 1990.
22. Roebroek AJM, Schalken JA Bussemakers MJG, van Heerikhuizen H, Onnekink C, Debruyne FMJ, et al.: Characterization of human c-fes/fps reveals a new transcription unit *(fur)* in the immediately upstream region of the proto-oncogene. *Mol Biol Rep* 11:117–125, 1986.
23. Van den Ouweland AMW, Van Duijnhoven HLP, Keizer GD, Dorssers LCJ, Van de Ven WJM: Structural homology between the human fur gene product and the subtilisin-like protease encoded by yeast KEX-2. *Nucleic Acids Res* 18:664, 1990.
24. Schalken JA, Roebroek AJM, Oomen PPCA, Wagenaar SS, Debruyne FMJ, et al.: *fur* gene expression as a discriminating marker for small cell and non small cell lung carcinomas. *J Clin Invest* 80:1545–1549, 1987.
25. Molloy SS, Bresnahan PA, Leppla SH, Klimpel KR, Thomas G: Human furin is a calcium-dependent serine endoprotease that recognises the sequence Arg-X-X-Arg and efficiently cleaves anthrax toxin protective antigen. *J Biol Chem* 267:16,396–16,402, 1992.
26. Wise RJ, Barr PJ, Wong PA, Kiefer MC, Brake AJ, Kaufman RJ: Expression of human proprotein processing enzyme: Correct cleavage of the von Willebrand factor precursor at a paired basic amino acid site. *Proc Natl Acad Sci USA* 87:9378–9382, 1990.
27. Bresnahan PA, Leduc R, Thomas L, Thorner J, Gibson HL, Brake AJ, et al.: Human fur gene encodes a yeast KEX-2-like endoprotease that cleaves pro-β-NGF *in vivo*. *J Cell Biol* 111:2851–2859, 1990.
28. Misumi Y, Oda K, Fujiwara T, Takami N, Tashiro K, Ikehara Y: Functional expression of furin demonstrating its intracellular localization and endoprotease activity for processing of proalbumin and complement pro-C3. *J Biol Chem* 266:16,954–16,959, 1991.

29. Hatsuzawa K, Hosaka M, Nakagawa T, Nagase M, Shoda A, Murakami K et al: Structure and expression of mouse furin, a yeast Kex2-related protease: Lack of processing of coexpressed prorenin in GH_4C_1 cells. *J Biol Chem* 265:22,075–22,078, 1990.
30. Oda K, Ikeda M, Tsuji E, Sohda M, Takami N, Misumi Y, et al.: Sequence requirements for proteolytic cleavage of precursors with paired basic amino acids. *Biochem Biophys Res Commun* 179:1181–1186, 1991.
31. Steiner DF, Smeekens SP, Ohagi S, Chan SJ: The new enzymology of precursor processing endoproteases. *J Biol Chem* 267:23435–23438, 1992.
32. Fricker LD, Das B, Hogue-Angeletti R: Identification of the pH-dependent membrane anchor of carboxypeptidase E (EC 341710). *J Biol Chem* 265:2476–2482, 1990.
33. Seidah NG, Gaspar L, Mion P, Marcinkiewicz M, Mbikay M, Chretien M: cDNA sequence of two distinct pituitary proteins homologous to Kex2 and furin gene products: Tissue-specific mRNAs encoding candidates for prohormone processing proteinases. *DNA Cell Biol* 9:415–424, 1990.
34. Schafer MK-H, Day R, Cullinan WE, Chretien M, Seidah NG, Watson, SJ: Gene expression of prohormone and proprotein convertases in the rat CNS: A comparative in situ hybridization analysis. *J Neurosci* 13:1258–1279, 1993.
35. Thomas L, Leduc R, Thorne BA, Smeekens SP, Steiner DF, Thomas G: Kex2-like endoproteases PC2 and PC3 accurately cleave a model prohormone in mammalian cells: Evidence for a common core of neuroendocrine processing enzymes. *Proc Natl Acad Sci USA* 88:5297–5301, 1991.
36. Bloomquist BT, Eipper BA. Mains RE: Prohormone-converting enzymes: Regulation and evaluation of function using antisense RNA. *Mol Endocrinol* 5:2014–2024, 1991.
37. Marriott D, Gillece-Castro B, Gorman CM: Prohormone convertase-1 will process prorelaxin, a member of the insulin family of hormones. *Endocrinology (Baltimore)* 6:1441–1450, 1992.
38. Nakayama K, Hosaka M, Hatsuzawa K, Murakami K: Cloning and functional expression of a novel endoprotease involved in prohormone processing at dibasic sites. *J Biochem* 109:803–806, 1991.
39. Nakayama K, Watanabe T, Nakagawa T, Kim WS, Nagahama M, Hosaka M, et al.: Consensus sequence for precursor processing at mono-arginyl sites: Evidence for the involvement of a Kex2-like endoprotease in precursor cleavages at both dibasic and mono-arginyl sites. *J Biol Chem* 267:16,335–16,340, 1992.
40. Shennan KIJ, Smeekens SP, Steiner DF, Docherty K: Characterization of PC2, a mammalian Kex2 homologue, following expression of the cDNA in microinjected *Xenopus* oocytes. *FEBS Lett* 284:277–280, 1991.
41. Bailyes EM, Shennan KIJ, Seal AJ, Smeekens SP, Steiner DF, Hutton JC et al.: A member of the eukaryotic subtilisin family has the enzymatic properties of the type 1 proinsulin-converting endopeptidase. *Biochem J* 285:391–394, 1992.

42. Bennett DL, Bailyes EM, Nielsen E, Guest PC, Rutherford NG, Arden SD et al.: Identification of the type 2 proinsulin processing endopeptidase as PC2, a member of the eukaryote subtilisin family. *J Biol Chem* 267:15,229–15,236, 1992.
43. Smeekens SP, Montag AG, Thomas G, Albiges-Rizo C, Carroll R, Benig M et al: Proinsulin processing by the subtilisin-related proprotein convertases furin, PC2 and PC3. *Proc Natl Acad Sci USA* 89:8822–8826, 1992.
44. Seidah NG, Day R, Hamelin J, Gaspar A, Collard MW, Chretien M: Testicular expression of PC4 in the rat: Molecular diversity of a novel germ cell-specific Kex2/subtilisin-like proprotein convertase. *Mol Endocrinol* 6:1559–1570, 1992.
45. Nakayama K, Kim W-S, Torii S, Hosaka M, Nakagawa T, Ikemizu J, Baba T et al.: Identification of the fourth member of the mammalian endoprotease family homologous to the yeast Kex2 protease: Its testis-specific expression. *J Biol Chem* 267:5897–5900, 1992.
46. Seidah NG, Day R, Marcinkiewicz M, Benjannet S, Chretien M: Mammalian neural and endocrine pro-protein and pro-hormone convertases belonging to the subtilisin family of serine proteinases. *Enzyme* 45:271–284, 1991.
47. Nakagawa T, Hosaka M, Torii S, Watanabe T, Murakami K, Nakagawa K: Identification and functional expression of a new member of the mammalian Kex2-like processing endoprotease family: Its striking structural similarity to PACE4. *J Biochem* 113:132–135, 1993.
48. Christie DL, Batchelor DC, Palmer DJ: Identification of Kex2-related proteases in chromaffin granules by partial amino acid sequence analysis. *J Biol Chem* 266:15,679–15,683, 1991.
49. Mackin RB, Noe BD, Speiss J: Identification of a somatostatin-14-generating propeptide converting enzyme as a member of the Kex2/furin/PC family. *Endocrinology (Baltimore)* 129:2263–2265, 1991.
50. Guest PC, Arden SD, Bennett DL, Clark A, Rutherford NG, Hutton JC: The posttranslational processing and intracellular sorting of PC2 in the islets of Langerhans. *J Biol Chem* 267:22,401–22,406, 1992.
51. Shennan KIJ, Seal AJ, Smeekens SP, Steiner DF, Docherty K: Site-directed mutagenesis and expression of PC2 in microinjected *Xenopus* oocytes. *J Biol Chem* 266:24,011–24,017, 1991.
52. Vindrola O, Lindberg I: Biosynthesis of the prohormone convertase mPC1 in AtT20 cells. *Mol Endocrinol* 6:1088–1094, 1992.
53. Alarcon C, Lincol, B, Rhodes CJ: The biosynthesis of the subtilisin-related proprotein convertase PC3, but not that of the PC2 convertase, is regulated by glucose in parallel to proinsulin biosynthesis in rat pancreatic islets. *J Biol Chem* 268:4276–4280, 1993.
54. Guest PC, Rhodes CJ, Hutton JC: Regulation of the biosynthesis of insulin secretory granule proteins: Co-ordinate translational control is exerted on some, but not all, granule matrix constituents. *Biochem J* 257:431–437, 1989.

55. Baekkeskov S, Aanstoot HJ, Christgau S, Reetz A, Solimena M, Cascalho M et al.: Identification of the 64K autoantigen in insulin-dependent diabetes as the gaba-synthesising enzyme glutamic acid decarboxylase. *Nature* 347:151–156, 1990.
56. Castano L, Russo E, Zhou L, Lipes MA, Eisenbarth GS: Identification and cloning of a granule autoantigen (Carboxypeptidase H) associated with type 1 diabetes. *J Clin Endocrinol Met* 73:1197–1201, 1991.
57. Roep BO, Kallan AA, Hazenbos WLW, Bruining GJ, Bailyes EM, Arden SD et al.: T-cell reactivity to 38kD insulin secretory granule protein in patients with recent onset type 1 diabetes. *Lancet* 337:1439–1441, 1991.
58. Temple RC, Carrington CA, Luzio SD, Owens DR, Schneider AE, Sobey WJ, Hales CN: Insulin deficiency in non-insulin-dependent diabetes *Lancet* 1:293–295, 1989.
59. Ward WK, LaCava EC, Paquette TL, Beard JC, Wallum BJ, Porte D Jr: Disproportionate elevation of immunoreactive proinsulin in type 2 (non-insulin-dependent) diabetes mellitus and in experimental insulin resistance. *Diabetologia* 30:698–702, 1987.
60. Rubenstein AH, Block MB, Starr J, Melani F, Steiner DF: Proinsulin and C-peptide in blood. *Diabetes* 21:661–672, 1972.
61. Gorden P, Roth J, Freychet P, Kahn R: The circulating proinsulin-like components. *Diabetes* 21:673–677, 1972.
62. Nishi M, Sanke T, Nagamatsu S, Bell GI, Steiner DF: Islet amyloid polypeptide: A new beta cell secretory product related to islet amyloid deposits. *J Biol Chem* 265:4173–4176, 1990.
63. Porte D Jr: Beta cells in type II diabetes mellitus. *Diabetes* 40:166–180, 1991.
64. Shibasaki Y, Kawakami T, Kanazawa Y, Akanuma Y, Takaku, F: Post-translational cleavage of proinsulin is blocked by a point mutation in familial hyperproinsulinaemia. *J Clin Invest* 76:378–380, 1985.
65. Yano H, Kitano N, Morimoto M, Polonsky KS, Imura H, Seino, Y: A novel point mutation in the human insulin gene giving rise to hyperproinsulinaemia (proinsulin Kyoto). *J Clin Invest* 89:1902–1907, 1992.
66. Chan SJ, Seino S, Gruppuso PA, Schwartz R, Steiner DF: A mutation in the B-chain coding region is associated with impaired proinsulin conversion in a family with hyperproinsulinaemia. *Proc Natl Acad Sci USA* 84:2194–2197, 1987.

Chapter 11

GTP and Its Binding Proteins in the Regulation of Insulin Exocytosis

Anjaneyulu Kowluru and Stewart A. Metz

Regulation of Islet Function by Purine Nucleotides

Despite considerable evidence for the involvement of the purine nucleotides GTP* and ATP in exocytosis, there is currently no consensus about their exact role(s). With regard to GTP (the focus of this chapter), our recent studies *(1)* have suggested that there is at least a permissive role for GTP in insulin release. Normal rat pancreatic islets were pretreated overnight with each of four structurally-dissimilar inhibitors of a rate-limiting step in the cytosolic production of GTP (inosine monophosphate dehydrogenase; IMPDH). When islet concentrations of GTP were inhibited by more than about 80% (to levels down to less than 0.6–0.7 pmol/islet), insulin release subsequently stimulated by nutrients (glucose or α-ketoisocaproate) or by a phorbol ester was reduced 40–60%. In contrast, insulin secretion induced by direct depolarization of β-cells (by 50 m*M* K^+) was refractory to inhibition. These results were attributed to a depletion of islet GTP stores, since repletion of GTP by coprovision of guanine (but not the normalization of both ATP and UTP content by the

**See* page 280 for a list of the abbreviations used in this chapter.

From: *Molecular Biology of Diabetes, Part I*
Edited by: B. Draznin and D. LeRoith © 1994 Humana Press Inc., Totowa, NJ

provision of adenine) reversed the inhibitory effects of the drugs both on GTP content and on insulin release. In subsequent studies, we observed that lesser degrees of inhibition of GTP, or, conversely, a stimulation of islet GTP content (by provision of guanine alone) to levels about 25% above basal, did not have any discernible negative or positive modulatory effects on secretion. These findings suggested that islet GTP content is normally saturating, and therefore mild to moderate changes in these levels do not alter secretion. Since the average islet content of GTP approximates 750–1000 μ*M*, it appears that a reduction in *total* islet GTP levels to less than 150–200 μ*M* (or, possibly, a comparable relative reduction of *free* GTP levels, which may be one-fifth to one-twentieth of total levels; ref. *2*) is needed to vitiate the effects of GTP on secretion. Such drastic changes are not likely to be induced by physiologic agonists (and in fact were not induced by glucose, which had relatively modest effects on total islet GTP content); therefore, we defined the effects of GTP as "permissive."

The site(s) at which GTP exerts this influence remain to be elucidated. The K_d of most classical GTP-binding proteins (GBPs) is in the nanomolar range, making it unlikely that the pharmacologic inhibitors had rendered GTP concentrations regulatory for typical GBPs. Furthermore, the inhibitory effect of epinephrine (which blunts insulin release largely by effects on G_i and/or G_o) was unaffected by prior drug treatment *(1)*. However, we have recently demonstrated *(see below)* that at least two GTPases exist in pancreatic islets or transformed β-cells that have an apparent K_m for GTP of 2 μ*M* and 700–800 μ*M*; this finding leaves open the possibility that high-K_m, low-affinity GTPases might be regulated by GTP concentrations relevant to the islet and could therefore subserve the permissive effect of GTP on secretion.*

Such speculations receive some support from the recent studies of Lillie and Gomperts *(4,5)*. These investigators, in their studies of secretion from permeabilized mast cells, observed that even calcium may not be required for secretion under certain circumstances, whereas GTP is both sufficient and possibly required to induce secre-

*There is some precedent for this: for example: ≥100 μ*M* GTP is needed for ADP-ribosylation factors (ARFs) to maximally activate cholera toxin (*3; see also below,* and Discussion in ref. *1*).

tion. Interestingly, in their studies, secretion was saturated by about 1 m*M* GTP, but fell off rather rapidly at concentrations under about 100 μ*M* GTP, supporting our estimations that, in islets, the effect of GTP on exocytosis is exerted in the high μ*M* range. Much lower concentrations of the nonhydrolyzable analogues of GTP (such as GTPγS) may suffice, owing to the persistence of the putative GBP of exocytosis ("G_E") in the GTP-liganded state; higher concentrations of GTP itself are needed since it can be hydrolyzed by the GTPase activity intrinsic to GBPs *(5)*. Agents which impede GTPase activity, therefore, such as insulinotropic lipids *(see below)* would be expected to potentiate secretion. (During these studies of lipid messengers, GTP, and secretion, we noted similarities between the exocytotic process and the generation of superoxide anion by NADPH oxidase in neutrophils, both of which involve complex roles for GBPs as well as phospholipase-derived lipid mediators [especially arachidonate and phosphatidic acid]). Interestingly, recent data, including some of our own, suggest that an exocytosis-inhibitory GBP may also exist ("G_{Ei}"); such a putative GBP, which may act very late in the cascade of stimulus-secretion coupling *(6)*, may also require high μ*M* levels of GTP *(6)*.

It is important to keep in mind that measurements of GTP provide data on islet content (and, thereby *average* concentrations throughout the cell); such determinations do not deal with the possibility of anatomical and/or functional compartmentalization of GTP within the cell, nor do they address "free" vs bound concentrations of GTP. (Since Mg^{2+} is needed for GTP binding to GBPs, one might presume that Mg^{2+}·GTP is one active form of GTP.) These concerns about the compartmentalization of (and "free" vs total) GTP concentrations have been previously discussed by us *(7)*. It is also worth keeping in mind that not only the anatomic location of GTP, but also its enzymatic derivation, might be important; these issues also would not be addressed in measurements of *total* islet GTP. We have observed that, whereas glucose increases the GTP content of islets over an 18-h incubation period by only 20–40%, it selectively stimulates cytosolic "compartments" of GTP up to 300% of basal. Specifically, glucose stimulated both the *de novo* synthetic pathway and especially the "salvage" of hypoxanthine, both of which proceed (via IMPDH) to form GTP *(8)*. This effect may be of clinical relevance since it could be readily observed at only slight increases in ambient glucose (115–140 mg/dL), which define impaired glucose tolerance or frank diabetes in humans. Since the "pools" of GTP stimulated by glucose are cytosolic and therefore presumably are in close proximity to the secretory granule, cytoskeleton, and plasma membrane, they may be located in a strategic location to modify exocytosis.

GTP (and ATP) may subserve a number of roles within the islet and other cells, beyond their roles in secretion. For example, nucleotides and deoxynucleotides have roles in RNA and DNA synthesis, and therefore in protein synthesis, cellular proliferation, and differentiation *(9,10)*. Even adult islet cells have some capacity to proliferate, and GTP could play an important role in this phenomenon. This possibility, in turn, could be important to the islet's response to chronic hyperglycemic stimulation. It also could be relevant to the regeneration of damaged islets in patients with incipient IDDM. For example, an adequate supply of purine nucleotides may be critical for damaged islet cells to proliferate and recover from a subtotal insult early in the natural history of insulin-dependent diabetes mellitus (IDDM); certain immunosuppressives that impede purine nucleotide synthesis could interfere in this process. On the other hand, GTP can be regulatory for the synthesis of nitric oxide (NO; *see* Table 1, #11); the latter has been recently implicated in the destruction of β-cells in IDDM, raising the possibility that perturbation of GTP levels could have *preventive* value in individuals at high risk for IDDM.

As indicated above, one site of action of GTP in insulin secretion may reside at novel GBPs ("G_E" and "G_{Ei}"). Our evidence for involvement of GBPs in insulin secretion, both stimulatory and inhibitory, are discussed in more detail below. However, one additional observation merits mention here, since it also suggests the involvement of one or more additional, inhibitory GBPs, that may have a high affinity for GTP yet that probably also acts late in the exocytotic cascade. When intact pancreatic islets were treated with pertussis toxin (which ADP-ribosylates the inhibitory G proteins G_i and G_o), the insulin secretion subsequently induced by a depolarizing concentration of K^+ was markedly augmented *(11)*. This might indicate a role for GBPs in modulating Ca^{2+} fluxes; however, pertussis toxin (PTX) treatment did not increase (and in fact slightly decreased) K^+-induced $^{45}Ca^{2+}$ efflux (S. Metz, unpublished data). Indirect effects

Table 1
Potential Cellular Roles for GTP[a]

Effector or site	Action	Effective GTP concentration	Involves GTP hydrolysis?	Comments; ref.
1. GTP-binding proteins (GBPs) a. Heterotrimeric b. Low molecular weight c. Miscellaneous (*see* #14) NB: Some effects of #2–15 (below) could be mediated via GBPs	Conformational change‡ or allosteric effect‡ and/or GTP hydrolysis,§ leading to effects on cell traffic, ion flux, phospholipases, cyclic nucleotides, receptor affinity, NADPH oxidase, and so on.	Us. n*M* to low μ*M* but note possible exceptions, re.: adenylate cyclase,[1] exocytosis[2], phospholipase D[3], K^+ currents[4]; NADPH oxidase[5], phospholipase C[6], ?other, which may require high μ*M* GTP	‡No (GTP or GTPγS effective) §Yes (requires GTP)	[1]*J Biol Chem* 254:95, 1979 [2]*J Biol Chem* 267:12517, 1992 [3]*Eur J Biochem* 77:113, 1977, *Biochem J* 278:81, 1991; 271:693, 1990; *Cell Regul* 2:1011, 1991; *J Biol Chem* 267:9826, 1992, 262:15309, 1987, 264:8847, 1989. [4]*J Physiol* 408:313, 1989 [5]*J Biol Chem* 266:20990, 1991 [6]*Biochem J* 291:235, 1993
2. Protein Synthesis a. RNA synthesis and translation i. Initiation factors ii. Elongation factors iii. Translocation to ER iv. Termination	Initiates polypeptide chain, directs mRNA to and along ER, translocates nascent peptide to ER lumen, displaces SRP from ribosomes and signal sequence, dissociates SRP from its receptor	*P* (? low μ*M* to high μ*M*)[c]	Yes, at least in part (? not for SRP dissociation from signal sequence; yes for SRP dissociation from SRP receptor)	*Biochem J* 275:23, 1991; *Science* 258:931, 1992 (*see also* refs. in #3)

(continued)

Table 1 *(continued)*

Effector or site	Action	Effective GTP concentration	Involves GTP hydrolysis?	Comments; ref.
b. Secretory granule or vesicle biogenesis and traffic (*see also* #1 and 6), e.g., ER to Golgi, SG or SV			Prob. Yes (at least for multiple cycles of traffic) but SG biogenesis may involve an inhibitory GBP able to use GTPγS	*FEBS Lett* 294:239, 1991 (GTP may also act as substrate for some H^+-pumping ATPases)
c. Formation of GDP mannose, GDP-fucose	Needed for dolichol-dep't N-linked protein glycosylation	μM^b	Yes	*Cancer Res* 46:2314, 1986; *Mol Pharmacol* 28:567, 1985
d. ? Other (? stabilize RNA, RNA capping, r-RNA polymerase, ribonucleotide reductase [GDP], mitochondrial protein synthesis)				
3. DNA synthesis; post-mitotic nuclear assembly and nuclear transport; Nucleolar localization of nucleophosmin/B23		prob. μM^b ? μM^b high μM^b	Yes	*Biochem J* 37:736, 1977, 113:515, 1969; 234:263, 1986; *J Biol Chem* 256:8713, 1981; *Science* 258:942, 1992 (GBPs may be involved: cf. *PNAS* 87:7080, 1990; *Nature* 358:512, 1992) NB: dGTP may be involved: *J Biol Chem* 268:5823, 1993

4. Adenine and Pyrimidine Nucleotide Synthesis (*see also* 7c)				
a. Adenylosuccinate synthetase	Converts inosine-P to AMP	low μ*M*[b]	Yes	a. *Biochim Biophys Acta* 437:87, 1976
b. Mitochondrial uncoupling protein (brown fat only; GDP also effective)	Recouples respiration, displaces acyl CoA	high μM	No	b. *Eur J Biochem* 19:276, 1971; *Biochim Biophys Acta* 549:1, 1979
c. Adenylate (AMP) deaminase	GTP inhibits AMP →inosine-P	low μ*M* (>100 μ*M* activates		c. *J Biol Chem* 254:8994, 1979; 253:8728, 1978
d. ? PRPP synthetase, PRPP-glutamine amidotransferase, other enzymes of ATP/GTP synthesis				
e. CTP synthetase		high μ*M*[b]		
5. Cytoskeletal Function a. Tubulin b. Dynamin	Assembly and disaggregation of microtubules via reversible polymerization	*P* (low μ*M*)[c]	Yes (on β subunit) (? also allosteric effects)	a. *Biochem J* 277:239, 1991 b. *Nature* 355:733, 1992

(continued)

Table 1 *(continued)*

Effector or site	Action	Effective GTP concentration	Involves GTP hydrolysis?	Comments; ref.
6. Exocytosis (see also #1,2b,4,7,9d,12)				*J Cell Biol* 105:191, 1989; *J Biol Chem* 267:12517, 1992
a. Fusion		high μM^b	Possibly	a. *Biochem J* 286:747, 1992; *Biochim Biophys Acta* 1070:274, 1991; *J Histochem Cytochem* 39:363, 1991
b. PIP kinase	Maintenance of polyphosphoinositides	high μM^b	No	b. *J Biol Chem* 264:3206, 1989; *Biochem J* 237:25, 1986, 271:591, 1990
c. Direct" effects on ion channels (e.g., K^+ (ATP channel); Ca^{2+} mobilization)		P (low-high μM)^c low μM	? No; Yes (see #11a,b)	c. *Phlug Arch Pharm* 407:564; 1986; *Biochem J* 242:137, 1987 NB: 6(c) may reflect action on GBPs (*see* #1) or phosphorylation (*see* #10a)
d. Direct" effects on phospholipases	Activate Ca^{2+}-indep't phospholipase A_2 (ATP is preferred), independently of GBPs (see also #1)	P (high μM-mM)^c	No	d. *J Biol Chem* 266:14526, 1991, 265:10622, 1990; *Biochim Biophys Acta* 1165:167, 1992
7. Primary or alternative substrate for NTP hydrolysis	Hormone processing and secretion; high energy P transfer			
a. P transfer to water (hydrolysis)				
i. Secretory granule anion-sensitive ATPase		high μM^b	Yes	*J Biol Chem* 256:12802, 1981 *Biochem J* 287:423, 1992

ii. Vesicular H^+-ATPases		*P* (n*M* to high μ*M*)[c]	Yes	NB: GTP has same ΔG^{o1} (free energy change) as ATP
iii. Other		m*M*[b]	Yes	
b. P transfer to peptide				
i. Protein kinases (esp. casein kinase II-like activity)	Phosphorylation	*P* (low to high μ*M*)	Yes	i. *J Biol Chem* 267:23894, 1992; *Blood* 75:479, 1990; *Biochem J* 277:811, 1991; 234:311, 1986; *Diabetologia* 29:808, 1986; *BBRC* 87:757, 1979
ii. Protein phosphatases	Phosphorylation			ii. *Trends Neurosci* 15:403, 1992
iii. Potentiate cAMP-dep't binding	Phosphorylation	low-high μ*M*[b]		iii. *Am J Physiol* 246:C131, 1984; *Diabetes* 36:37, 1987
c. P transfer to intermediary metabolites				
i. Fructokinase, phosphorylase kinase (inhibition), other		high μ*M* to m*M*	Yes	i. *Biochem J* 228:667; 1985; *J Biol Chem* 266:16524, 1991; 263;5543, 1988
ii.P transfer to diglyceride	? Activation of diglyceride kinase	low μ*M*		ii. *BBRC* 164:1060, 1989
iii.*See* 6b				

(continued)

Table 1 *(continued)*

Effector or site	Action	Effective GTP concentration	Involves GTP hydrolysis?	Comments; ref.
d. P transfer to nucleotides (transphosphorylation)				
i. Nucleoside diphosphokinase	Nucleotide triphosphate regeneration	low-mid μ*M* to m*M*[b]	Yes (but GTPγS can transphosphorylate)	i. *J Biol Chem* 259:11297, 1984; *FEBS Lett* 107:198, 1979; *IRCS Med Sci* 14:354, 1986; *Biochem Pharm* 39:1399, 1990
ii. GTP-AMP phosphotransferase	Mitochondrial ADP synthesis	*P* (high μ*M*)[c]	Yes	ii. *Eur J Biochem,* 1:199, 1967, 93:263, 1979; *Biochim* Biophys Acta 438:310, 1976
8. Substrate for Guanylate Cyclase (See #11)	cGMP formation	*P* (low-high μ*M*)[c]	(Substrate)	*Biochim Biophys Acta* 438:310, 1976; 718:49, 1982; *BBRC* 183:312, 1992; *J Biol Chem* 250:374, 1975; 249:6910, 1974
9. Enzyme Activity				
a. Glutamate dehydrogenase	Allosteric inhibitor	*P* (*nM to low μM; ?* high μ*M* in presence Mg^{2+})[c]	No	a. *J Biol Chem* 263:13610, 1988; *Biochem* 31:10544, 1992; *Biochem J* 220:853, 1984
b. Succinyl thiokinase	Activates succinic acid; ? modulates ketone metabolism	*P* (low μ*M*)[c]	Yes	b. *J Biol Chem* 264:12303, 1989, 263:13610, 1988 (Reaction to OAA transphosphorylates GDP to GTP)

c. PEP carboxykinase	Control of gluconeogenesis (promotes interconversion of PEP and OAA)	*P* (low-high μ*M*)[c] *P* (low-high μ*M*)[c]		c. *Biochem J* 285:767, 1992; *J Biol Chem* 241:2421, 1966, 251:37, 1976
d. Transglutaminase	Protein cross-linking and amine incorporation; ? exocytosis (GTP is inhibitory)	*P* (low-high μ*M*)[c]	? No (but enz. has GTPase activity)	d. *FEBS Lett* 307:177, 1992; *J Biol Chem* 267:13267, 1992, 262:1901, 1987; *BBRC* 162:1370, 1989
e. Acyl CoA synthetase	Lipid metabolism			e. *J Biol Chem* 242:2111, 1967
f. CDP-diglyceride synthetase (phosphatidate cytidylyl-transferase)	Phospholipid synthesis (stimulate microsomal, ? inhibits mitochondrial enz.)	m*M*[b] high μ*M*[b]	Yes	f. *BBRC* 79:749, 1977; *FEBS Lett* 312:236, 1992; *J Histochem Cytochem* 39:363, 1991
g. Ornithine decarboxylase (bacteria)		n*M*	No	g. *BBRC* 114:779, 1983
h. Other (? acetyl CoA carboxylase, ATP sulfurase, glycerol-3-P-acyltransferase, glycosyl-phosphatidylinositol biosynthesis)		low-high μ*M* (GDP = GTP in some enzymes)	Yes	h. *J Biol Chem* 256:8573, 1981; 267:542, 1992; 268:9718, 1993
10.				
a. Sarcoplasmic Reticulum GTPase	Ca^{2+} accumulation	Two forms (n*M*; high μ*M*)[b]	Yes	a. *J Biol Chem* 264:7809, 1989

(continued)

Table 1 *(continued)*

Effector or site	Action	Effective GTP concentration	Involves GTP hydrolysis?	Comments; ref.
b. ER Ca^{2+} binding and release	Ca^{2+} mobilization	P (low μ*M*)	Yes	b. *Biochem* J 234:311, 1986; 244:87, 1987; 248:741, 1987; 242:137, 1987 (islets); *Nature* 320:461, 1986; *Biochim Biophys Acta* 945: 185, 1988; *J Biol Chem* 266: 19599, 1991 NB: ? related to GBP or protein phosphorylation [see 6b and 7b (i)]
11. Substrate for GTP Cyclohydrolase	Tetrahydrobiopterin synthesis (and thereby NO formation)	High μ*M*[b]	(Substrate)	*J Biol Chem* 267:20734, 1992
12. Carboxymethyltransferase Activity				
a. Protein	Increased hydrophobicity, membrane association	P (? high μ*M*)	No	a. *J Biol Chem* 267:18432, 1992, 263:15864, 1988; 266:4387, 1991; *Biochim Biophys Acta* 1136:150, 1992
b. Phospholipid	Converts PE to PC (? unique pool)	high μ*M*[b]		b. *BBRC* 114:425, 1983 NB: GTP inhibits methyltransferase I and stimulates methyltransferase II
13. Protein Nucleotidylation				*J Biol Chem* 266:20525, 1991

14. ADP Ribosylation of GBPs (incl. ADP Ribosylation Factor)	*P* (variable: n*M*[c] to high μ*M*[b])	? (ARF may have GTPase activity) No	*J Biol Chem* 267:17766, 1992, 268:7064, 1993
15. Miscellaneous a. Pregnenelone synthesis b. ? Cytochrome C reduction c. Prccessing of PI-glycan-anchored proteins or PI-glycan synthesis	high μ*M*	Yes	a. *J Biol Chem* 264:17674, 1989 b. *Free Radic Biol Med* 11:187, 1991 c. *PNAS* 89:6124, 1992; *J Biol Chem* 268:9718, 1993

[a]for overview, *see* M. Pall, *Curr Top Cell Regul* 25:1–20, 1985.

[b]indicates GTP requirement that likely makes this action amenable to pharmacologic manipulation and, possibly, physiologic regulation.

[c]*p* indicates GTP requirement that is possibly subject to pharmacologic manipulation.

Abbreviations: SG = secretory granule; SV - secretory vesicle; ER = endoplasmic reticulum; AMP = adenosine monophosphate; K^+ (ATP) = ATP-sensitive potassium channel; OAA = oxaloacetate; PEP = phosphoenolpyruvate; NO = nitric oxide; ARF = ADP-ribosylation factor; *PNAS = Proc Natl Acad Sci USA*; P = phosphate; BBRC = *Biochem Biophys Res Commun;* SRP = signal recognition particle; dGTP=deoxy-GTP of PTX (e.g., an increase in cellular cyclic AMP content) were not excluded as the cause of the increase in secretion. Nonetheless, this rather dramatic effect on Ca^{2+}-induced secretion (apparently occurring distal to the mobilization of Ca^{2+} itself), in conjunction with the failure of GTP synthesis inhibitors to impede K^+-induced secretion despite reducing that induced by glucose or a phorbol ester *(1)*, raises the possibility that there is at least one GBP that selectively modulates Ca^{2+}-induced secretion. This protein, we feel, may be a substrate for PTX, has a K_m for GTP substantially below the levels that can be reached via the use of inhibitors of cytosolic GTP synthesis, and may mediate an inhibition of Ca^{2+}-induced exocytosis distal in the cascade of events in secretion. This effect likely involves G_i and/or G_o, at least in part. As indicated above, a second GBP appears to have a much higher K_m(GTP) and mediates (a part of) the effect of nutrients and phorbol esters to *stimulate* secretion independently of increases in cytosolic free Ca^{2+} levels. Such an effect of glucose at fixed levels of cytosolic free Ca^{2+} levels has recently been demonstrated *(12)*; we speculate that this effect of glucose may itself be modulated by its own stimulatory and inhibitory GBPs. The formulation that nutrients may stimulate more than one GBP, as well as activating pathways both dependent on, *and* independent of, changes in $[Ca^{2+}{}_i]$, may be supported by the findings that inhibitors of GTP synthesis, or of the posttranslational modification of GBPs *(see below)*, inhibit fuel-induced insulin release by only about 50–60% each. Furthermore, Ullrich et al. *(13)* have observed that $[Ca^{2+}{}_i]$-activated insulin release may not require exogenous addition of GTP; the low levels of cellular GTP that persist even after plasma membrane permeabilization *(14)* may suffice.

It should be noted that we have only been able to achieve an 80–85% depletion of islet GTP through pharmacologic inhibition; one might ask whether even K^+-induced secretion (i.e., Ca^{2+}-activated release) might be blocked if GTP content were to be reduced more completely. Most of the residual 15 or 20% of GTP that persists after inhibition of the major cytosolic biosynthetic pathways probably does *not* have such a permissive effect on secretion for the following reasons. Unlike cytosolic and mitochondrial pools of ADP and ATP, which are probably in equilibrium owing to their transport in and out of mitochondria via the ADP/ATP translocase, guanine nucleotides are not transported by this translocase *(15)*. How much GTP, then, resides in mitochondria and what is its role there? Based on our preliminary studies, we feel that only 20–35% of the GTP content of intact islets resides in mitochondria,* and probably comprises most of the residual GTP that is not blockable by the cytosolic inhibitors. It is unlikely that this mitochondrial "compartment" of GTP directly promotes insulin secretion. It has been shown, and we have confirmed (Meredith M, Rabaglia M, Metz S, unpublished observations) that the provision of succinic acid methyl esters promotes insulin secretion *(16)*; these esters are hydrolyzed within the cell to free succinic acid, which is then metabolized (by the enzyme succinate thiokinase) to its CoA-ester derivative. This latter step, which utilizes (and thereby depletes the mitochondria of) GTP, is associated with a *stimulation* of secretion; thus, it seems likely that, mitochondrial GTP is *inhibitory* for secretion, probably because GTP is an allosteric inhibitor of glutamate dehydrogenase *(17)*. Thus, Ca^{2+}-induced secretion probably requires only extremely low cellular levels of GTP (presumably the small amount of cytosolic GTP not reduced by the pharmacologic inhibitors); this conclusion is in accord with other observations cited above.

There are many roles for GTP, and some of these may not involve classical GBPs. Table 1 summarizes known cellular actions of GTP derived from studies of many different cell types; the table indicates whether or not these actions involve the hydrolysis of GTP or only the presence of an appropriate GTP analog (i.e., allosteric effects). Table 1 also summarizes the cellular "concentrations" of GTP required for these effects. GTP may have roles in exocytosis that are direct or that are mediated by effects on GBPs that in turn modulate ion channels, phospholipase activation, cyclic AMP generation, and other signal transduction mechanisms. As indicated in Table 1, there are also a number of sites at which GTP is critical for the (re)synthesis of the major anionic or cationic phospholipids, which may in turn be critical for secretion. Additionally, in addition to effects on phospho-

*This figure is based on two findings: 1. That 20% of islet GTP is not removed by inhibitors of cytosolic IMPDH; and 2. That provision of succinic acid methyl esters (which deplete mitochondrial GTP stores; *see below*) cause only a small decline in total GTP levels in islets. (Meredith M, Kowluru A, Rabaglia M, Metz S, unpublished, preliminary data.)

lipases via GBPs or synthesis of substrates, GTP may directly activate one or more phospholipases allosterically *(18)*. Another interesting effect of cellular GTP that might have relevance to exocytosis is the activation of one or more protein kinases that may preferentially utilize GTP as substrate for phosphorylation; we have termed these, generically, "protein kinase G." These could be relevant to exocytosis in other cells, since, for example, a "protein kinase G" (probably a casein kinase) can phosphorylate synaptotagmin, a secretory vesicle-associated peptide that may have an intrinsic role in secretion *(19)*. We have recently identified the presence of an apparent protein kinase in islets that utilizes GTP but not ATP (Kowluru A, Metz S, unpublished observations). Another relevant enzyme is transglutaminase, the activity of which is inhibited by GTP. This enzyme can posttranslationally modify a number of proteins potentially relevant to secretion, including phospholipases *(20)* and some secretory vesicle proteins *(21)*. In addition, GTP modulates a number of processes (such as protein carboxyl methylation and ADP-ribosylation) that, in turn, regulate other proteins, including GBPs. GTP may also have direct effects on membrane fusion and on the cytoskeleton; it also modulates the synthesis of hormones as well as their processing, packaging, trafficking, and diversion into the secretory vesicle or granule that stores them (Table 1). Future studies will be required to elucidate which of these potential roles of GTP are relevant to the pancreatic islet.

Although ATP is not the focus of this chapter, one could question whether the role of GTP is not merely to act as a high energy phosphate donor to maintain cellular stores of ATP, which until the recent past was widely regarded as *required* for exocytosis. However, some recent studies have suggested that ATP may not have a mandatory, direct role in secretion, although it also may serve a permissive, priming role. In fact, studies of Lillie and Gomperts have suggested that, under certain circumstances, ATP may not be required at all *(4,5)*. Perhaps, then, the major role of ATP might be to maintain cellular stores of GTP (i.e., by the action of nucleoside diphosphokinase, an enzyme present [Kowluru A, Rabaglia M, Metz S, submitted for publication] in pancreatic islets; 22). Others have also raised this possibility *(4)*. We have been able to deplete the islet content of ATP by approximately 40% through a number of different pharmacologic maneuvers under which GTP content was preserved. Under these circumstances, no inhibitory effect upon insulin secretion was observed. This cannot be construed as excluding a role for ATP in exocytosis (especially one that may be acute in onset and not relevant to such subacute studies). Furthermore, the role of ATP may be associated with changes in the ATP/ADP ratio (which have not been examined yet in our studies); additionally, effects of ATP may involve cellular levels lower than those reached after a 40% inhibition. Nonetheless, these studies suggest that, as a candidate mediator or modulator of endocrine secretion, GTP merits at least the same degree of consideration as that previously afforded to ATP.

GTP Binding Proteins in Insulin-Secreting Cells

Insulin secretion from the pancreatic β-cell is regulated principally by the concentration of D-glucose in the interstitial fluid surrounding the islet cells. However, the molecular and cellular mechanisms underlying stimulus-secretion coupling in pancreatic islets remain poorly understood. It is widely accepted that changes in Ca^{2+} concentrations lead to regulation of various cellular enzymes or effectors resulting in facilitated insulin secretion. A growing body of evidence also suggests that certain hormones and neurotransmitters elicit insulin release via GBPs. In a recent review Robertson et al. *(23)* summarized the existing body of evidence in support of a putative role for heterotrimeric GBPs in insulin secretion. In this section, we describe the existing data on the presence (and tentative identification) of some of these GBPs (especially, the low molecular weight GBPs) in insulin-secreting cells. We also present some of the recent experimental evidence obtained in our laboratory on the functional regulation of these proteins by various (positive as well as negative) modulators of insulin secretion.

At least three classes of GBPs have been identified in eukaryotic cells. The first group of GBPs are heterotrimeric in nature, comprised of α (39–53 kDa), β (ca. 37 kDa), and γ (7–10 kDa) subunits. These proteins are generally involved in coupling plasma membrane receptors to their intracellular effectors such as ion channels, phospholipases, adenyl cyclase, and cGMP-dependent phosphodiesterase *(24)*. The α subunits of these heterotrimers undergo ADP-ribosylation catalyzed by ribosyl-transferases endogenous to bacterial toxins, such as cholera and PTX. Apart from immunologic characterization, bacterial toxin-mediated ribosylation of the a subunits of these proteins is generally used as a tool to quantitate heterotrimeric GBPs.

The second group is comprised of a large group of monomeric (17–30 kDa) GBPs which have been shown to play a regulatory role(s) in protein sorting and trafficking as well as vectorial transport of secretory vesicles in yeast. These proteins possess unique C-terminal amino acid sequences, which render them suitable candidates for posttranslational modifications (i.e., isoprenylation, carboxyl methylation, and palmitoylation) such modifications increase their association with membranes and/or with their downstream effectors. Unlike the heterotrimeric GBPs, most of the low molecular weight GBPs (with the possible exception of *rho* and CDC42) retain their ability to bind GTP even after SDS-PAGE and nitrocellulose transfer. Therefore, the GTP overlay technique is widely used to quantitate this class of proteins.

The third group of GBPs, such as elongation factor and Tu factor are involved in protein synthesis. Although these proteins are characterized in several cell types, very little is known about this group of proteins in endocrine cells. We will focus on the first two groups of GBPs and their role in stimulus-secretion coupling in insulin-secreting cells.

Heterotrimeric GBPs in Insulin-Secreting Cells

The involvement of PTX-sensitive GBPs in insulin secretion was first demonstrated by Katada and Ui *(25)*, who showed that treatment of rats with (or prior exposure of isolated islets to) PTX prevented the adrenergic inhibition of glucose-induced insulin secretion, suggesting an involvement of a PTX-sensitive mechanism(s) underlying insulin secretion. These observations were confirmed by several investigators using isolated islets *(26)*, intact pancreas *(27)*, and insulin-secreting transformed β-cell (HIT or RINm5F) lines *(23)* employing different adrenergic agents such as epinephrine or clonidine or, alteratively, the secretory inhibitors somatostatin or PGE_2 *(23)*. More recent studies have, indeed, identified the presence of PTX-sensitive heterotrimeric GBPs in normal rat and human islets as well as in RIN and HIT cell membranes (Table 2). It is interesting to note that although these proteins are present in all insulin-secreting cells studied, there seem to be subtle differences in their number as

Table 2
Heterotrimeric GBPs in Insulin-Secreting Cells

Cell type(s)	Toxin used	Number of GBPs identified[a]	Ref.
Rat islets	Pertussis	3 (G_{i2} and G_o)	*J Mol Endocrinol* 8:103, 1992
Rat islets	Pertussis	1 (G_o)	*Brain Res* 417:190, 1987
Rat islets	Pertussis	1 (39 kDa)	*Diabetologia* 35(suppl 1): A12, 1992
Rat islets	Pertussis	1 (41 kDa)	*Biochem J* 258:669, 1989
RINm5F cells	Pertussis	2 (39 and 40 kDa)	*J Biol Chem* 262:5049, 1987
RINm5F cells	Pertussis	5 (3 of G_i and 2 of G_o)	*Diabetes* 40:1170, 1991
HIT cells	Pertussis	7 (G_{i1}, G_{i2} and G_o)	*Diabetologia* 35(suppl 1): A118, 1992
HIT cells	Pertussis	6 (3 of G_i and 3 of G_o)	*Diabetes* 41:1390, 1992
HIT cells	Pertussis	3 (36–39 kDa)	Kowluru et al. *Biochim Biophys Acta,* 1994, in press
Rat islets	Cholera	3 (22–48 kDa)	*Cell Biochem Funct* 3:25, 1985
RINm5F cells	Cholera	1 (45kDa)	*J Biol Chem* 262:5049, 1987

[a]Immunologic identity or the apparent molecular weights of the identified GBPs is provided in parentheses.

well as abundance as reported by different investigators (Table 2). While such differences may be owing partly to differences in experimental approaches (i.e., gel separations of proteins involving different detergents such as SDS vs urea), but there seem to be true qualitative and quantitative differences in the presence and abundance of some GBPs in normal rat islets compared with HIT cells (Table 2 and ref. *28a,b)*, even when quantitated under identical experimental conditions using similar probes. There seem to be subtle differences in the abundance of cholera toxin-sensitive GBPs (presumably the G_s type) between rat islets and RIN cells (Table 2). These data may imply that the physiology of GBPs in insulin-secreting transformed cell lines may be different from normal rat islets.

Table 3
Low Molecular Weight GBPs (Identified by Overlay) in Insulin-Secreting Cells

Cell Type	Subcellular Locus	Number[a] of GBPs Identified[b]	Ref.
Rat islets	Homogenate	6 (14–28 kDa)	*Biochem Soc Trans* 18:485, 1989
Rat islets	Secretory granules	1 (24 kDa)	*Diabetes* 41(suppl 1) 103A, 1992
Rat islets	Secretory granules, membranes and cytosol	4 (21–28 kDa)	*Diabetologia* 35(suppl 1) A12, 1992
Human islets	Membranes and cytosol	2 (21–28 kDa)	Kowluru et al. *Biochim Biophys Acta,* 1994, in press
HIT cells	Homogenate	5 (20–27 kDa)	*Biochem J* 289:379, 1993
HIT cells	Membranes and cytosol	6 (21–27 kDa)	Kowluru et al. *Biochim Biophys Acta,* 1994, in press
RINm5F cells	Secretory granules	2 (23–27 kDa)	*Eur J Biochem* 208:729, 1992
RINm5F cells	Homogenate	13 (20–30 kDa)	*Horm Metab Res* 23:304, 1991

[a]Values in parentheses represent apparent molecular weight range of the GBPs identified.
[b]Some may not be separate GBPs but multiple (differently processed or precursor) forms of GBPs

Low Molecular Weight GBPs in Insulin-Secreting Cells

Table 3 summarizes some of the data on the presence and the subcellular location of these proteins in insulin-secreting cell lines. Once again, like the heterotrimeric GBPs, there are some differences in the abundance of these low weight GBPs between normal islets and transformed cell lines (Table 3). This may partly be a result of the fact that the metabolism of low molecular weight *ras*-like GBPs seem to be altered by transformation *(29)*. Some of these proteins are associated with the secretory granule fraction of rat islets *(28a* and *30a)* as well as HIT and RIN cells *(31)*. This raises the possibility that GBPs are candidates to mediate insulin packaging and the vectorial transport of secretory granules toward plasma membrane for fusion and exocytosis. Fortunately, with the availability of specific antisera directed toward some of these proteins, it has become possible to

Table 4
Low Molecular Weight GBPS Immunologically Identified in Insulin-Secreting Cells

Cell type(s)	GBPs identified	Ref.
Rat islets	*rab*3a	Kowluru et al. *Biochim Biophys Acta,* 1994, in press
	CDC42Hs	
	*rac*2	
HIT cells	*rab*3a	Kowluru et al. *Biochim Biophys Acta,* 1994, in press
	CDC42Hs	
	*rac*2	
HIT cells	*rab*3a	*Eur J Biochem* 208:729, 1992
	CDC42Hs	*J Biol Chem* 267:17,512, 1992
	rho	
RINm5F cells	*rab*3a	*J Biol Chem* 267:17,512, 1992
	ADP-ribosylation factor	*Biochem J* 275:639, 1991

identify some of these proteins in insulin-secreting cells (Table 4), including those that do not bind GTP after nitrocellulose transfer. There is a close *qualitative* similarity between islets and HIT cells, since *rab*3a, CDC42Hs, and *rac*2 are all detectable in these cell types studied. However, recent studies from our laboratory *(28b)* and by Regazzi et al. *(31)* have clearly shown that the abundance *rab*3a is several times higher in normal rat islets than in HIT cells. Taken together, the data presented in Tables 2 and 3 dictate caution in using transformed insulin-secreting cell lines to study the normal physiology of GBPs, since both qualitative and quantitative differences exist between such cell lines and intact islets.

Quantitation of GBP (GTPase) Activity

GBPs possess an intrinsic GTPase activity that catalyzes the removal of the terminal phosphate from the bound GTP (active configuration of the GBP) to an inactive GDP-bound form (Fig. 1). It has been postulated that the "cycling" between the active and inactive configuration of GBPs not only determines their ability to regulate various effector functions, but also controls their translocation back and forth between the membrane and the cytosolic fractions *(32)*. In characterizing GTPase activities intrinsic to islet endogenous GBPs, we observed that islet and HIT cell homogenates have high activities

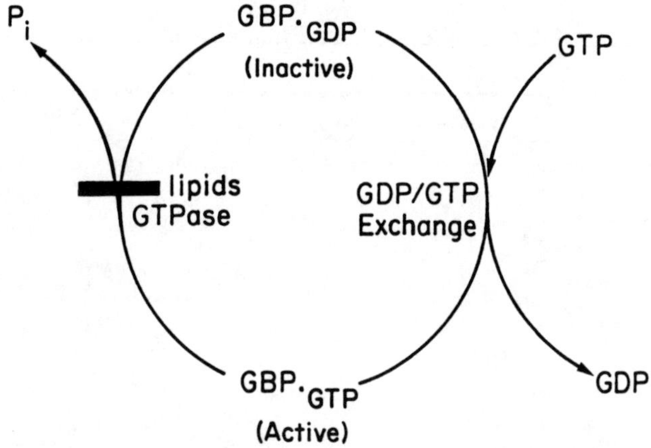

Fig. 1. Schematic representation of the regulation of GBP function by insulinotropic lipids in islets. We propose that biologically active (and insulinotropic lipids) maintain the putative GBPs in their GTP-bound active configuration to elicit their effects on insulin secretion. This is achieved by inhibiting the GTPase activity intrinsic to GBPs as well as by increasing the GTP binding and GDP/GTP exchange activities *(see text).*

of nonspecific nucleotide triphosphatase activities. Therefore, optimized GTPase assay conditions included millimolar concentrations of ATP, App(NH)p (a nonhydrolyzable analog of ATP), and an ATP regenerating system to saturate the nonspecific nucleotide triphosphate binding sites. Under these conditions, islet homogenates contained three specific GTPase activities with K_m values for GTP of 370 n*M*, 2.2 μ*M*, and 720 μ*M (28b)*. Similar GTPases are also present in HIT cells with minimally higher apparent K_m (for GTP). Further quantitation of these activities indicated that a high affinity GTPase activity (Table 5 and Fig. 2) was present in the membrane and secretory granule fraction. The lowest affinity, high K_m activity (Fig. 3) was present in the membrane, secretory granules, and in cytosolic fractions, whereas the GTPase with K_m of 2.2 μ*M* was absent from the secretory granule fraction *(28b)*. The presence of both high and low affinity GTPase activities has been reported in several cell types, including insulin-secreting RIN cells (Table 5), although such low affinity GTPases has generally been dismissed as physiologically irrelevant. However, our studies (cited above) suggested that a K_m of

Table 5
Specific GTPase Activities and Their Regulation in Some Cell Types

Fraction studied	K_m for GTP of High affinity GTPase	K_m for GTP of Low affinity GTPase	Simulator(s) of high affinity GTPase	Ref.
Erythrocyte membranes	100 n*M*	ND	Catecholamines	*Biochim Biophys Acta* 452:538, 1976
Brain membranes	350 n*M*	619 µ*M*	Muscarinic agents	*J Pharm Sci* 77:353, 1988
Pancreatic membranes	100–200 n*M*	>30 µ*M*	Pancreozymin	*FEBS Lett* 99:303, 1979
Liver membranes	200–500 n*M*	150-350 µ*M*	Glucagon	*FEBS Lett* 117:172, 1980
Adipocyte membranes	200 n*M*	180 µ*M*	PGE_1 and nicotinic acid	*Biochem Biophys Res Commnn* 174:600, 1991
RINm5F membranes	225 n*M*	>60 µ*M*	Galanin	*Diabetes* 42:74, 1993
Islet heavy membranes and secretory granules	370 n*M*	2.2 µ*M* 720 µ*M*	Epinephrine Clonidine PGE_2	Kowluru et al. *Biochim Biophys Acta,* 1994, in press

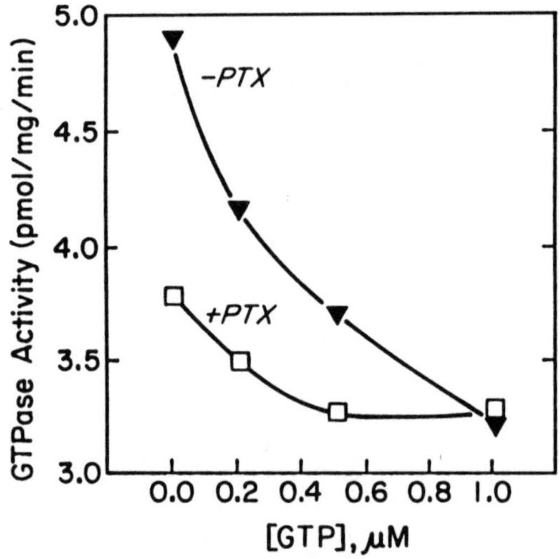

Fig. 2. Pertussis toxin-sensitive, high-affinity (low K_m) GTPase activity in secretory granule fraction of rat islets. GTPase activity was assayed at various GTP concentrations (0–1 µ*M*) in the secretory granule fraction pretreated with activated pertussis toxin (□—□) or with diluents (▼—▼). It was observed that pertussis toxin pre-treatment significantly reduced the GTPase activity (at low nM GTP concentrations), suggesting the presence of pertussis toxin-sensitive, high-affinity GTPase activity in the islet secretory granule fraction.

720 µ*M* GTP could be quite relevant to β-cell function; furthermore, this islet GTPase is regulated by biologically-active lipid messengers *(see below)*.

GTPase as a Negative Modulator of Insulin Secretion

The GTPase activity intrinsic to GBPs requires Mg^{2+} for its activity. Using permeabilized mast cells, Lillie and Gomperts *(4)* have recently demonstrated that depletion of Mg^{2+} from the incubation media results in a dramatic increase in mast cell secretion. This may, in part, be caused by inhibition of the GTPase activity (via Mg^{2+} depletion), thereby maintaining the putative GBPs in their GTP-bound (active) configuration (Fig. 1). Recent data obtained in our laboratory are compatible with this formulation. We observed a close relationship between the GTPase activity of normal rat islets and their insulin release. Inhibitors of glucose-induced insulin secretion,

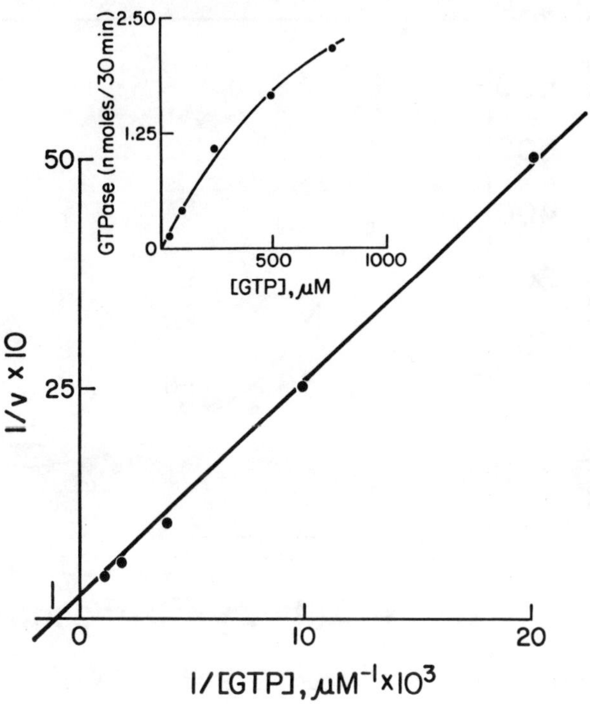

Fig. 3. Kinetic characterization of low-affinity (high K_m) GTPase activity in rat islet secretory granule fraction. GTPase activity was assayed in the secretory granule fraction in the presence of various concentrations of GTP as indicated. Reaction velocities are plotted against GTP concentration (inset) or the inverse of the reaction velocities are plotted against 1/GTP concentration (main panel). Data are representative of 2–3 individual determinations at each substrate concentration performed in triplicate.

such as epinephrine, clonidine, or PGE_2, stimulate GTPase activity, whereas stimulators of insulin secretion (such as arachidonic acid, lysophosphatidylcholine, and phosphatidic acid) inhibited the GTPase activity *(30a,b)*. Other (lyso)lipids and fatty acids that do not promote insulin secretion also failed to exert appreciable effects on GTPase activity (ref. *30b* and Fig. 4). Similar GTPase-stimulatory effects of inhibitors of insulin secretion have been reported in RIN and HIT cell membranes by several investigators (Fig. 4 and Table 6).

However, mastoparan, an amphiphilic peptide, stimulated both insulin secretion, as well as GTPase activity in the secretory granule

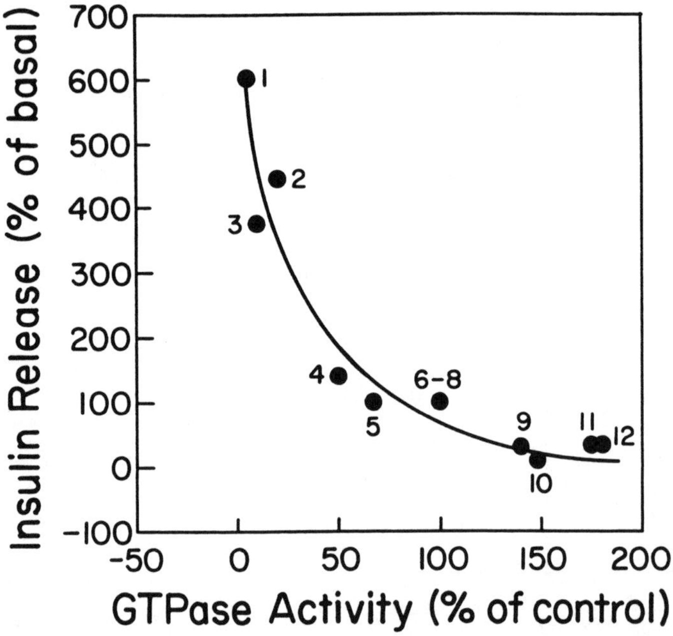

Fig. 4. Inverse relationship between GTPase activity and insulin secretion in normal islets and insulin-secreting cell lines. Based on the information existing in the literature (Table 6) and the data obtained from our laboratory, effects of both positive and negative modulators of insulin secretion were compared to their effects on GTPase activity. Insulin secretion data were observed from the existing literature *(11,23,37,40–47)*. Identities of various modulators represented numerically in the figure are as follows: 1: arachidonic acid; 2: phosphatidic acid; 3: lysophosphatidylcholine; 4: linoleate; 5: oleate; 6: control; 7: lysophosphatidylethanolamine; 8: palmitate; 9: clonidine; 10: epinephrine; 11: PGE_2; 12: galanin. Insulin release studies utilized rodent islets (for agents 1–5 and 7–10), HIT cells (for PGE_2), or RIN cells (for galanin). Effects of agents on insulin secretion were studied either at substimulatory (<2 m*M* glucose; for 1–5, 7, and 8) or at stimulatory (11.1–20 m*M* glucose; for 9–11) glucose concentrations. Phorbol ester (30 n*M*) was the agonist used in studies of galanin. In each case, insulin release obtained in the absence of modulators was taken as 100%. Inhibitors of agonist-induced insulin secretion (such as epinephrine, clonidine, PGE_2, or galanin) stimulate GTPase activity, whereas stimulators of insulin secretion (such as AA, PA, or LPC) inhibit GTPase activity. These data indicate the presence of both inhibitory and stimulatory GBPs in insulin-secreting cells *(see text)* which are differentially regulated by modulators of insulin secretion.

Table 6
Regulation of GTPase Activity by Modulators of Insulin Secretion

			Effects on		
Cell type(s)	Modulator(s)	Subcellular locus	GTPase	Insulin secretion	Ref.
Rat islets clonidine PGE2	Epinephrine membrane	Secretory granule,	Stimulatory	Inhibitory	*Biochem J*
RINm5F	Galanin	Membrane	Stimulatory	Inhibitory	*Diabetes* 42:74, 1993
RINm5F cells	Epinephrine clonidine	Membrane	Stimulatory	Inhibitory	*J Biol Chem* 266:18,025, 1991
Rat islets cells	AA, LPC, PA	Membrane, secretory granule, cytosol	Inhibitory	Stimulatory	*Diabetologia* 35(suppl 1):12A, 1992
Human	AA islets	Cytosol	Inhibitory	Not known in this preparation	Kowluru et al. *Biochim Biophys Acta,* 1994, in press
HIT cells	AA, LPC, PA	Homogenates	Inhibitory	Not known in this preparation	Kowluru et al. *Biochim Biophys Acta,* 1994, in press

Abbreviations: AA: arachidonic acid; LPC: lysophosphatidylcholine; PA: phosphatidic acid; PGE_2: prostaglandin E_2

fraction *(30b)*. This observation possibly suggests the requirement for more than one GTPase (possibly, a stimulatory and an inhibitory) activity associated with the putative GBPs involved in exocytosis. Furthermore, in most systems including pancreatic islets, the nonhydrolyzable analogs of GTP, such as GTPγS, are more potent than GTP itself in promoting secretion. Therefore, based on the effects on GTPase activity of lipids, mastoparan, clonidine, or PGE_2 *(see above)*, it is reasonable to postulate the presence of both stimulatory (G_E) and inhibitory (G_{Ei}) GBPs in islets. This is consistent with other data cited in the previous sections. In order to reconcile the effects on the GTPase activity by both the positive and negative modulators of insulin secretion, we propose the following two models.

GBPs that Require "Cycling"

Multiple steps in secretion may be promoted by GBPs, but only some of these may require hydrolysis of the GTP bound to GBPs. This may be true in the case of mastoparan, which stimulates the GTPase activity (as well as GTP binding owing to augmentation of GDP/GTP exchange activity). Under such conditions, there is increased "cycling" of the putative stimulatory GBP (G_E) culminating in secretion. Likewise, the "cycling" of an inhibitory GBP (G_{Ei}) may be increased by agents such as PGE_2 or clonidine that increase GTPase activity (presumably of G_{Ei}) concomitant with inhibition of insulin secretion. It may also be possible that GTPγS could prevent "cycling" of G_{Ei}, leading to increased insulin secretion *(see above)*.

GBPs that Can Be "Permanently" Activated

Another group of GBPs seems not to require GTP hydrolysis and may be maintained in their GTP-bound (i.e.,m"permanently"-activated) configuration by modulators of insulin secretion such as lipids (or GTPγS) and thereby might elicit an insulin secretory response. We have observed that insulinotropic lipids inhibit GTPase activity while stimulating the GTP binding as well as GDP/GTP exchange *(30b)*.

Another possibility that we cannot exclude is that both mastoparan and GTPγS activate one or more heterotrimeric GBPs, leading to release of its α subunit from the complex with βγ; the latter could have direct stimulatory effects on effectors of exocytotic cascade *(33,34)*.

Does PLA_2 Represent the "Pseudoreceptor" Protein for the Activation of "G_E"?

Recently, it has been proposed by Lillie and Gomperts *(4)* that the rate of nucleotide exchange onto "G_E" is stimulated by Ca^{2+} subsequent to its binding to a Ca^{2+}-binding "pseudoreceptor" protein ("C_E"). These investigators proposed that the activation of G_E in such a manner not only reduces its requirement for Mg^{2+}, but also increases secretion severalfold. A similar system may be operable in pancreatic islets. It is reasonable to postulate that a increase in intracellular Ca^{2+} concentration stimulated by glucose results in stimulation of a Ca^{2+}-sensitive "pseudoreceptor" protein endogenous to islets. These proteins could include some annexin and 14-3-3 protein family members *(35,36)*; phospholipase A_2 (or other phospholipases) that generate soluble mediators of insulin secretion, such as AA and LPC, might also represent such candidate proteins. We have observed that these lipids inhibit the GTPase activity intrinsic to several of islet GBPs; this effect might maintain "G_E" in its active configuration to regulate secretion *(30a,b)*. Alternatively, as observed in several other systems, AA and PA may mimic receptor stimulation and promote Ca^{2+} mobilization and flux through one or more ion channels *(37)*, again perhaps via reduction of GTPase activity.

Requirement for Posttranslational Modifications of GBPs in Insulin Exocytosis

Most low molecular weight GBPs, as well as the γ subunits of heterotrimeric GBPs, undergo posttranslational modifications, such as isoprenylation, carboxyl methylation, and palmitoylation, all on C-terminal cysteine residues *(29)*. These modifications increase the hydrophobicity of the GBPs and thus facilitate their translocation from cytosol to the membrane fraction *(29)*. Recent studies from our laboratory have shown that at least some of the low molecular weight GBPs in islets undergo isoprenylation and carboxyl methylation. Furthermore, specific inhibitors of these reactions impaired nutrient-induced insulin secretion from pancreatic islets *(38,39)*. Using [^{14}C]mevalonic acid as a precursor for the isoprene groups, we observed that at least five proteins in the molecular weight range of 18.5 - 27.5 kDa underwent isoprenylation in normal rat pancreatic islets *(38,39)*. These proteins seem to be similar to the GBPs we identified by the [α-^{32}P]GTP overlay method. Pretreatment of islets with lovastatin (15-30 µ*M*), a blocker of HMG-CoA reductase and therefore of endogenous mevalonic acid production, inhibited the localization of low molecular weight GBPs to the membrane (Fig. 5), leading to their accumulation in cytosol; at the same time glucose-induced insulin secretion was inhibited. The latter effect was reversed by exogenous mevalonic acid *(38)*. These data imply that glucose-induced insulin secretion from pancreatic islets may require the membrane association of certain isoprenylated low molecular weight GBPs. Using S-adenosyl[^{3}H]methionine as a methyl donor, we also observed that two proteins in the molecular weight region of 21–23 kDa, underwent carboxyl methylation in normal rat and human pancreatic islets, as well as in HIT cell homogenates *(38)*. GTPγS (10 µ*M*) stimulated the methylation of these proteins. Acetyl farnesyl cysteine (AFC, 100 µ*M*), a competitive inhibitor of methyl group transfer to prenyl-cysteine residues on GBPs, inhibited the stimulation by GTPγs of the methylation of GBPs in islets. Moreover, AFC (but not its inactive analog, acetyl geranyl cysteine, 100 µ*M*) inhibited nutrient-induced insulin secretion from normal rat islets by 50–65% *(38,39)*. These data further support the requirement for carboxyl methylation of specific proteins in insulin exocytosis. Further studies are underway to characterize this protein(s) in rat islets as well as in HIT cells; initial studies suggest that CDC42 may play a significant role here (Kowluru A, Rabaglia M, Metz S, submitted). Additional recent studies from our laboratory have also indicated that an inhibitor of palmitoylation (cerulenin, 90–135 µ*M*) also reduces nutrient-induced insulin secretion from normal rat islets *(38)*. Thus, taken together, there is emerging evidence to suggest that posttranslational modifications of GBPs are required for nutrient-induced insulin secretion. Furthermore, lovastatin or AFC (100 µ*M*) *potentiated* the insulinotropic effects of mastoparan or TPA *(38)*, which are *nonnutrient* secretagogues probably acting distally in the cascade culminating in exocytosis. These observations suggests that carboxyl methylation is needed also for the function of inhibitory GBPs ("G_{Ei}"; *see above*); therefore, blockade of their prenylation and/or carboxyl methylation would impede their inhibitory functions, leading to *increased* secretion. Further studies of GTP and GBPs in islets are

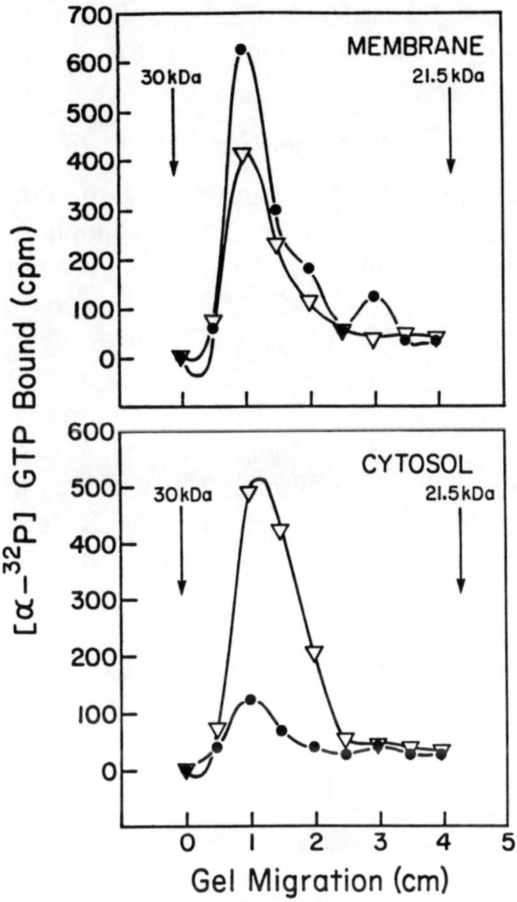

Fig. 5. Inhibition of isoprenylation results in the cytosolic accumulation of GBPs. Islets (300–350) were cultured for 18 hrs in the absence (●—●) of presence (Δ—Δ) or 15 μ*M* lovastatin. The total membranous and cytosolic fractions were isolated by centrifugation (105,000*g* for 60 minutes) and the GBPs were identified by [α-^{32}P]GTP overlay method *(38)*. Following autoradiography, the nitrocellulose membranes were sliced into 0.5 cm sections and the radioactivity bound to GBPs was quantitated by scintillation spectrometry. Pre-treatment of islets with lovastatin resulted in accumulation of GBPs in the cytosolic fraction, suggesting that selective blocking of the synthesis endogenous mevalonic acid (a precursor for isoprenoid groups), results in the cytosolic accumulation of nonisoprenylated proteins *(see text)*.

likely to provide insights into both positive and the negative modulators of exocytosis, and to place these steps in the sequence of events leading to insulin secretion.

Abbreviations

GTP, guanosine triphosphate; ATP, adenosine triphosphate; UTP, uridine triphosphate; IMPDH, inosine monophosphate dehydrogenase; GBPs, GTP-binding proteins; G_i, a Pertussis toxin-sensitive heterotrimeric G-protein; G_0, a Pertussis toxin-sensitive heterotrimeric G-protein; G_E, A putative GBP of exocytosis; G_{Ei}, An inhibitory GBP of exocytosis; GTPγS, guanosine 5'-O-(3-thiotriphosphate); AA, arachidonic acid; LPC, lysophosphatidylcholine; PA, Phosphatidic acid; GTPase, Guanosine triphosphatase; IDDM, Insulin-dependent diabetes mellitus; PTX, Pertussis toxin; SDS-PAGE, sodium dodecyl sulfate polyacrylamide gel electrophoresis; ARF, ADP-ribosylation factor; PGE_2, Prostaglandin E_2.

Acknowledgments

The studies of the authors were supported by the Veterans Administration and the National Institutes of Health (DK 37312).

References

1. Metz SA, Rabaglia ME, Pintar TJ: Selective inhibitors of GTP synthesis impede exocytotic insulin release from intact rat islets. *J Biol Chem* 267:12,517–12,527, 1992.
2. Otero A deS: Transphosphorylation and G protein activation. *Biochem Pharmacol* 39:1399–1404, 1990.
3. Haun RS, Tsai S-C, Adamik R, Moss J, Vaughan M: Effect of myristoylation on GTP-dependent binding of ADP-ribosylation factor to Golgi. *J Biol Chem* 268:7064–7068, 1993.
4. Lillie THW, Gomperts BD: Guanine nucleotide is essential and Ca^{2+} is a modulator in the exocytotic reaction of permeabilized rat mast cells. *Biochem J* 288:181–187, 1992.
5. Lillie THW, Gomperts BD: Kinetic characterization of guanine-nucleotide-induced exocytosis from permeabilized rat mast cells. *Biochem J* 290:389–394, 1993.
6. Ahnert-Hilger G, Dayanithi G, Spicher K, Nordmann JJ: G-proteins mediate inhibition and activation of Ca^{2+}-induced exocytosis from SLO-permeabilized peptidergic nerve endings. *Biosci Rep* 12:463–469, 1992.
7. Metz SA, Meredith M, Kowluru A: Purine nucleotide metabolism and GTP-binding proteins in the pancreatic β-cell. In *Frontiers of Pancreatic β-Cell Research* (Flatt PR, ed.), 1994, in press.

8. Metz SA, Meredith M, Rabaglia ME, Kowluru A: Small elevations of glucose concentration re-direct and amplify the synthesis of GTP in rat islets. *J Clin Invest* 92:872–882, 1993.
9. Welsh N, Sandler S, Welsh M, Hellerström: Regulation of RNA metabolism in relation to insulin production and oxidative metabolism in mouse pancreatic islets in vitro. *Biochim Biophys Acta* 887:58–68, 1986.
10. Liang Y, Najafi H, Smith RM, Zimmerman EC, Magnuson MA, Tal M, Matschinsky FM: Concordant glucose induction of glucokinase, glucose usage, and glucose-stimulated insulin release in pancreatic islets maintained in organ culture. *Diabetes* 41:792–806, 1992.
11. Metz SA: Epinephrine impairs insulin release by a mechanism distal to calcium mobilization. Similarity to lipoxygenase inhibitors. *Diabetes* 37:65–73, 1988.
12. Gembal M, Detimary P, Gilon P, Gao Z-Y, Henquin J-C: Mechanisms by which glucose can control insulin release independently from its action on adenosine triphosphate-sensitive K^+ channels in mouse B cells. *J Clin Invest* 91:871–880, 1993.
13. Ullrich, S, Prentki, M, Wollheim, CB: Somatostatin inhibition of Ca^{2+}-induced insulin secretion in permeabilized HIT-T15 cells. *Biochem J* 270:273–276, 1990.
14. Koffer A: Calcuim-induced secretion from permeabilized rat mast cells: requirements for guanine nucleotides. *Biochim Biophys Acta* 1176:231–239, 1993.
15. Lauquin GJM, Villiers C, Michejda JW, Hryniewiecka LV, Vignais PV: Adenine nucleotide transport in sonic submitochondrial particles. Kinetic properties and binding of specific inhibitors. *Biochim Biophys Acta* 460:331–345, 1977.
16. MacDonald MJ, Fahien LA: Glyceraldehyde phosphate and methyl esters of succinic acid. Two "new" potent insulin secretagogues. *Diabetes* 37:997–999, 1988.
17. Fahien LA, MacDonald MJ, Kmiotek EH, Mertz RJ, Fahien CM: Regulation of insulin release by factors that also modify glutamine dehydrogenase. *J Biol Chem* 263:13,610–13,614, 1988.
18. Miyake R, Gross RW: Multiple phospholipase A_2 activities in canine vascular smooth muscle. *Biochim Biophys Acta* 1165:167–176, 1992.
19. Davfetov B, Marie-Sontag J-M, Hata Y, Petrenko AG, Fykse EM, Jahn R, Sudhof TC: Phosphorylation of synaptotagmin I by casein kinase II. *J Biol Chem* 268:6816–6822, 1993.
20. Cordella-Miele E, Miele L, Beninati S, Mukherjee AB: Transglutaminase-catalyzed incorporation of polyamines into phospholipase A_2. *J Biochem (Tokyo)* 113:164–173, 1993.
21. Facchiano F, Benfenati F, Valtorta F, Luini A: Covalent modification of synapsin I by a tetanus toxin-activated transglutaminase. *J Biol Chem* 268:4588–4591, 1993.
22. Zünkler BJ, Lenzen S, Panten U: D-glucose enhances GTP content in mouse pancreatic islets. *IRCS Med Sci* 14:354,355, 1986.

23. Robertson RP, Seaquist ER, Walseth TF: G proteins and modulation of insulin secretion. *Diabetes* 40:1–6, 1991.
24. Helper JR, Gilman AG: G-proteins. TIBS 17:383–387, 1992.
25. Katada T, Ui M: Islet activating protein. Enhanced secretion and cyclic AMP accumulation in pancreatic islets due to activation of native calcium ionophores. *J Biol Chem* 254:469–479, 1979.
26. Nakakki G, Nakadate T, Ishili K, Kato R: Postsynaptic alpha 2 adrenergic receptors in isolated rat islets of Langerhans: Inhibition of insulin release and cyclic 3' 5' adenosine monophosphate accumulation. *J Pharmacol Exp Ther* 216:607–614, 1981.
27. Hillaire-Buys D, Gross R, Roye M, Ribes G, Loubatieres-Mariani M-M: Adrenergic inhibition of insulin secretion involves pertussis toxin-sensitive and -insensitive mechanisms. *Eur J Pharmacol* 218:3359–3362, 1992.
28a. Morgan NG, Berrows NS: Immunological characterization of pertussis toxin-sensitive G-proteins in isolated islets and cultured insulinoma cells. *Diabetologia* 35(supp 1):A118, 1992.
28b. Kowluru A, Rabaglia ME, Muse KE, Metz SA: Subcellular localization and kinetic characterization of guanine nucleotide binding proteins in normal rat and human pancreatic islets and transformed beta cells. *Biochim Biophys Acta* 1994, in press.
29. Takai Y, Kaibuchi K, Kikuchi A, Kawata M: Small GTP-binding proteins. *Int Rev Cytol* 133:187–230, 1992.
30a. Kowluru A, Metz SA: Stimulation by prostaglandin E_2 of a high affinity GTPase in the secretory granules of normal rat and human pancreatic islets. *Biochem J* 297:399–406, 1994.
30b. Kowluru A, Metz SA: Regulation of guanine-nucleotide binding proteins in islet subcellular fractions by phospholipase-derived lipid mediators of insulin secretion. *Biochim Biophys Acta* 1994, in press.
31. Regazzi R, Vallar L, Ullrich S, Ravazzola M, Kikuchi A, Takai Y, Wollheim CB: Characterization of small-molecular-mass guanine nucleotide-binding regulatory proteins in insulin-secreting cells and PC 12 cells. *Eur J Biochem* 208:729-737, 1992
32. Bourne HR, Sanders DA, McCormick F: The GTPase superfamily: a conserved switch for diverse cell functions. *Nature* 348:125–132, 1990.
33. Boyer JL, Waldo GL, Harden TK: βγ-subunit activation of G-protein-regulated phospholipase C. *J Biol Chem* 267:25,451–25,456, 1992.
34. Katz A, Wu D, Simon MI: Subunits βγ of heterotrimeric G protein activate β2 isoform of phospholipase. *Nature* 360:686–689, 1992.
35. Creutz CE: The annexins and exocytosis. *Science* 258:924–931, 1992.
36. Zupan LA, Steffans DL, Erry CA, Landt M, Gross RW: Cloning and expression of a human 14-3-3 protein mediating phospholipolysis. *J Biol Chem* 267:8707–8710, 1992.
37. Dunlop ME, Larkins RG: Effect of phosphatidic acid on islet cell phosphoinositide hydrolysis, Ca^{2+}, and adenylate cyclase. *Diabetes* 38:1187–1192, 1989.

38. Metz SA, Rabaglia ME, Stock J, Kowluru A: Modulation of insulin secretion from normal rat islets by inhibitors of the posttranslational modifications of GTP-binding proteins. *Biochem J*, 295:31–40, 1993.
39. Kowluru A, Rabaglia ME, Stock J, Metz SA: A requirement in exocytotic insulin secretion for GTP-dependent carboxyl methylation of specific islet proteins. *Diabetes* 42:76A, 1993.
40. Metz SA: Ether-linked lysophospholipids initiate insulin secretion. Lysophospholipids may mediate effects of phospholipase A_2 activation on hormone release. *Diabetes* 35:808–817, 1986.
41. Metz SA: Exogenous arachidonic acid promotes insulin release from intact or permeabilized rat islets by dual mechanisms. *Diabetes* 37:1453–1469, 1988.
42. Metz SA, Draznin B, Sussman KE, Leitner JW: Unmasking of arachidonate-induced insulin release by removal of extracellular calcium. *Biochem Biophys Res Commun* 142:251–258, 1987.
43. Seaquist ER, Walseth TF, Nelson DM, Robertson RP: Pertussis toxin-sensitive G-protein mediation of PGE_2 inhibition of cAMP metabolism and phasic glucose-induced insulin secretion in HIT cells. *Diabetes* 38:1439–1445, 1989.
44. Sharp GWG, Merchand-Brustel YL, Yada T, Russo LL, Bliss CR, Cormont M, Monge L, Van Obberghen E: Galanin can inhibit insulin release by a mechanism other than membrane hyperpolarization or inhibition of adenylate cyclase. *J Biol Chem* 264:7302–7309, 1989.
45. Persaud SJ, Jones PM, Howell SL: Effects of Bordetella pertussis toxin on catecholamine inhibition of insulin release from intact and electrically permeabilized rat islets. *Biochem J* 258:669–675, 1989.
46. Basudev H, Jones PM, Persaud SJ, Howell SL: Arachidonic acid-induced insulin secretion from rat islets of Langerhans is not mediated by protein phosphorylation. *Mol Cell Endocrinol* 91:193–199, 1993.
47. Vara E, Tamarit-Rodriguez J: Glucose stimulation of insulin secretion in islets of fed and starved rats and its dependence of lipid metabolism. *Metabolism* 35:266–271, 1986.

Chapter 12

β-Cell Receptors

Mechanisms of Signal Transduction

Joseph S. Dillon, Ming Lu, Michael B. Wheeler, and Aubrey E. Boyd III

Introduction

The secretion of insulin is closely regulated in vivo in order to maintain the plasma glucose concentration in a narrow range despite long periods of fasting and intermittent food intake. The regulation of insulin secretion has been studied extensively and involves a complex interaction of glucose and other nutrients, and endocrine, paracrine, and neurohumoral factors. The effects of these factors on insulin secretion are transduced by their interaction with specific receptor molecules on the surface of the β-cell. The physiologic role of many of these ligand–receptor interactions in altering insulin secretion has been clarified recently and their distal signaling mechanisms characterized.

Most hormonal insulin secretagogues have relatively small effects on insulin secretion in the absence of glucose and thus act as modulators of glucose stimulated insulin secretion. Glucose is the major physiologic stimulator of insulin secretion. The mechanism of glucose stimulated insulin secretion involves glucose transport into the β-cell by GLUT 2 (a glucose transporter specific to the β-cell and liver). Glucose is then phosphorylated by glucokinase and the ATP

From: *Molecular Biology of Diabetes, Part I*
Edited by: B. Draznin and D. LeRoith

produced during subsequent glucose metabolism closes the ATP-dependent potassium channels, causing the retention of positive charge, leading to cell depolarization *(1)*. The change in membrane potential opens voltage-dependent calcium channels (VDCCs) and increases the free cytosolic calcium concentration $[Ca^{2+}]_i$, triggering a host of distal steps and finally insulin release (Fig. 1A). In general, factors modulating insulin secretion interact with their specific receptors on the β-cell and alter the intracellular cAMP or calcium concentrations (Fig. 1B,C). Certain hormones and neuropeptides may also alter insulin secretion by effects on the ATP sensitive potassium channel and membrane polarity or direct effects on insulin exocytosis (Fig. 1D).

It is difficult to experimentally determine the exact physiologic role of specific hormonal and neurohumoral agents on β-cell insulin secretion in intact animals, whole pancreases, or intact islets. Factors such as indirect hormonal action on β-cell mediated by paracrine or neurocrine factors and cosecretion of multiple neurohumoral agents by autonomic nervous stimulation, complicate the assessment. For example, apart from a direct action on pancreatic β-cells, GLP-1 stimulates somatostatin secretion from pancreatic δ-cells that may inhibit both α- and β-cell function. The sympathetic nerves innervating the islets of Langerhans show colocalization and cosecretion of catecholamines, neuropeptide Y, and galanin, making it difficult to determine the physiologic role of each of these hormones during sympathetic stimulation. Studies using isolated β-cells or β-cell derived lines simplify this problem. Beta cell lines offer advantages of being a uniform population of β-type cells and thus free of problems of tissue or whole animal studies, i.e., neurocrine and paracrine influences and easily grown and prepared for binding studies or analysis of second messenger systems. It must be remembered, however, that β-cell lines may differ significantly from native β-cells. The drawbacks of these cell lines for studying the mechanism of hormonal regulation of insulin secretion include:

1. Cell lines may not respond to glucose in a physiologic fashion;
2. Cell lines may lack certain receptors found on native β-cells;
3. The intracellular signal transduction machinery may be different from the native state; and
4. Characteristics of cell lines may be passage dependent.

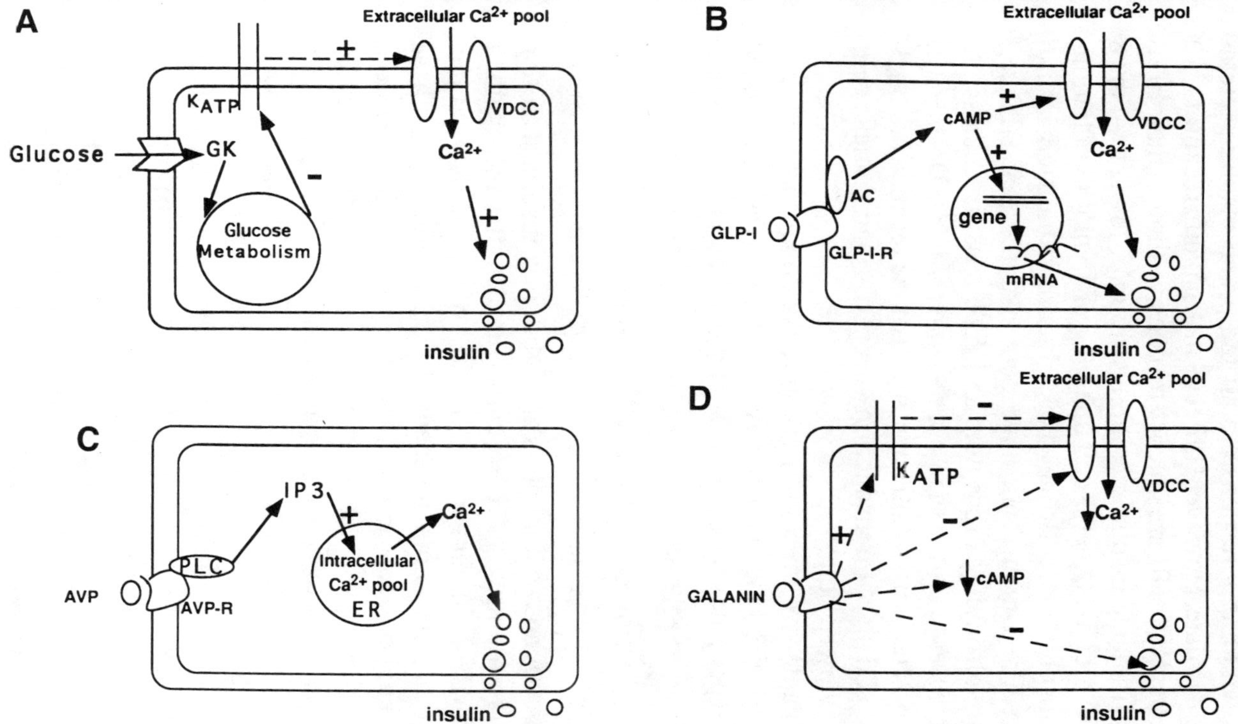

Fig. 1. Models for the signal transduction pathways of **(A)** glucose; **(B)** GLP-1, an adenylyl cyclase coupled β-cell receptor; **(C)** AVP, a phospholipase C coupled β-cell receptor; and **(D)** Galanin, a receptor coupled to effects on ion channels, cAMP, and insulin exocytosis. GK, Glucokinase; K_{ATP}, ATP sensitive potassium channel; VDCC, voltage dependent calcium channel; GLP-1R, GLP-1 receptor; AC, adenylyl cyclase; AVP-R, AVP receptor; PLC, phospholipase C; IP3, Inositol trisphosphate; ER, endoplasmic reticulum.

For example, the HIT cell line, an SV40 transformed hamster islet cell line retains many of the differentiated functions of pancreatic β-cells, including a response to all the β-cell insulin secretagogues studied to date. However HIT cells lack galanin receptors *(2)*. Like the β-cells, HIT cells are glucose responsive though their ED_{50} for glucose stimulated insulin secretion is 1.5 m*M*, lower than the 8 m*M* of normal β-cells. Other β-cell lines, e.g., RINm5f (a radiation-induced rat insulinoma cell line) lack glucose stimulated insulin secretion. Aguilar-Bryan et al. have demonstrated that HIT cell expression of sulfonylurea receptors and ATP sensitive potassium channels decreases with passage number over 75 *(3)*. Despite the problems associated with β-cell lines, much of the recent work on β-cell receptors and signal transduction was performed in these cells and will be reviewed here.

In this chapter we will summarize information regarding β-cell receptors categorized mechanistically according to their associated second messenger pathway and funtionally as potentiators or inhibitors of insulin secretion.

Potentiators of Insulin Secretion

β-Cell Receptors Linked to Adenylyl Cyclase

Many endogenous potentiators or inhibitors of insulin secretion act through G-protein coupled receptors to alter the intracellular content of cAMP or calcium or both. Typical of the β-cell G-protein coupled receptors that stimulate adenylyl cyclase activity are those of the potent incretins gastric insulinotropic polypeptide (GIP) and glucagon like peptide-1 (GLP-1). Incretins are hormones secreted from endocrine cells of the gastrointestinal tract in response to ingested nutrients especially carbohydrates. They increase insulin biosynthesis and release in a glucose dependent manner.

The β-cell receptor for GIP has been defined by binding analysis and cross linking studies in hamster β-cell lines. The receptor is 59 kDa in size and the K_d for GIP binding is 1.9 n*M* *(4)*. The GLP-1 receptor on RIN cells has an apparent molecular weight of 63 kDa and a K_d of 0.25 n*M* *(5)*. We have recently cloned two human pancreatic islet GLP-1 receptor cDNAs *(6)*. Both of these cDNAs encode a 463 amino acid sequence, which is 90% homologous with the rat receptor sequence isolated by Thorens *(7)*. The cDNAs differ in their

3' untranslated regions suggesting alternate splicing of the receptor. There is a high degree of polymorphism in this region of the GLP-1 receptor gene (Tanizawa et al., manuscript in press). Conformational analysis of the encoded protein shows the characteristic structure of a G-protein-coupled receptor with seven potential transmembrane spanning domains.

A hallmark of many hormonal or neurohumoral modulators of insulin secretion is the dependence of their effects on the ambient glucose levels. In the hamster insulinoma (HIT) cell line, Lu et al. *(8)* have demonstrated that GIP stimulates insulin secretion and activates adenylyl cyclase in the presence of glucose over the same concentration range with ED_{50}s of 0.3 and 0.8 n*M*, respectively. GLP-1 has also been shown to activate adenylyl cyclase in a RIN cell line, in a glucose dependent manner *(9)*. Neither GIP nor GLP-1 altered cAMP content or insulin secretion in the absence of glucose. Thus, glucose must be present for both peptides to increase cAMP content and potentiate insulin secretion.

The glucose dependence of GLP-1 stimulated insulin secretion is a property of the milieu of the β-cell rather than intrinsic to the receptor itself since transfection of GLP-1 receptor to COS cells (a monkey kidney cell line) does not confer glucose sensitivity *(10)*. Fig. 2 shows that there was no significant difference in GLP-1 stimulated COS cell cAMP content in the absence of glucose.

Similar to the situation with cAMP, GIP and GLP-1 stimulate increases in $[Ca^{2+}]_i$ only in the presence of glucose. Lu et al *(8)* have shown that neither peptide had an effect on $[Ca^{2+}]_i$ in fura 2 loaded HIT cells in the absence of glucose (Fig. 3A) but in the presence of 4 m*M* glucose they increased $[Ca^{2+}]_i$ in a concentration dependent manner. The GIP stimulated calcium influx passes through VDCCs since GIP failed to elicit a rise in $[Ca^{2+}]_i$ in the absence of extracellular calcium or in the presence of a VDCC blocker, nimodipine (Fig. 3B,C). Neither GIP nor GLP-1 altered the levels of inositol 1,4,5-trisphosphate, at stimulatory glucose concentrations, during 3 second to 3 minute incubations in HIT cells. Thus, neither agent activates phospholipase C or mobilizes intracellular calcium in HIT cells.

The influx of calcium and increase in $[Ca^{2+}]_i$, but not the increase in cAMP content determines the potentiation of glucose-stimulated insulin secretion by GIP and GLP-1. L-type calcium channel blockers

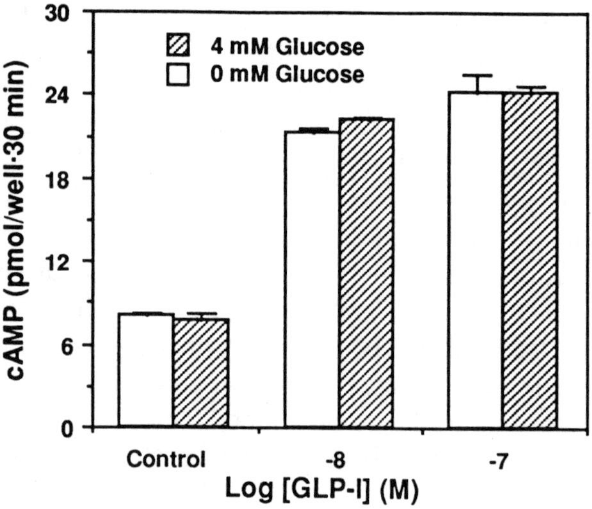

Fig. 2. Effects of GLP-1 on cAMP accumulation in rat GLP-1 receptor transfected COS cells are not glucose dependent. Seventy-two hours after transfection COS cells, preincubated in either 0 or 4 m*M* glucose, were stimulated with 10 or 100 n*M* GLP-1(7–37) at 0 or 4 m*M* glucose for 30 min. Mean ± SE (n = 3–7).

reduce the basal level of insulin secretion but have no effect on the basal levels of cAMP at stimulatory glucose concentrations. The potentiation of glucose-stimulated insulin secretion by both GIP and GLP-1 is blocked by L- type calcium channel blockers yet the same increase in cAMP levels is seen in the presence of these compounds. Furthermore, omission of calcium from the treatment buffer also inhibited the potentiation of glucose-stimulated insulin secretion by GIP and GLP-1 despite unchanged or even greater increments in cAMP accumulation *(8)*. Thus, calcium not cAMP is the true second messenger for GIP and GLP-1 stimulated insulin secretion.

Though the GIP stimulated increase in $[Ca^{2+}]_i$ is the signal for insulin secretion the change in cAMP is the modulator of GIP stimulated insulin gene expression *(11)*. In HIT cells, at 4 mM glucose, a maximum concentration of GIP increased proinsulin mRNA levels 2.9 ± 0.3-fold over basal without altering actin mRNA levels. HIT cells were transiently transfected with a plasmid containing 410 base pairs of the rat insulin I gene promoter fused to the transcriptional

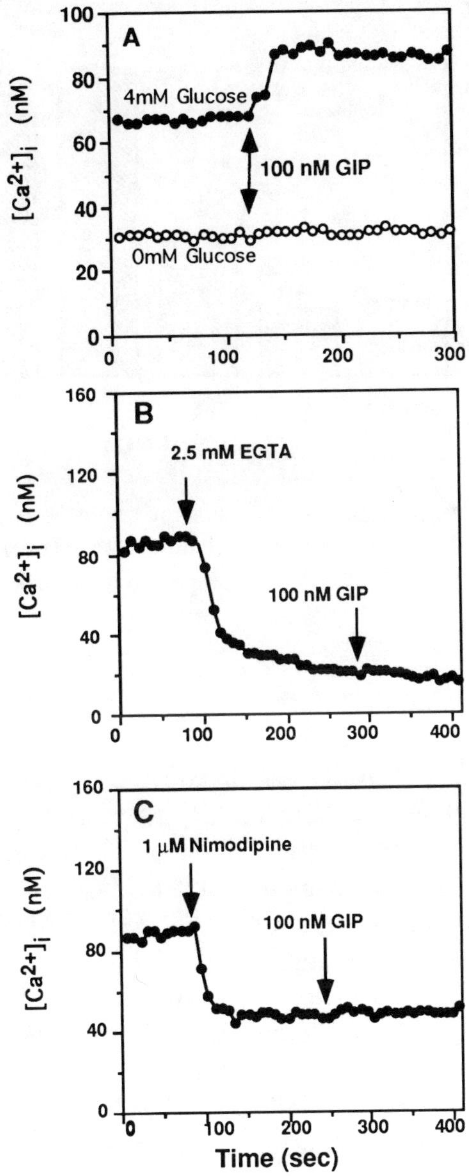

Fig. 3. (**A**) Effects of GIP on $[Ca^{2+}]_i$ in HIT cells, (**B**) effect of EGTA and (**C**) nimodipine on GIP stimulated $[Ca^{2+}]_i$. Fura 2 loaded HIT cells were stimulated with 100 nM GIP (A) or pretreated with EGTA 2.5 m*M* (B) or Nimodipine 1 m*M* (C) before GIP stimulation.

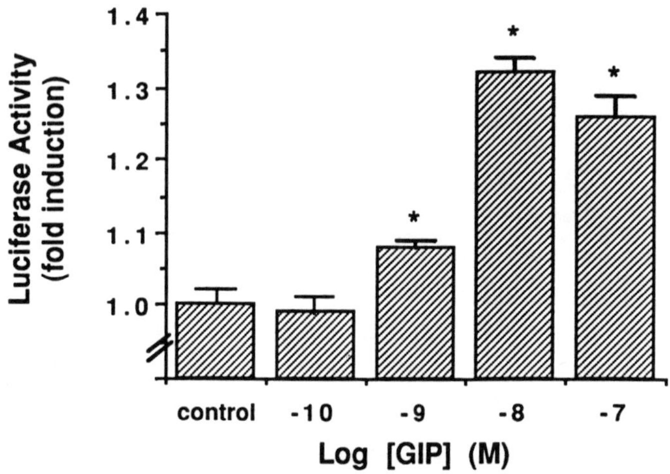

Fig. 4. The induction of proinsulin gene promoter driven luciferase activity by GIP in HIT cells transfected with the –410 bp Insulin promoter-Luciferase chimera. Mean ± SE for six independent experiments, each in triplicate.

reporter gene encoding the firefly luciferase enzyme (LUC). This 410 base promoter contains a single cAMP response element (CRE) (184·-TGACGTCC- 177). GIP stimulated LUC expression in a concentration dependent manner (ED_{50} of 1.6 n*M*) to a maximum of 1.32 ± 0.02-fold (Fig. 4). Thus the GIP induced change in proinsulin mRNA level was partially owing to increased proinsulin gene transcription, in addition to an alteration in the processing or stability of the proinsulin mRNA. GIP-stimulated LUC expression was not affected by nimodipine at a concentration that blocked the GIP-induced increase in $[Ca^{2+}]_i$ and potentiation of insulin secretion. However, when HIT cells were transfected with the chimera luciferase gene containing a mutated CRE (184· · -GTCCGTCC- 177) within the insulin promoter, GIP did not affect the expression of the reporter luciferase gene. These data suggest that GIP, like GLP-1 *(12)*, enhances insulin gene expression mainly through the cAMP-CRE pathway, and not through the elevation of $[Ca^{2+}]_i$.

The information presented thus far suggests that the adenylyl cyclase linked receptors potentiate insulin secretion by stimulating calcium influx through VDCC and increase proinsulin gene expression by the effect of cAMP on the CRE of the proinsulin gene. These receptors do not activate phospholipase C in HIT cells. The GLP-1 receptor, however, is related structurally to the parathyroid hormone and glucagon receptors, which signal through both adenylyl cyclase and phospholipase C *(13)*. In order to study the mechanism of signal transduction of the recombinant GLP-1 receptor, and to determine whether it activates phospholipase C as well as adenylyl cyclase, both the rat and human receptors were transfected into COS-7 cells. Both of the recombinant receptors signal by the same mechanism in COS cells, equipotently activating phosphoinositide turnover and adenylyl cyclase *(10)*. When the rat GLP-1 receptor was transfected to COS-7 cells GLP-1 increased $[Ca^{2+}]_i$ in these cells with a pattern quite characteristic of the release of calcium from an intracellular pool followed by a sustained elevation of $[Ca^{2+}]_i$. Chelation of extracellular calcium did not significantly change the GLP-1 stimulated increase in $[Ca^{2+}]_i$ suggesting that the transient increase of $[Ca^{2+}]_i$ came primarily from an intracellular Ca^{2+} pool. Associated with the increase in $[Ca^{2+}]_i$ in GLP-1 receptor transfected COS-7 cells GLP-1 increased the Ins(1,4,5)-P_3 levels 2.0-fold. These data indicate that GLP-1(7-37) rapidly activates phospholipase C in COS cells expressing the recombinant receptor.

The COS cells do not possess VDCCs that are present in the HIT cells and important in GLP-1 potentiated insulin secretion in these cells. To determine whether the difference in second messenger pathways between the native GLP-1 receptor in HIT cells and the recombinant receptor in COS cells might be related to differential VDCC expression, the rat GLP-1 receptor was transfected into INR1-G9 cells, a hamster α-cell line that does have VDCC. In this cell line the GLP-1 receptor was also coupled to the activation of adenylyl cyclase and liberation of calcium from an intracellular pool *(11)*. The basis for the cell specific differences in second messenger pathways associated with recombinant receptors is still unclear. The difference in signaling pathways used by the GLP-1 receptor in HIT and transfected COS cells may depend on the G-protein milieu of the cell in which the receptor is expressed. Amatruda et al. *(14)* have shown that the COS cell response to chemoattractant is only present when the cells are cotransfected with a hematopoietic cell specific G-protein cDNA in addition to the chemoattractant receptor cDNA. Alternatively there might be variant GLP-1 receptors each with different signaling pathways.

Receptors Linked to Phospholipase C

The cholinergic *(15)*, CCK *(16)* and arginine vasopressin (AVP) *(17)* receptors on the β-cell are coupled to insulin secretion by G-protein-mediated activation of phospholipase C. Phospholipase C activation generates phosphoinositides, including inositol trisphosphate (IP_3) which stimulates calcium release from the intracellular calcium stores, and the production of diacylglycerol which stimulates protein kinase C formation. The role of protein kinase C generation in the insulin secretory pathway is unclear at present *(18)*.

Arginine vasopressin stimulates insulin secretion from HIT cells in a concentration dependent fashion in the presence of glucose *(17)*. Insulin secretion occurs as early as 30 s after stimulation with AVP and shows a biphasic pattern in perifusion experiments with an early peak (3–15 min) and a sustained plateau (15–30 min).

Low concentrations of AVP (0.1-1 n*M*) cause a monophasic sustained increase of $[Ca^{2+}]_i$. At higher concentrations (10-100 n*M*), AVP triggers a biphasic increase of $[Ca^{2+}]_i$ with an immediate acute rise and a sustained plateau phase (Fig. 5). This pattern in $[Ca^{2+}]_i$ closely resembles the insulin secretory pattern at high AVP concentrations. The immediate increase in $[Ca^{2+}]_i$ (determined from the peak maximal net increase) is dose-dependent with an ED_{50} of 6 n*M*, whereas the sustained increase (determined when $[Ca^{2+}]_i$ has reached a steady level 160 sec after AVP addition) has an ED_{50} of 0.2 n*M*. The biphasic insulin secretion stimulated by AVP was mediated by biphasic changes in $[Ca^{2+}]_i$ *(17)*.

The AVP stimulated increase in $[Ca^{2+}]_i$ originates from both the intracellular and the extracellular calcium pools *(17)*. After the chelation of extracellular calcium by the addition of EGTA, AVP evoked a rapid transient increase in $[Ca^{2+}]_i$ not significantly different from cells without EGTA, suggesting the transient increase of $[Ca^{2+}]_i$ came primarily from the intracellular calcium pool. Consistent with this was evidence of early activation of phospholipase C by AVP. AVP (100 n*M*) stimulated a significant increase in Ins-1,4-P_2, Ins-1,3,4-P_3, Ins-1,4,5-P_3, and Ins-1,3,4,5-P_4 levels within 3 sec. Although the AVP stimulated increases in $[Ca^{2+}]_i$ and insulin secretion are glucose

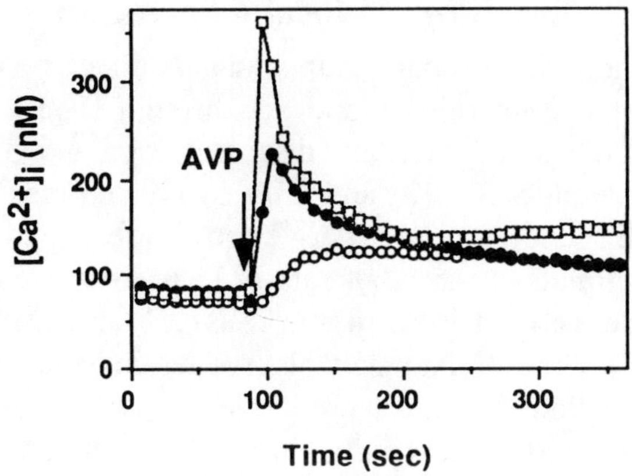

Fig. 5. Effect of AVP on HIT cell $[Ca^{2+}]_i$ (s, 1 n*M*; d, 10 n*M*; h, 100 n*M*).

dependent the AVP stimulated phospholipase C activation is not altered by ambient glucose concentration.

The sustained plateau phase of $[Ca^{2+}]_i$ was lost with EGTA or L-type calcium channel blocker treatment, indicating that the plateau phase of the $[Ca^{2+}]_i$ increase came from the extracellular medium through VDCCs. In contrast to our studies, Li et al. *(19)* found that the second phase of calcium entry triggered by AVP was abolished by EGTA or diazoxide treatment but not blocked by nimodipine, verapamil, or nickel. The difference in these results may be owing to the use of different cell lines. Unlike HIT cells the RIN cells are not glucose responsive.

In HIT cells, glucose depolarizes the plasma membrane as monitored by bisoxonol fluorescence or patch clamp techniques. Consistent with the activation of VDCC by AVP in HIT cells, AVP causes further membrane depolarization in the presence of glucose *(17)*. This effect of AVP on depolarization was not inhibited by L-type calcium channel blockers, which suggested that membrane depolarization induced by AVP occurred before calcium influx through VDCCs, possibly by an effect of closing the ATP-sensitive potassium channel *(20)*. The AVP-induced depolarization was not observed at nonstimulatory glucose concentrations, suggesting that glucose is required for AVP to induce membrane depolarization.

Inhibitors of Insulin Secretion

Norepinephrine, somatostatin, and galanin are potent negative regulators of insulin release and act through G-protein coupled receptors on the β-cells. Galanin decreases basal and GIP-, GLP-1-, glucagon-, arginine-, CCK-, and VIP- stimulated insulin secretion and proinsulin gene expression *(21–23)* in a variety of studies involving whole animals (dogs *[24]*, rats *[25]*, and mice *[26]*) isolated perfused pancreas *(27)*, isolated islet cells *(28)*, and insulin secreting cell lines *(29)*. The cellular mechanism of action of galanin to inhibit basal and stimulated insulin secretion involves the specific interaction of galanin with high affinity galanin receptors on the beta cell. These receptors have been characterized by binding studies to hamster insulinoma and RIN cell lines *(30,31)*. The K_d of the receptor in RINm5F cells is 0.3 nM *(30)*. Sharp estimated the receptor number to be 30,000/RINm5F cell *(32)*. The molecular weight of the receptor has been estimated by chemical crosslinking and polyacrylamide gel electrophoresis to be 54 kDa in RINm5F cells *(33)*.

Galanin acts at multiple sites (ion channels, adenylyl cyclase and on the exocytotic event) to inhibit insulin release. A high affinity interaction between galanin and its receptor on β-cells is followed by opening of the ATP-sensitive potassium channels *(34)*. Channel opening increases potassium efflux from the cells *(35)*, causing cellular hyperpolarization *(36)* with a consequent decrease in VDCC activity, and a fall in $[Ca^{2+}]_i$. Galanin may directly effect closure of the VDCC *(37)* and thus further decrease $[Ca^{2+}]_i$. We have shown that both α2 adrenergic stimulation and somatostatin decrease insulin secretion by closing the VDCC, a G-protein linked action *(38,39)*.

Galanin also inhibits the activity of the adenylyl cyclase enzyme decreasing intracellular cAMP concentrations *(40)*. Cyclic AMP is an important modulator of glucose-induced proinsulin gene expression by the interaction of the cAMP-binding protein with the insulin promoter *(41)* and also modulates insulin secretion, perhaps by the effect of cAMP-dependent protein kinases on the calcium channel *(42)*.

Using RINm5F cells, Sharp *(32)* demonstrated that, in the absence of extracellular calcium, galanin inhibited insulin release in the presence of 8-bromo cAMP and 12-*o*-tetradecanoylphorbol-13-acetate (TPA) (an activator of protein kinase C). This study suggests that, in addition to the effect of membrane hyperpolarization (with decreased calcium influx through the VDCCs) and decreased adenylyl cyclase activity, there are additional mechanisms for inhibition of insulin secretion by galanin. Galanin is thought to inhibit insulin secretion at a distal step in the secretory pathway and is presumed to be related to the insulin secretory granule exocytotic event *(43)*.

Like other negative regulators of insulin secretion (α_2 adrenergic agonists and somatostatin), the effects of galanin on insulin secretion appear to be mediated through inhibitory G proteins (G_i) *(44)*. Pertussis toxin (PTX) pretreatment of RINm5F cells abolished the galanin-induced suppression of forskolin and GIP-stimulated insulin secretion and cAMP generation *(40)*. In addition, pertussis toxin pretreatment also blocked the galanin-induced cell hyperpolarization and the decrease in intracellular calcium in dispersed beta cells isolated from obese hyperglycemic mice *(45)* and RINm5F cells *(46)*. Cormont *(47)* further demonstrated that RINm5F cells contain three forms of G_i (G_{ia1}, $_{a2}$, and $_{a3}$) and two forms of G_o. The G_{ia2} is the most abundant in the cell. Antibodies with specificity for a common epitope on G_{ia1} and G_{ia2} diminished the binding of galanin to the galanin receptor suggesting that the receptor was coupled to either G_{ia1} or G_{ia2}.

Summary and Conclusions

Insulin secretion is closely regulated by the plasma concentration of glucose and other nutrients and its secretion is further modulated by the interplay of various hormones, neuropeptides, and paracrine factors. These factors modulate the glucose stimulated insulin secretion by interacting with β-cell surface receptors to:

1. Change the intracellular concentrations of second messengers such as cAMP and calcium;
2. Alter the membrane potential; or
3. Directly affect the insulin secretory apparatus at the level of exocytosis.

Acknowledgments

This work was funded by grants DK34447 and RR00054 from the National Institute of Health (to AEB), a grant from the Juvenile Diabetes Foundation (to AEB and MBW) and an American Diabetes Association Mentor Based Fellowship Award (to JD).

References

1. Rajan AS, Aguilar-Bryan L, Nelson DA, Yaney GC, Hsu WH, Kunze DL, et al.: Ion channels and insulin secretion. *Diabetes Care* 13:340–363, 1990.
2. Boyd AE, Aguilar-Bryan L, Bryan J, Kunze D, Moss LG, Nelson DA, et al.: Sulfonylurea signal transduction. *Rec Prog Horm Res* 47:299–317, 1991.
3. Aguilar-Bryan L, Nichols C, Rajan A, Parker C, Bryan J: Co-expression of Sulfonylurea receptors and KATP channels in hamster insulinoma tumor (HIT) cells. *J Biol Chem* 267:14,934–14,940, 1992.
4. Maletti M, Portha B, Carlquist M, Kergoat M, Laburthe M, Marie J, et al.: Evidence for and characterization of specific high affinity binding sites for the gastric inhibitory polypeptide in pancreatic β cells. *Endocrinology* 115:1324–1331, 1984.
5. Goke R, Cole T, Conlon J: Characterization of the receptor for glucagon-like peptide-1(7-37)amide on plasma membranes from rat insulinoma-derived cells by covalent cross-linking. *J Mol Endocrinol* 2:93–98, 1989.
6. Dillon JS, Tanizawa T, Wheeler MB, Leng X-H, Ligon BB, Rabin DU, et al.: Cloning and functional expression of the human glucagon-like peptide-1 (GLP-1) receptor. *Endocrinology* 133:1907–1916, 1993.
7. Thorens B: 1992 Expression cloning of the pancreatic beta cell receptor for the gluco-incretin hormone glucagon-like peptide 1. *Proc Natl Acad Sci USA* 89:8641–8645.
8. Lu M, Wheeler M, Leng X-H, Boyd AE: The role of the free cytosolic calcium level in beta-cell signal transduction by gastric inhibitory polypeptide and glucagon-like peptide I(7-37). *Endocrinology* 132:94–100, 1993.
9. Drucker DJ, Philippe J, Mojsov S, Chick WL, Habener JF: Glucagon-like peptide I stimulates insulin gene expression and increases cyclic AMP levels in a rat islet cell line. *Proc Natl Acad Sci USA* 84:3434–3438, 1987.
10. Wheeler M, Lu M, Dillon J, Leng X-H, Chen C, Boyd AE: Functional expression of the glucagon-like peptide-1(7-37) receptor: evidence for coupling to phospholipase C as well as adenylyl cyclase. *Endocrinology* 133:57–62, 1993.
11. Lu M: *Signal transduction of the endogenous and recombinant glucagon-like peptide 1(7-37) receptor.* Baylor College of Medicine: PhD Thesis in Cell Biology, 1993.
12. Fehmann HC, Habener JF: Insulinotropic hormone glucagon-like peptide-I(7-37) stimulation of proinsulin gene expression and proinsulin biosynthesis in insulinoma beta TC-1 cells. *Endocrinology* 130:159–166, 1992.
13. Jelinek LJ Lok, S., Rosenberg, G.B., Smith, R.A., Grant, F.J., Biggs, S., et al.: Expression cloning and signaling properties of the rat glucagon receptor. *Science* 259:1614–1616, 1993.
14. Amatruda T, Gerard N, Gerard C, Simon M: Specific interactions of chemoattractant factor receptors with G-proteins. *J Biol Chem* 14:10,139–10,144, 1993.

15. Wolf B, Florholmen J, Turk J, McDaniel M: Studies of the calcium requirement for glucose and carbachol induced augmentation of inositol trisphosphate and inositol tetrakisphosphate accumulation in digitonin permeabilized islets. *J Biol Chem* 263:3565–3575, 1988.
16. Zawalich W: Modulation of insulin secretion from β cells by phosphoinositide derived second messenger molecules. *Diabetes* 37:137–141, 1988.
17. Lu M, Soltoff S, Yaney G, Boyd AE: The mechanisms underlying the glucose dependence of arginine vasopressin induced insulin secretion in β cells. *Endocrinology* 132:2141–2148, 1993.
18. Metz S: Is protein kinase C required for physiologic insulin release. *Diabetes* 37:3–7, 1987.
19. Li G, Pralong W, Pittet D, Mayr G, Schlegel W, Wollheim C: Inositol tetrakisphosphate isomers and elevation of cytosolic Ca^{2+} in vasopressin-stimulated insulin-secreting R1Nm5F cells. *J Biol Chem* 267:4349–4356, 1992.
20. Martin S, Yule D, Dunne M, Gallacher D, Petersen O: Vasopressin directly closes ATP sensitive potassium channels evoking membrane depolarization and an increase in the free intracellular calcium concentration in insulin secreting cells. *EMBO J* 8:3595–3599, 1989.
21. Miralles P, Peiro E, Silvestre RA, Villanueva ML, Marco J: Effects of galanin on islet cell secretory responses to VIP, GIP, 8-CCK, and glucagon by the perfused rat pancreas. *Met Clin Exp* 37:766–770, 1988.
22. Tajiri Y, Sako Y, Umeda F, Hisatomi A, Nawata H: Effect of galanin on arginine-stimulated pancreatic hormone release from isolated perifused rat islets. *Horm Metab Res* 22:1–6, 1990.
23. Fehmann HC, Habener JF: Galanin inhibits proinsulin gene expression stimulated by the insulinotropic hormone glucagon-like peptide-I(7-37) in mouse insulinoma beta TC-1 cells. *Endocrinology* 130:2890–2896, 1992.
24. Greenberg GR, McDonald TJ: Effect of galanin and vagal integrity on insulin release in dogs. *Pancreas* 3:122–127, 1988.
25. Lindskog S, Ahren B: Effects of galanin on insulin and glucagon secretion in the rat. *Int J Pancreatol* 4:335–344, 1989.
26. Lindskog S, Ahren B: Galanin and pancreastatin inhibit stimulated insulin secretion in the mouse: comparison of effects. *Horm Res* 29:237–240, 1988.
27. Yoshimura T, Ishizuka J, Greeley GJ, Thompson JC: Effect of galanin on glucose-, arginine-, or potassium-stimulated insulin release. *Am J Physiol* 256:E619–E623, 1989.
28. Ahren B, Ar'Rajab A, Bottcher G, Sundler F, Dunning BE: Presence of galanin in human pancreatic nerves and inhibition of insulin secretion from isolated human islets. *Cell Tis Res* 264:263–267, 1991.
29. McKnight GL, Karlsen AE, Kowalyk S, Mathewes SL, Sheppard PO, O'Hara PJ, et al.: Sequence of human galanin and its inhibition of glucose-stimulated insulin secretion from RIN cells. *Diabetes* 41:82–87, 1992.

30. Lagny PI, Amiranoff B, Lorinet AM, Tatemoto K, Laburthe M: Characterization of galanin receptors in the insulin-secreting cell line Rin m 5F: evidence for coupling with a pertussis toxin-sensitive guanosine triphosphate regulatory protein. *Endocrinology* 124:2635–2641, 1989.
31. Amiranoff B, Servin AL, Rouyer FC, Couvineau A, Tatemoto K, Laburthe M: Galanin receptors in a hamster pancreatic beta-cell tumor: identification and molecular characterization. *Endocrinology* 121:284–289, 1987.
32. Sharp GW, Le M, Brustel Y, Yada T, Russo LL, Bliss CR, et al.: Galanin can inhibit insulin release by a mechanism other than membrane hyperpolarization or inhibition of adenylate cyclase. *J Biol Chem* 264:7302–7309, 1989.
33. Amiranoff B, Lorinet AM, Laburthe M: Galanin receptor in the rat pancreatic beta cell line Rin m 5F. Molecular characterization by chemical cross-linking. *J Biol Chem* 264:20,714–20,717, 1989.
34. deWeille J, Schmid AH, Fosset M, Lazdunski M: ATP-sensitive K+ channels that are blocked by hypoglycemia-inducing sulfonylureas in insulin-secreting cells are activated by galanin, a hyperglycemia-inducing hormone. *Proc Natl Acad Sci USA* 85:1312–1316, 1988.
35. Drews G, Debuyser A, Nenquin M, Henquin JC: Galanin and epinephrine act on distinct receptors to inhibit insulin release by the same mechanisms including an increase in K+ permeability of the B-cell membrane. *Endocrinology* 126:1646–1653, 1990.
36. Ahren B, Arkhammar P, Berggren PO, Nilsson T: Galanin inhibits glucose-stimulated insulin release by a mechanism involving hyperpolarization and lowering of cytoplasmic free Ca2+ concentration. *Biochem Biophy Res Commun* 140:1059–1063, 1986.
37. Homaidan FR, Sharp GW, Nowak LM: Galanin inhibits a dihydropyridine-sensitive Ca^{2+} current in the RINm5f cell line. *Proc Natl Acad Sci USA* 88:8744–8748, 1991.
38. Hsu W, Xiang H, Rajan A, Boyd AE: Activation of alpha 2 adrenergic receptors decreases calcium influx to inhibit insulin secretion in a hamster β cell line: an action mediated by guanosine triphosphate binding protein. *Endocrinology* 128:958–964, 1991.
39. Hsu W, Xiang H, Rajan A, Kunze D, Boyd AE: Somatostatin inhibits insulin secretion by a G-protein mediated decrease in Ca^{2+} entry through voltage dependent Ca2+ channels in the beta cell. *J Biol Chem* 266:837–843, 1991.
40. Amiranoff B, Lorinet AM, Lagny PI, Laburthe M: Mechanism of galanin-inhibited insulin release. Occurrence of a pertussis-toxin-sensitive inhibition of adenylate cyclase. *Eur J Biochem* 177:147–152, 1988.
41. Philippe J, Missotten M: Functional characterization of a cAMP-responsive element of the rat insulin I gene. *J Biol Chem* 265:1465-1469, 1990.
42. Osterrieder W, Brum A, Hescheler J, Trautwein W: Injection of subunits of cAMP - dependent protein kinase into cardiac myocytes modulates calcium current. *Nature* 298:576–578, 1982.
43. Ullrich S, Wollheim CB: Galanin inhibits insulin secretion by direct interference with exocytosis. *FEBS Lett* 247:401–404, 1989.

44. Robertson RP, Seaquist ER, Walseth TF: G proteins and modulation of insulin secretion. *Diabetes* 40:1–6, 1991.
45. Nilsson T, Arkhammar P, Rorsman P, Berggren PO: Suppression of insulin release by galanin and somatostatin is mediated by a G-protein. An effect involving repolarization and reduction in cytoplasmic free Ca^{2+} concentration. *J Biol Chem* 264:973–980, 1989.
46. Rokaeus A: Galanin: a newly isolated biologically active neuropeptide. *Trends Neurosci* 10:158–164, 1987.
47. Cormont M, Le M, Brustel Y, Van OE, Spiegel AM, Sharp GW: Identification of G protein alpha-subunits in RINm5F cells and their selective interaction with galanin receptor. *Diabetes* 40:1170–1176, 1991.

Chapter 13

Molecular Biology of the Ion Channels in the Pancreatic β-Cell

Illani Atwater, Manuel Kukuljan, and Elia Martha Pérez-Armendariz

Introduction

The pancreatic β-cell acts as a glucose sensor that secretes insulin at a rate dependent on the extracellular glucose concentration. This capability depends critically on the ability of the metabolic processing of glucose and other substrates to modulate the β-cell plasma membrane electrical activity. Similarly, the action of many physiological regulators of insulin secretion is exerted through the alteration of the electrical activity of the β-cell. Clinically, pharmacological modulation of this activity is used to increase the insulin output from the pancreatic islets of individuals with type II diabetes mellitus. Thus, the knowledge of the cellular and molecular basis of the electrical activity of the β-cell is central to the understanding of its function in physiological and pathological states.

Ion channels are the protein molecules that determine the selective flow of ions through otherwise impermeable membranes, and consequently change the electrical potential across these membranes; the activity of channels can be modulated by factors such as the

From: *Molecular Biology of Diabetes, Part I*
Edited by: B. Draznin and D. LeRoith

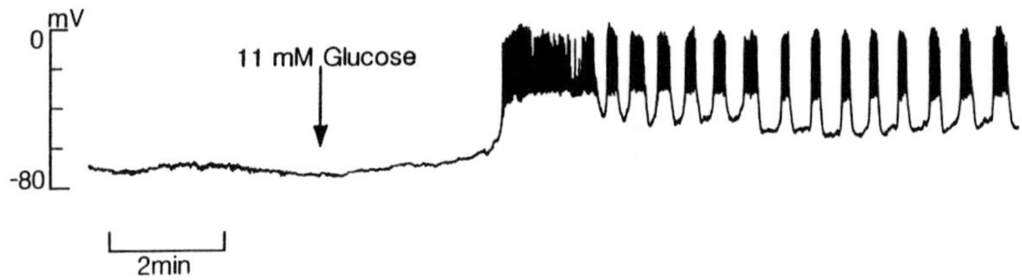

Fig. 1. Glucose-induced biphasic electrical activity from a β-cell in a microdissected, perifused mouse islet of Langerhans.

electric field in the membrane, intracellular or extracellular ligands, or covalent modification. Even though the study of the ion channels provides one of the closest views of the function of a cell or organ, we must remember that the function of the ensemble many times can not be understood merely by adding up the parts, and that the opposite process of starting with the function of the ensemble and trying to fit the parts in it may be required. This is particularly true in the study of the β-cell electrical activity (and insulin release) in response to glucose. Therefore, before introducing the ion channels expressed in the β-cell and the processes that control their activity, we will trace the path that has lead to our current knowledge of the subject and describe the pattern of electrical activity induced by glucose in the β-cells within the whole islet of Langerhans, keeping in mind that what the whole cell membrane actually "sees" are the changes in membrane potential (V_m) rather than the localized currents flowing through ion channels that underlie these changes in V_m.

Most of the studies on the electrical properties of β-cells have been carried out in V_m mouse islets of Langerhans, using V_m recording through an intracellular electrode. Thus, it was learned that β-cells are electrically excitable, firing action potentials in the presence of glucose *(1)*. Extensive work characterized this property of the islet of Langerhans and demonstrated that the firing of action potentials occurs following a complex pattern of bursts, which is modulated by the extracellular glucose concentration *(2)*. In the absence of glucose, the V_m remains very negative, close to –70 mV; on introduction of glucose, the plasma membrane depolarizes to the threshold for the firing of action potentials (Fig. 1). After several of these action potentials, the plasma membrane repolarizes spontaneously, and then slowly depolarizes again to start a new burst of action potentials. This process is repeated under steady glucose concentrations giving rise to an oscillatory pattern characteristic of each glucose concentration. The relative duration of the bursts of action potentials is directly related to the extracellular concentration of glucose; thus, higher glucose concentrations are associated with higher numbers of action potentials over a given period of time, in other words, a higher fraction of time is spent in the "active phase" (Fig. 2). Very high glucose concentrations lead to continuous firing of action potentials (i.e., 100% active phase).

The Electrical Activity of the Islet of Langerhans Is Closely Related to Insulin Secretion

The glucose concentration vs active phase duration or insulin secretion curves have very similar slopes, the half maximal point for electrical activity falling at slightly lower glucose concentrations than the half-maximal point for insulin secretion (Fig. 3A). Also, action potentials have been observed to occur at least 20 s before detectable glucose stimulated insulin release can be measured (Fig. 3B). Furthermore, most experimental conditions that increase the firing of action potentials in the islet, also increase insulin output and the blockade of electrical activity is associated with diminished insulin secretion. Simultaneous measurements of pulsatile insulin secretion and bursting electrical activity from a single islet showed that both occur in phase *(3)* (also illustrated in Fig. 11D). Since the β-cell action potentials reflect an increase in calcium permeability, and insulin secretion is dependent on extracellular calcium, these observations prompted the idea that the action potentials are causally related to insulin secretion and that the transduction of the glucose signal for insulin secretion includes modulation of electrical activity. Recently, oscillatory changes in the intracellular calcium concentration, presumably resulting from the calcium entry through voltage-gated channels, have been shown to occur in phase with oscillations in electrical activity *(4)* (also illustrated later in Fig. 11C) and with oscillations in insulin secretion *(5)*.

Glucose Modulation of V_m and Electrical Activity Requires Its Metabolism

Metabolic uncouplers such as 2,4-dinitrophenol or sodium azide induce hyperpolarization. Nonmetabolizable glucose derivatives,

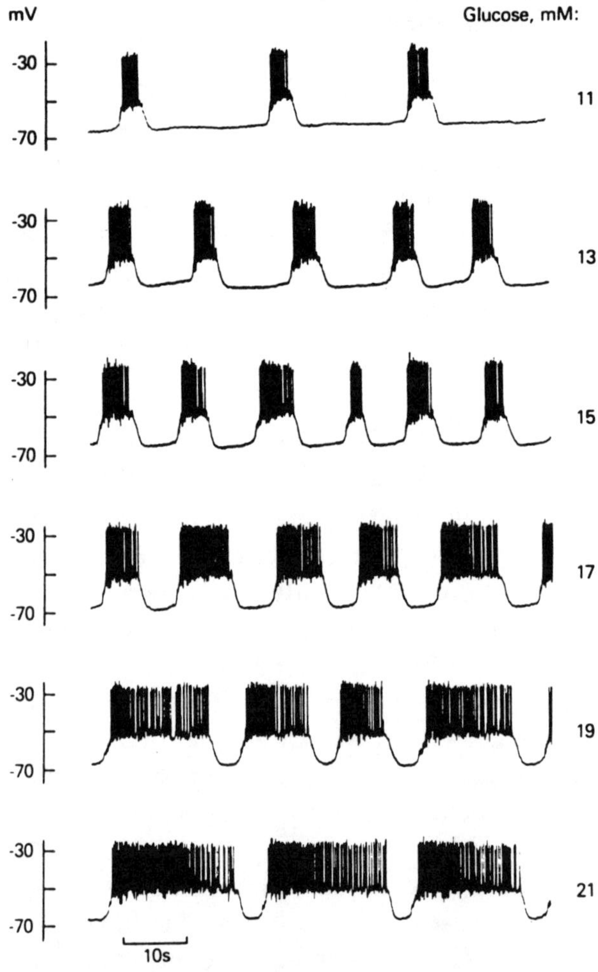

Fig. 2. Burst pattern of electrical activity induced by graded increases in glucose concentration *(59)*.

such as 2-deoxyglucose, do not induce depolarization or electrical activity. These agents antagonize the effects of glucose. Moreover, nonglucose metabolic substrates, such as α-keto isocaproic acid can mimic glucose effects on the V_m of islets of Langerhans. The important message here is that the β-cell recognizes glucose as a metabolic substrate, not as a structure; in other words, there is no discrete glucose receptor, but rather the whole cell with its metabolic pathways acts as the sensor.

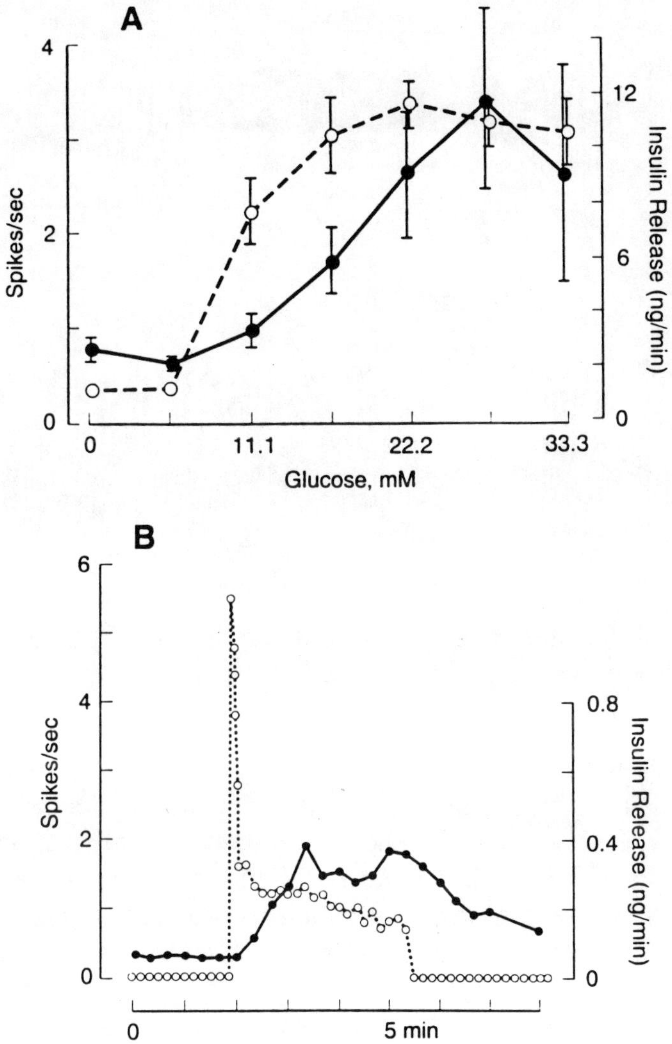

Fig. 3. Insulin secretion measured from single mouse islets of Langerhans and compared with electrical activity measured from a β-cell within the islet. Measurements were made simultaneously. Dashed lines indicate average spike frequency, solid lines represent insulin. **(A)** Data pooled from six islets; parameters measured over last three minutes of a ten minute exposure to each glucose concentration, given in the horizontal axis. More variability was measured in insulin secretion than in electrical activity from islet to islet. **(B)** Data from a single islet, illustrating time dependence of responses, electrical activity always preceded detectable insulin secretion by at least 20 s *(2)*.

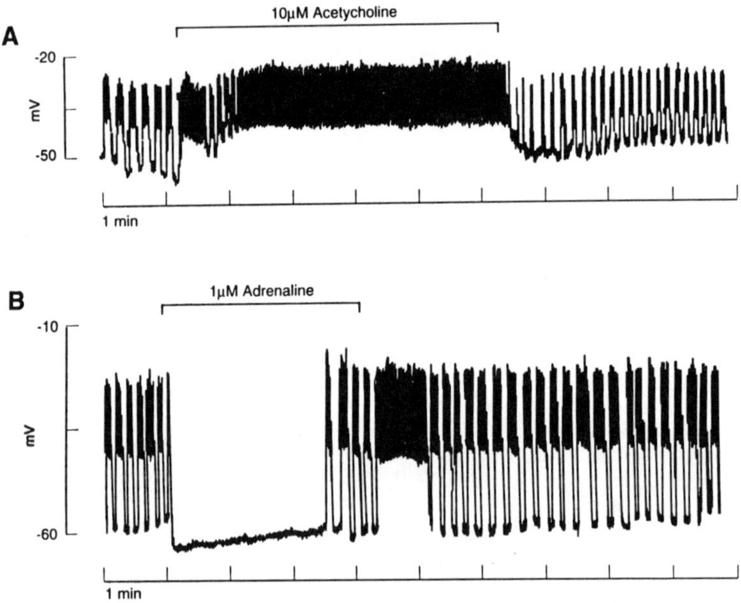

Fig. 4. Modulation of glucose-induced electrical activity by acetylcholine and adrenaline. Reprinted from ref. *5a* with permission.

Besides glucose, other physiological modulators of insulin secretion also affect cell membrane potential in the islet of Langerhans. Classical examples are cholinergic agonists which act on muscarinic type receptors to depolarize β-cells and stimulate electrical activity, and adrenergic agonists which act on α-receptors to induce a transient hyperpolarization and suppress spike activity (Fig. 4). These responses correlate with the action of these agonists on insulin secretion, except that the inhibition of insulin secretion by adrenergic agonists is sustained, whereas inhibition of electrical activity is only transient *(5)*. This is one condition during which there is a clear dissociation between electrical activity and insulin secretion. Another condition under which the electrical activity may continue while insulin secretion is inhibited is lowering the experimental temperature to below 27°C *(6)*.

Initially, the identity of the ionic currents involved in the cycle of electrical activity of the islet of Langerhans was defined by the combined approaches of measuring isotope fluxes, observing the effects of ion substitutions on V_m, measuring input resistance, and blocking

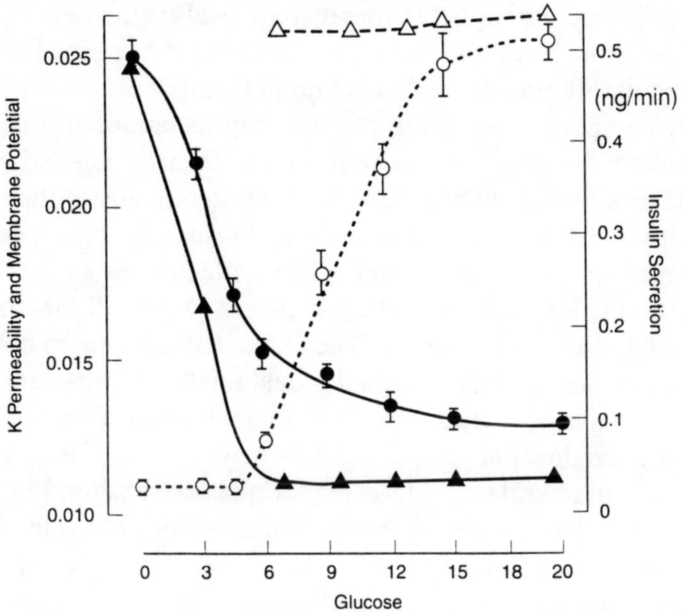

Fig. 5. Potassium permeability, insulin release, and membrane potential as a function of glucose concentration. Filled circles represent the dependence of Rb efflux on glucose concentration *(7)*. *Open* circles represent insulin secretion *(7)*. Filled triangles represent the membrane potential during the resting and silent phases, open triangles represent membrane potential during the active phase. Reduction of K permeability, as measured by Rb efflux, is associated with changes in the silent phase potential of the membrane, whereas insulin secretion is associated with the oscillation in the membrane potential between silent and active phases.

specific ion channel activity pharmacologically *(7–9)*. Thus it was determined that in the absence of glucose, the permeability to potassium predominates (as in the vast majority of animal cells), and that addition of glucose reduces potassium permeability and increases the permeability to calcium (Fig. 5). With this basic information, β-cell signal transduction can be understood: At rest potassium permeability is high, keeping V_m close to the equilibrium potential for this ion. Glucose metabolism leads to the closing of pathways selective for potassium (i.e. blocks potassium channels), and the cell membrane depolarizes. The depolarization activates calcium channels (i.e., increases permeability to calcium) and the resultant increase in cytosolic calcium triggers exocytosis of insulin granules. This simple scheme is the result of interactions between many ion channels and the regulatory processes that act upon them.

The application of the patch-clamp technique to the study of pancreatic β-cells in primary culture and from tumor-derived β-cell lines has allowed the precise identification of many of the ion channels involved in signal transduction of insulin secreting cells. This information has clarified some of the molecular processes underlying stimulus-secretion coupling in β-cells, especially the processes involved in glucose sensing. The challenge remains to construct a total correlate between information obtained in patch-clamp studies with that from V_m measurements in intact islets. A further challenge will be to engineer an artificial β-cell, incorporating the essential ion channels and regulatory elements for glucose sensing. For this purpose, we will need to know the molecular biology of the ion channels expressed in normal β-cells. Below, we describe the ion channels so far identified in pancreatic β-cells and mention some of the work accomplished in the study of their molecular characteristics. Since most of the searches for the molecular identity of ionic channels are based on homology, it is not surprising that those channels found in the β-cell so far are similar or identical to known channels in other tissues. Nevertheless, β-cell electrical activity is likely not to be determined by a unique type of ion channels, but rather by the expression of a unique assortment of channels.

Potassium Channels

As stated above, the existence of a potassium permeability that can vary as a function of extracellular glucose concentration is instrumental for the glucose signal transduction. Several classes of potassium channels have been described in the β-cells; only one of them shows an activity with clear dependence on glucose metabolism, the adenosine triphosphate (ATP) sensitive potassium channel ($K_{(ATP)}$).

ATP Sensitive Potassium Channels

In the absence of extracellular glucose, the most frequently observed potassium selective channel is a ca 80 pS, voltage-independent, channel that opens in bursts separated by longer closed periods. The open time probability of this channel, studied with the whole cell metabolism intact, diminishes when glucose is added to the extracellular medium; this effect is dose-dependent, with a K_i of near 3 m*M* glucose *(10)* (Fig. 6A). The effect of extracellular glucose on $K_{(ATP)}$ channels fulfills the role of the glucose metabolism-regulated potassium conductance that determines the basal permeability for this ion. Furthermore, it was demonstrated that ATP, acting from the intracellular side of the membrane, reversibly diminishes this channel open time probability *(11)*. The K_i for the intracellular ATP effects is in the micromolar range (Fig. 6B). This contrasts with the millimolar level expected in the cytosol of living β-cells (Fig. 6C); millimolar ATP would keep all channels closed. Also difficult to reconcile is the observation that between about 5–20 m*M* glucose all $K_{(ATP)}$ channels appear to be closed and islet ATP content appears to be constant. These facts would preclude an important role for the $K_{(ATP)}$ in the range of glucose concentrations within which modulation of the electrical activity is observed.

In spite of the discrepancies, it is accepted that $K_{(ATP)}$ channels constitute the main glucose metabolism modulated potassium channels present in the β-cell. Explanations that try to close the gap include the suggestion that indeed most of the $K_{(ATP)}$ channels are closed under physiological conditions and that the change in the state of just a few of them could account for the changes in V_m; an alternative view is that $K_{(ATP)}$ channels are actually completely closed at these glucose levels, their modulation contributing to set the threshold for the initiation of the electrical activity and insulin secretion. In other words, channel closure would bring V_m from the very hyperpolarized level recorded at zero glucose to the V_m from which action potentials are fired. This role would attribute to $K_{(ATP)}$ channels the control of the fasting plasma glucose concentration. Still another possibility is that differences in the environment for single channel records and whole islet experiments *(see below)* may underlie these apparent discrepancies and that under physiological conditions modulation of the activity of $K_{(ATP)}$ channels could account for the whole range of changes of the islet electrical activity in response to glucose.

In addition to glucose metabolism, through the modulation of cytosolic ATP concentration, other factors influence the $K_{(ATP)}$ open state probability. These include intracellular pH, extracellular HCO_3^- *(12)*, and the relationship between ATP and other adenine nucleotides *(13)*.

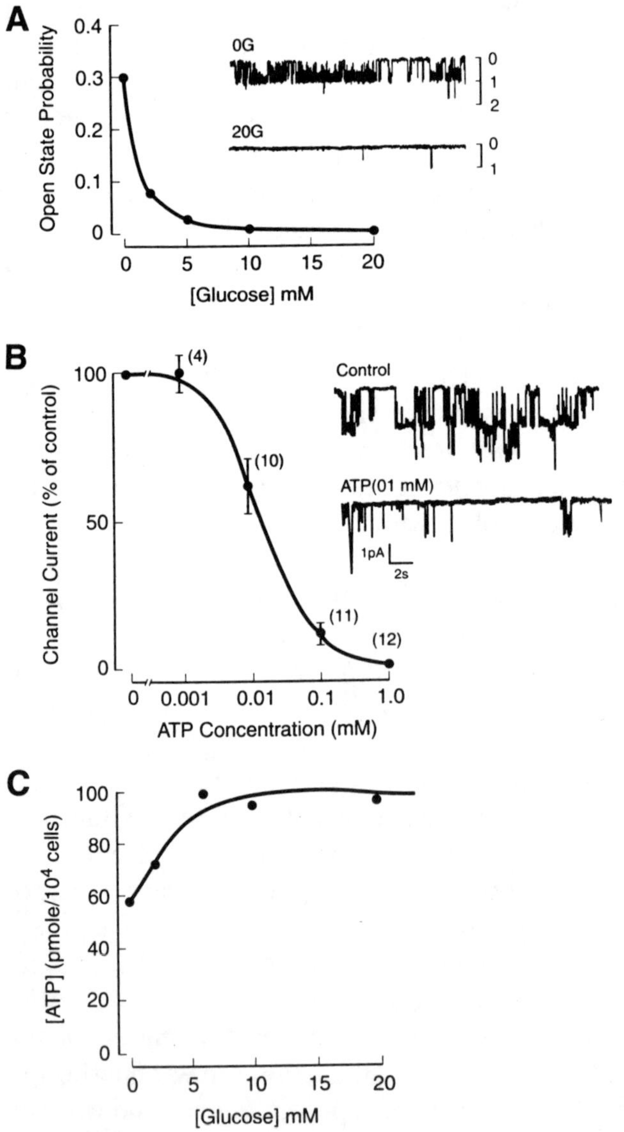

Fig. 6. Relatively high sensitivity of the $K_{(ATP)}$ channel to ATP compared to ATP in the β-cell. **(A)** Inset illustrates $K_{(ATP)}$ channel activity in a cell-attached patch and inhibition by glucose. Graph indicates that most of the channel activity is inhibited by glucose concentrations below 5 m*M* *(10)*. **(B)** Inset illustrates $K_{(ATP)}$ channel activity in an excised patch and partial inhibition by ATP applied to the inner side *(11)*. **(C)** Total ATP measured in islets in response to glucose.

$K_{(ATP)}$ channels also display some interesting pharmacological properties. In addition to being blocked by "classical" potassium channel blockers, such as tetraethylammonium, cesium and barium ions, they are the target of a class of drugs, the sulfonylureas, used since long before the discovery of these channels as oral hypoglycemic agents. Glyburide, tolbutamide, and clorpropamide, among others, diminish the open state probability of the $K_{(ATP)}$ channels and thus depolarize the β-cell plasma membrane; the depolarization leads to the firing of action potentials. The related compound diazoxide, opens $K_{(ATP)}$ channels, hyperpolarizing the membrane of the β-cell and inhibiting the electrical activity. This action provides the rational for the use of diazoxide in the treatment of insulinoma tumors and may explain the hyperglycemia observed in some individuals after the administration of diazoxide as an antihypertensive drug.

The search for the gene or genes coding for the $K_{(ATP)}$ has not yet yielded positive results, in spite of intense work aimed to purify the channel as a sulfonylurea binding protein *(14,15)*. Strategies based on search for sequence homology seem unlikely to work for the moment, since genes for channels of similar properties are not known. The recent cloning of another type of ATP-regulated potassium channel from kidney could prove useful in this search *(16)*, even though the product of this gene does not appear to be a "sulfonylurea receptor," as does the $K_{(ATP)}$ appears to constitute. However, the characterization of this gene, a rat brain inward-rectifier potassium channel, and even a plant *(Arabidopsis taliana)* potassium channel *(17)*, makes it possible to envision at least the conservation of the motifs in the pore-forming region well studied in the Shaker family of channels and well conserved in all the potassium channels so far characterized at the molecular level. Another important lesson is that a structure quite different from previously characterized potassium channels may be expected, with far fewer membrane spanning domains (two in the case of the inward rectifier). Of course, it is possible to propose the existence of important regulatory structures such as nucleotide binding sites and sulfonylurea binding domains. Such regulatory structures have been described for the CFTR chloride channel *(18,19)*. Thus, important questions at the molecular and biophysical level, such as the mechanism by which ATP binding is linked to channel gating and the structural basis of the action of sulfonylureas will be open to solution once the genetic encoding for this channel is characterized. Besides these questions at the molecular level, the role of each type of channel in the complex bursting pattern could be approached once gene transfer or gene knockout technologies are applied to the study of ion channels in the β-cell.

Calcium Activated Potassium Channels ($K_{(Ca)}$)

The study of the V_m in whole islets of Langerhans led to a proposal that the cyclic change in activity of the calcium-activated potassium channel could underlie most of the pattern of electrical activity observed in response to glucose. In this model, calcium entry during the active phase would lead to the increase in cytosolic calcium concentration $[Ca^{2+}]i$ and to the opening of $K_{(Ca)}$, which results in the repolarization of the membrane that creates the bursting pattern *(20)*. Glucose metabolism, through the modulation of the rate of calcium removal from the cytosol would determine the timing for the closure of the channels and the new phase of depolarization. This hypothesis was based on experimental observations that the burst pattern includes a calcium feedback mechanism; the active phases are shortened by increasing the extracellular calcium concentration (Fig. 7A) and a substantial silent phase follows a depolarization induced by raising the extracellular potassium concentration (Fig. 7B).

Three Types of $K_{(Ca)}$ Have Been Discovered

The apamin sensitive $K_{(Ca)}$ was ruled out, since apamin failed to affect the burst pattern *(21)*. Patch clamp recording identified a high conductance, calcium and voltage gated potassium channel in the membrane of β-cells, similar to the one found in many other cell types *(22)*. Modulation of this "maxi" $K_{(Ca)}$ channel open time probability by glucose in HIT-T15 cells supported its role in the genesis of the bursting pattern in whole islets *(23)*. However, experiments using charybdotoxin, a selective blocker of this channel, demonstrated that it is not involved in the oscillations of V_m recorded in whole islets *(24)*. Moreover, "maxi" $K_{(Ca)}$, when studied in cell attached patches, open at very depolarized V_m (i.e., positive to 0 mV), a condition that is not reached during the physiological electrical activity of the islet of Langerhans. As occurs in most of the other cell types in which this "maxi" potassium channel has been described, its function remains elusive. Possibly, it plays a role in the transduction of signals other than glucose.

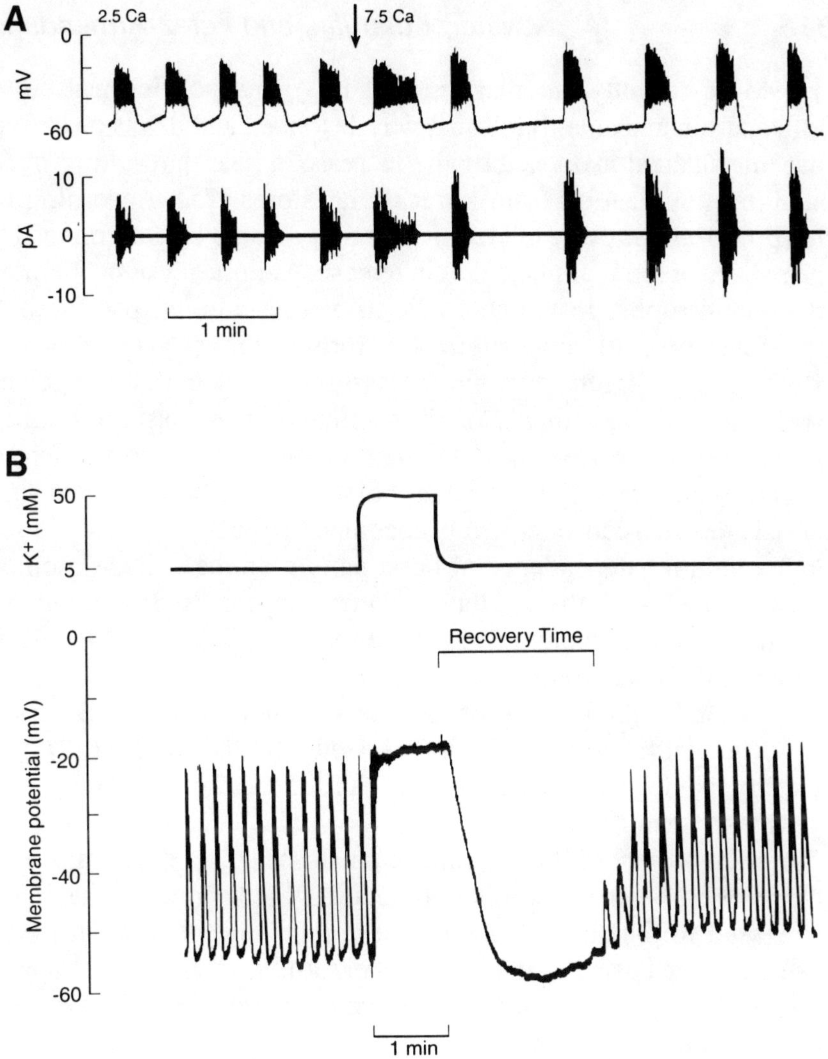

Fig. 7. Evidence for a Ca-feedback mechanism in β-cell electrical pattern. **(A)** Upper trace shows the effect of raising Ca in the perifusion medium on membrane potential fluctuations, after an initial increased burst of action potentials, high Ca increases the duration of the silent phases. Lower trace illustrates the instantaneous currents calculated during the action potential rising phases. The increased silent phases are associated with increased Ca-currents *(2)*. **(B)** Upper trace indicates the K concentration in the perifusion medium and the lower trace represents the membrane potential oscillations in the presence of 11 m*M* glucose. High K depolarizes the membrane, effectively bypassing the physiological feedback mechanism, and thus loads the cell with Ca. A prolonged silent phase follows the return to normal K. *(2)*.

More recently, another class of $K_{(Ca)}$ channel, insensitive to both apamin and charybdotoxin, was described and it was proposed that this channel is opened by the increase in $[Ca^{2+}]_i$ resulting from calcium mobilization from intracellular stores *(25)*. According to this proposal, the cycle of electrical activity would be determined by the pattern of intracellular calcium release. A similar system operates in gonadotrophs, in which $InsP_3$-triggered calcium oscillations determine an oscillatory pattern of V_m through the activation of small conductance calcium-sensitive potassium channels that are selectively blocked by apamin *(26)*. The oscillations in potassium conductance continue, however, under voltage clamp or blockade of calcium influx, conditions which inhibit the burst pattern in β-cells. Thus, this model does not seem completely adequate for the β-cell, since it does not explain the dependence of burst pattern on the voltage oscillations. In the β-cell, the oscillatory pattern appears to depend on the voltage sensitive calcium entry more than on calcium mobilization from intracellular stores.

Recently, the cloning of the "maxi" calcium activated potassium channel from mouse brain has been reported (mSlo) *(27)*; the strategy that lead to this was the search for genes homologous to the previously identified product of the slowpoke locus in *Drosophila*. The expression of mSlo was detected in tissues other than brain, and it may well be that a similar molecule is identified as the $K_{(Ca)}$ expressed in β-cells. The molecular architecture of Slo and mSlo resembles the basic motif of the Shaker family, six membrane spanning domains, a remarkably conserved pore region, a putative voltage sensor situated in the fourth transmembrane domain and a long carboxyterminal domain with a myriad of possible regulatory sites, including a proposed calcium binding domain that constitutes the distinctive attribute of this class of channels. This information may prove useful to the understanding of the physiological role of the $K_{(Ca)}$.

Delayed Rectifier Potassium Channels

In common with many excitable cells, β-cells express a depolarization-activated potassium current that remains active for a long time provided the cell remains depolarized *(28)*. The range of V_m at which these channels are active makes them suitable candidates for controlling the repolarization of the action potentials fired during the active phase of the electrical cycle of the β-cells *(29)*. Polymerase chain reaction using cDNA prepared from a β-cell derived cell line has shown that these express a channel structurally similar to delayed rectifier potassium channels found in brain, cardiac muscle, and other tissues, all of them members of the Shaker related family of genes *(30)*. Again, homology was used as a search method. The primary structure predicts the conserved features for these channels: six membrane spanning domains, one of which bears a string of positively charged residues, thought to act as the voltage sensor and a partially hydrophobic segment that accounts for ion conduction *(31,32)*.

Other Potassium Channels

The expression of a small conductance, voltage-insensitive potassium current which is modulated by adrenergic agonists was described in mouse β-cells *(33)*. This current is activated by adrenaline, presumably through the direct interaction of an activated β-subunit of a G-protein with the channel. This effect would account for the transient inhibition of the electrical activity of the islet of Langerhans associated with the exposure to adrenergic agonists *(34)* (Fig. 4B). More details about the physiological and pharmacological properties of this novel channel are required before asserting its role in the response to adrenergic agonists.

Calcium Channels

Calcium channels play a critical role in the coupling of the glucose signal to the insulin secretory response, allowing the calcium entry that triggers the exocytosis of the insulin containing granules. The action potentials recorded from pancreatic beta cells, like most other secretory cells, are generated by the activation of Ca-channels. Upon depolarization of the membrane the channels open, allowing the influx of calcium from the extracellular space. The pattern of the electrical activity of the β-cell ultimately determines the activity of these channels and thus the calcium influx and $[Ca^{2+}]_i$. The correlation between the cycle of electrical activity in whole islets and the $[Ca^{2+}]_i$ has been determined by measuring both parameters simultaneously in isolated islets *(4)* (also shown later in Fig. 11C).

Voltage-Gated Calcium Channels

Before the invention of the patch-clamp technique, noise analysis of current or voltage fluctuations was used to calculate single channel activity in excitable cells. Thus, β-cell calcium channels were measured to have a unitary conductance of about 5 pS with an extracellular concentration of calcium of 2.5 m*M* *(35)*. Such a small channel is difficult to dissociate from the noise level in single channel patch clamp studies, thus, most investigators have studied the calcium channels using either Ba^{2+} or high concentrations of Ca^{2+} on the extracellular face of the membrane patch, or by studying whole cell calcium currents. Whole cell patch-clamp recording of inward currents allowed the identification of two types of voltage-activated calcium channels: a long-lasting ("L" type) class and a transiently activated ("T" type) population *(28,36)*. They share the characteristics ascribed to these types of channels in other cell types, such as neurons, chromaffin cells, pituitary cells, and so on *(37)*.

Voltage-gated calcium channels may be modulated by signals other than changes in the electrical field across the plasma membrane in different cell types. Phosphorylation or direct interaction of activated α-subunits of G-proteins is an important regulatory mechanism of calcium currents in cardiac myocytes and in neurons. Given the influence of metabolism and neurotransmitters on β-cell electrical activity, calcium channel modulation by them is an attractive possibility. Several groups have approached this problem using electrophysiological techniques; glucose increases the magnitude of the "L" type calcium currents in rat β-cells (Fig. 8) *(38)*. Other substrates also seem to increase the opening of these channels. However, the mechanism has not yet been elucidated. Phosphorylation by cAMP-dependent protein kinase, an important modulator of calcium channels in cardiac muscle and chromaffin cells, among others, seems to be of secondary importance. The potentiating effect of cAMP on insulin secretion may be more owing to changes in the secretory machinery rather than an effect on calcium channels, calcium entry and increases in $[Ca^{2+}]_i$ *(39)*. The effect of glucose on the amplitude of the calcium currents follows a slow time course that does not support an important role for this phenomenon in the rapid changes of the electrical activity of the whole islet in response to changes in the concentration of the sugar. A longer term modulation of the functional status of these channels by the ambient glucose concentration could exist and may account for such phenomena as glucose priming.

The β-cell burst pattern of electrical activity may be the result of changes in potassium permeability (i.e., activation of a hyperpolarizing current—potassium channels—at the end of a burst) or as the

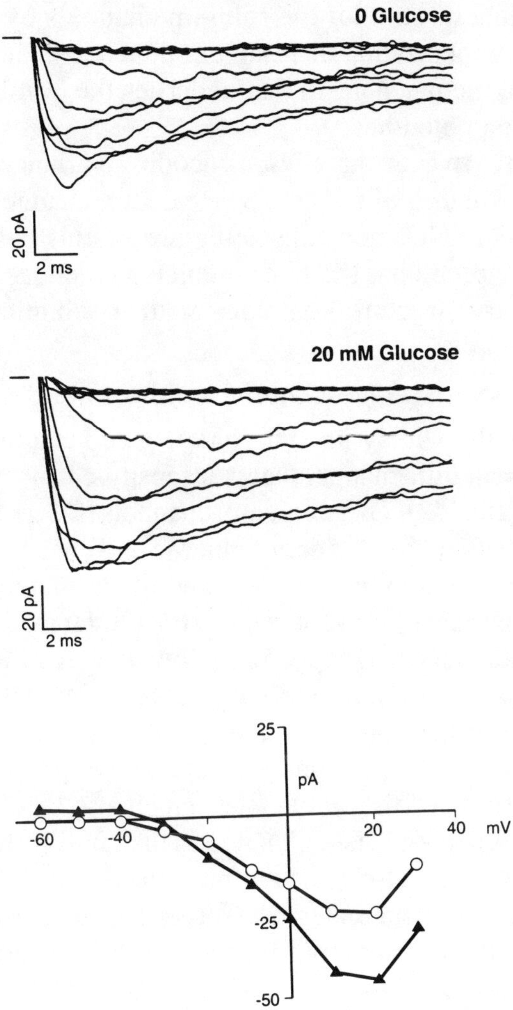

Fig. 8. Glucose increases voltage-gated Ca currents in whole cell nystatin permeabilized patch clamp experiments. Upper records show a family of currents in response to a series of progressive depolarizing voltage pulses. The lower graph summarizes the current-voltage relationship for steady-state currents before (open circles) and after (filled triangles) application of glucose.

consequence of changes in calcium permeability (i.e., inactivation of a depolarizing current—calcium channels—to end the burst), or as a combination of both processes. "L" type calcium currents inactivate slowly during a sustained depolarization, a phenomenon attributed to the inactivation of the calcium channels by calcium *(40)*. It has been proposed that this calcium-dependent channel inactivation could be the mechanism that underlies the termination of each burst of action potentials.

Recently, two of the cDNA encoding variants of the widely expressed α-subunit of the "L"-type calcium channel subunit were identified *(41)*. The molecular structure of this calcium channel subunit in the β-cell has the same predicted secondary structure and a 65% primary structure homology with α-subunits expressed in other tissues.

Nonvoltage-Gated Calcium Channels

Besides the widely known voltage-gated calcium channels, a new type of calcium channel that is insensitive to V_m was described in rodent β-cells *(42)*. These calcium channels ($Ca_{(g)}$), show very low open probability in the absence of glucose and open when the hexose or permeable metabolic intermediates of its metabolism (i.e., α ketoisocaproic acid) are added to the extracellular medium. Although of small conductance and apparently low density in the membrane, these channels could contribute to the depolarization that sustains the burst of action potentials. Selective agonists or antagonists for these channels have not been found yet; thus, their participation in the electrical activity of the whole islet remains to be elucidated. One interesting property of these channels is that, unlike the "L" and "T" type channels, they also conduct manganese ions. Manganese has been observed to accumulate in the β-cell in response to glucose, and to induce insulin secretion (presumably by blocking potassium channels and depolarizing the β-cell). The $Ca_{(g)}$ channels could provide a mechanism for Mn^{2+} entry.

Sodium Channels

Voltage activated sodium channels, crucial for the generation of the action potential in neurons and skeletal muscle, do not appear to be important in the generation of action potentials in islets of Langerhans from mouse since tetrodotoxin, a potent and specific blocker of sodium channels, does not significantly modify the burst pattern. However, in dog and human islets cells, sodium channels contribute to the inward currents (mainly carried by calcium) and determine the rising phase of the action potential *(43)*. It may be that in some β-cells, sodium channels contribute to the depolarization of the cells, thus contributing to the stimulus for the opening of voltage gated calcium channels. The cDNA sequence of voltage-gated sodium channels expressed in a wide variety of tissues is known, with all of them sharing a highly conserved primary structure. The primary structure of the Na-channel consists of two subunits, α and β. The α subunit contains the conductance pathway and the voltage sensor; the β subunit is required for the fast inactivation characteristics of the Na channel *(44,45)*. Even though the expression of similar molecules in pancreatic islets or β-cell derived cell lines has not been investigated using molecular biology approaches, it is highly possible that the sodium channels expressed in the islet are very closely related, if not identical, to the sodium channels expressed elsewhere.

Gap Junction Channels

The study of ion channels and their modulation during the generation of the burst pattern of electrical activity in the islet of Langerhans has been hampered by an unexpected complication—the difficulty to correlate the results obtained measuring V_m in whole, microdissected islets with the patch clamp studies carried out on dispersed cells in primary culture. The most distinctive feature of the whole islet electrical activity, the bursting pattern, is not reproducible in single cells or the patch clamp setting. Although firing of action potentials is observed in β-cells in culture, it occurs as more of a constant activity without a clearly defined temporal pattern. In only one report, a very slow burst pattern has been reported from isolated mouse β-cells *(46)*. At least two factors appear to be important in this difference: the temperature at which experiments are conducted (37°C for the V_m recording from whole islets and room temperature for patch-clamp), and the number of coupled β-cells. Lowering the temperature is associated with a lengthening of the burst period and a depolarization of the silent phase, continuous firing is reached at about room temperature. On the other hand, using a theoretical model of β-cell bursting, it has been demonstrated that the number of cells electrically coupled can influence the pattern of electrical activity of the ensemble, with a minimal number of communicated cells being necessary to originate the oscillatory activity (Fig. 9) *(47)*. Since the modulation of electrical activity by glucose

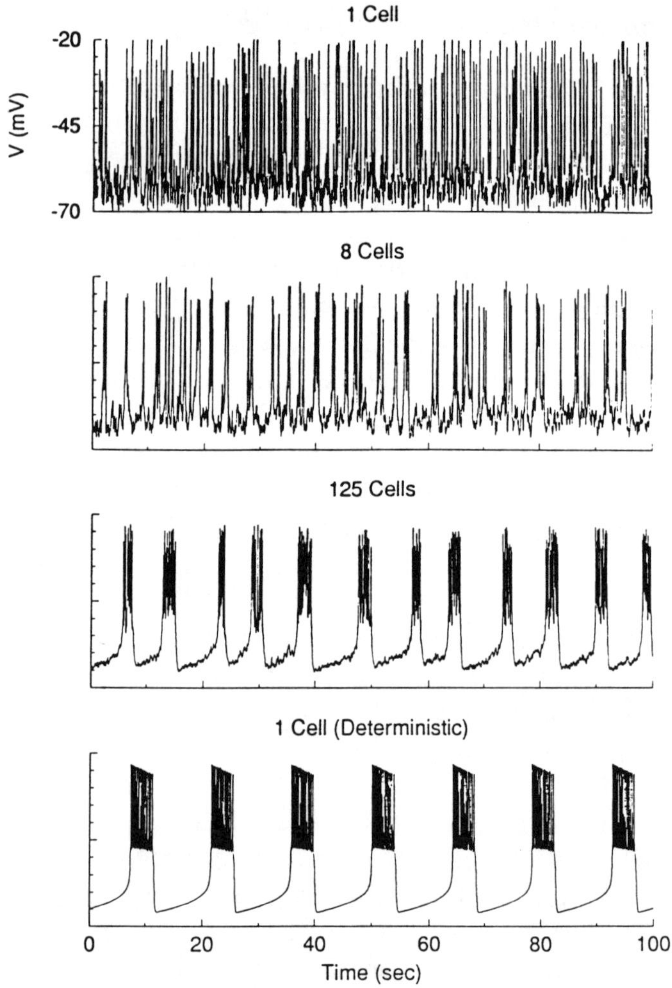

Fig. 9. Predicted glucose-induced membrane potential fluctuations from a single β-cell (upper trace), from 8 cells coupled (middle trace), and from 125 cells coupled (lower trace) in a cluster. As the number of cells coupled increases, the spikes become organized into bursts *(47)*.

is mostly by modulation of the oscillatory pattern, gap junctional channels (responsible for electrical coupling) probably play a key role in the mechanism of glucose sensing.

The presence of gap junctions between β-cells *(48)*, pulsatile insulin secretion from single islets *(49)*, and electrical syncrony in the islet *(50)* were early indications that each islet of Langerhans acts

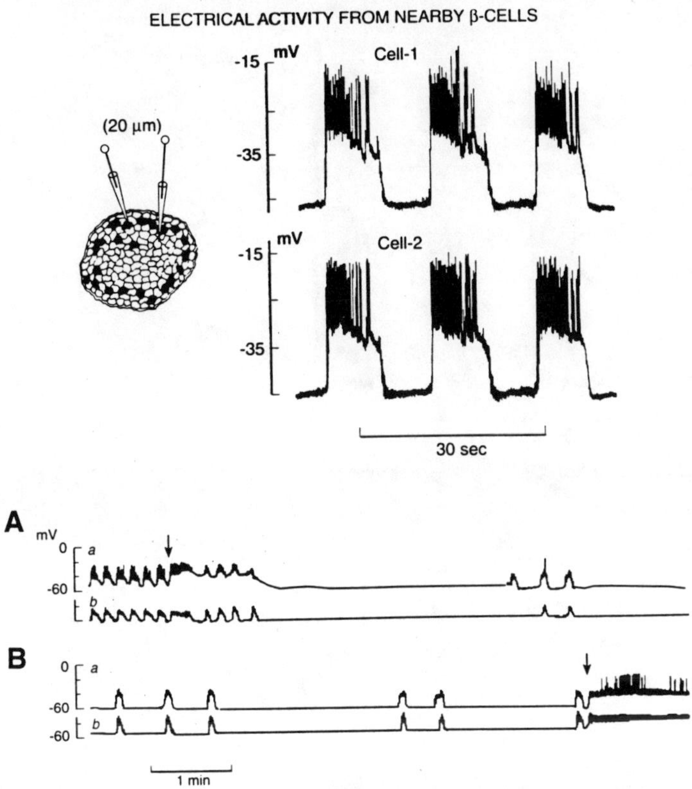

Fig. 10. Electrical synchrony among β-cells in the same islet. The inset at upper right part of Fig. 10 illustrates the position of two electrodes placed in the islet, the recording represents the membrane potential recorded from separate cells, cell 1 and cell 2. The lower panel illustrates the degree of synchrony between two cells when glucose concentration is changed. Note that as the glucose was lowered from 11.1 m*M* to 5.6 m*M* (at arrow over panel A), syncrony is less tight. One cell has an extra burst. In panel B, glyburide was applied at the arrow, both cells became electrically continuous, only one showed large action potentials *(50)*.

as a coupled domain. Thus, each burst of action potentials is synchronous with the bursts of other β-cells in the same islet (Fig. 10), and with an accumulation of extracellular potassium *(51)* (Fig. 11A), with a depletion of extracellular calcium *(52)* (Fig. 11B), with an increase in cytoplasmic calcium *(4)* (Fig. 11C) concentration, and with insulin secretion (Fig. 11D). Paradoxically, dye transfer through gap junctional coupling among the β-cells of an islet is limited *(53)*.

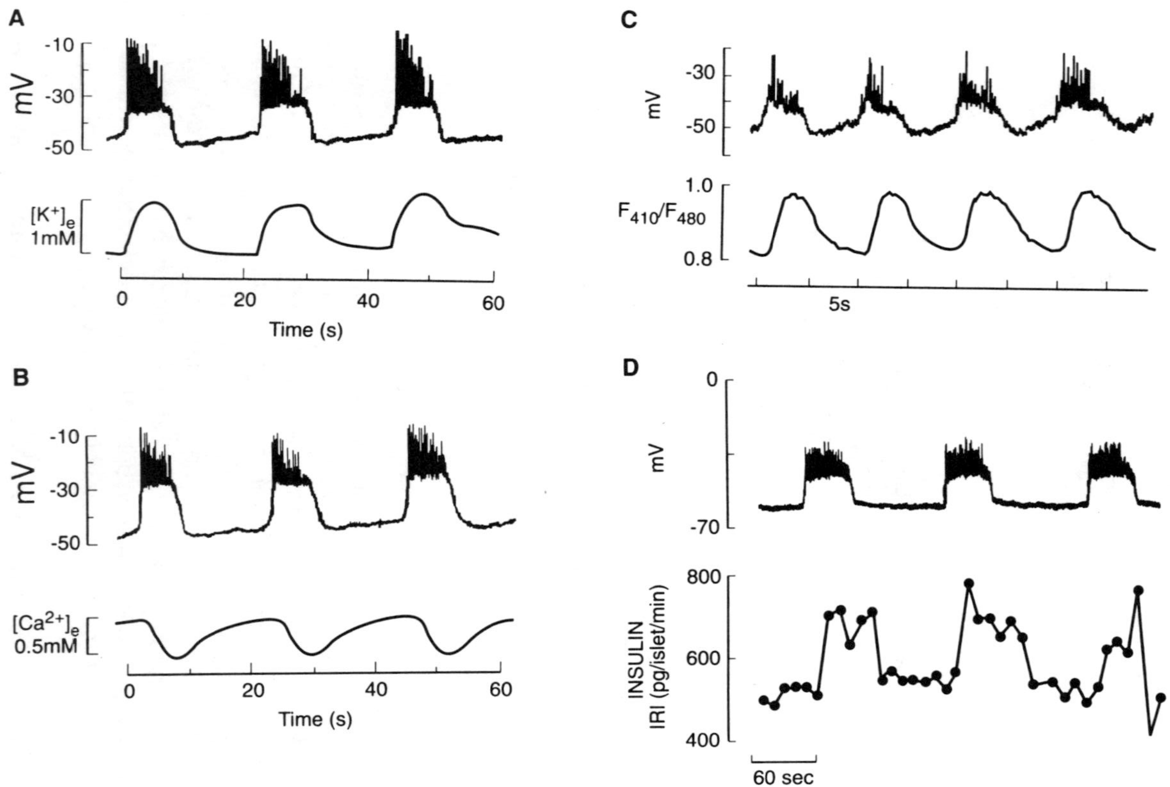

Fig. 11. Synchrony of the oscillations in extracellular ionic concentrations (**A** and **B**), intracellular Ca (**C**) and insulin release (**D**) with electrical burst pattern *(54)*. A *(51)*, B *(52)*, C *(4)*, D *(2)*.

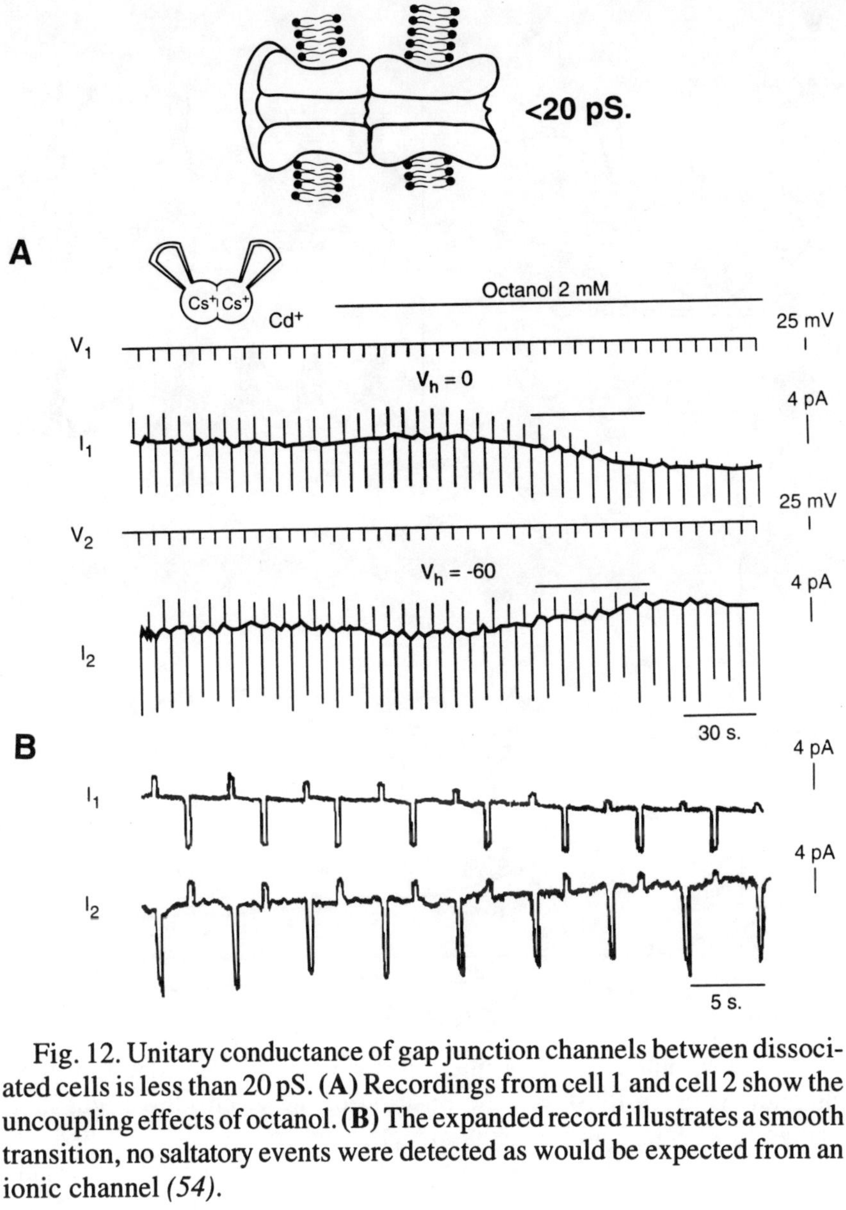

Fig. 12. Unitary conductance of gap junction channels between dissociated cells is less than 20 pS. **(A)** Recordings from cell 1 and cell 2 show the uncoupling effects of octanol. **(B)** The expanded record illustrates a smooth transition, no saltatory events were detected as would be expected from an ionic channel *(54)*.

The molecular biology of the β-cell gap junction channels is considered in depth in Chapter 15 of this book. Each channel is formed by 12 gap junction proteins, called connexins. The single gap junctional channel conductance is very small, less than 20 pS *(54)* (Fig. 12). Connexin 43 has been identified in pancreatic islet cells (*see* Chap-

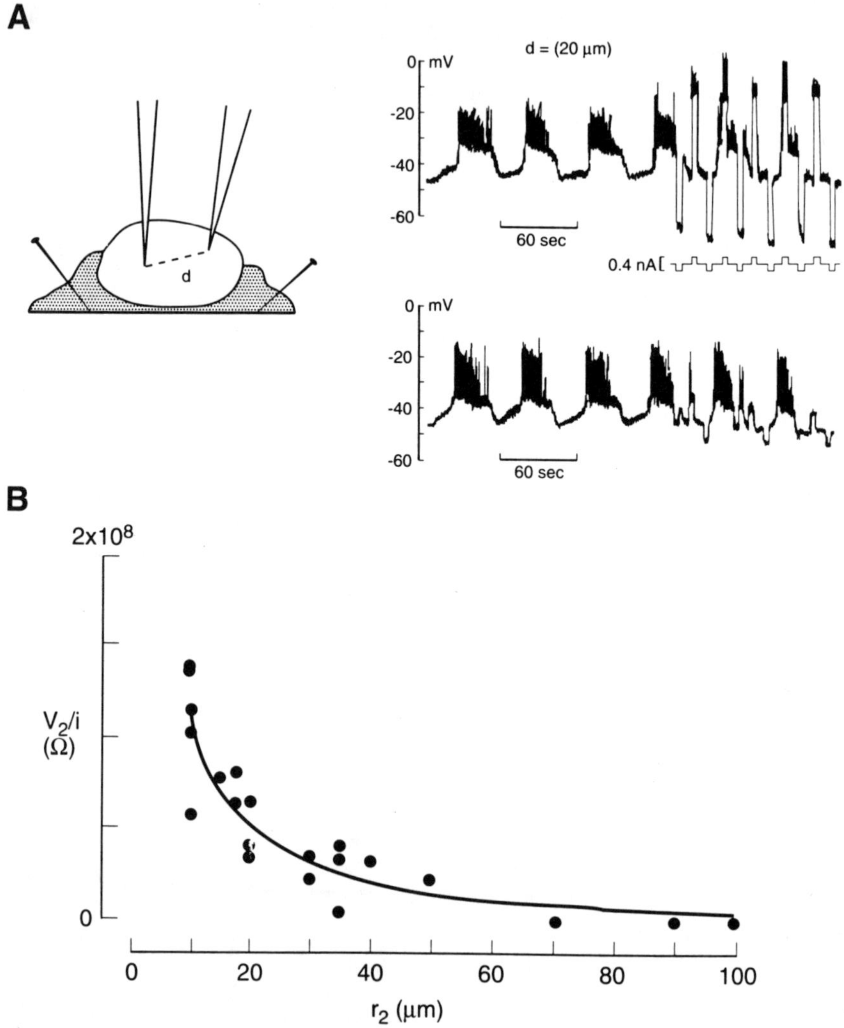

Fig. 13. Limited spread of injected current within the islet. Left inset diagrammatically illustrates the position of the electrodes. Right inset shows detail of the current injection regime, where current is injected into the upper one and small deflections can by recorded in a neighboring cell. Lower panel summarizes the decay of current deflections with distance between the cells being monitored *(55)*.

ter 15). Studies of islet cell junctional conductance indicate limited electrical coupling across the islet; injected current into one cell is barely detected four cells away (about 40 μm) *(50,55)* (Fig. 13). Further-

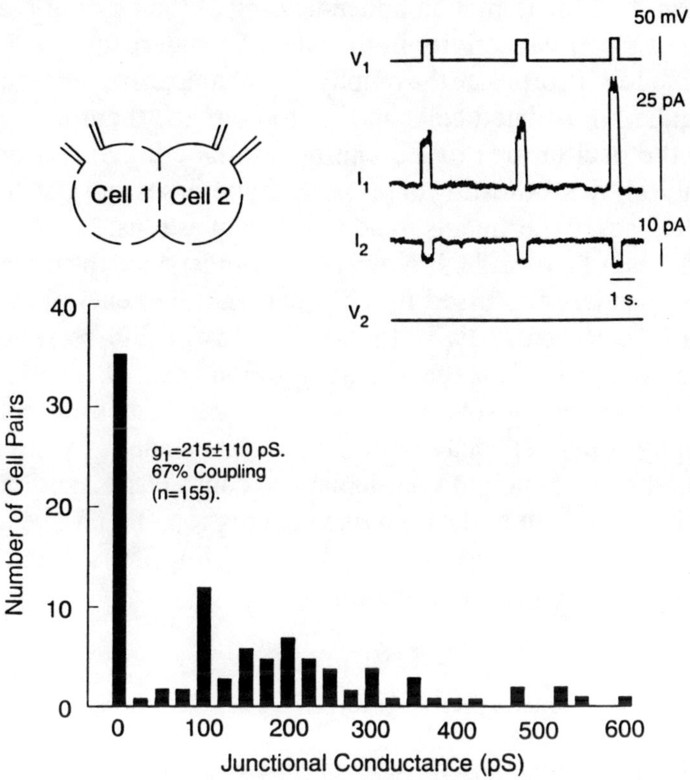

Fig. 14. Average gap junctional conductance between pairs of β-cells. The inset on the upper left of the figure illustrates the pair of cells. The inset on the right shows how the measurements were made. The lower panel indicates a large variability in the cell to cell conductance, with an average around 200 pS *(54)*.

more, the total junctional conductance, as measured between isolated cell pairs is relatively low, averaging only about 200 pS; about 30% of the cell pairs are not electrically coupled *(54)* (Fig. 14). These observations have led to the hypothesis that islet synchrony may also be driven in part by extracellular factors, such as the oscillations in the extracellular potassium concentrations (Fig. 11A) *(56)*.

Given the difficulties to correlate electrophysiological experiments on whole islets with patch clamp experiments on isolated cells, and the near impossibility to obtain ionic current records under voltage clamp in whole islets, mathematical modeling has become an important tool to attempt an understanding of the basis of the burst pattern of electrical activity in the islet of Langerhans *(47,56–59)*. These models incorporate the biophysical characteristics of the channels studied in isolated cells and try to combine them in a way in which the oscillations of V_m can be simulated. This theoretical approach allows the testing of proposed hypotheses and also helps to formulate new experiments to address the questions.

The use of molecular biology tools to understand the function of the ion channels expressed in the β-cell and the generation of the pattern of electrical activity that commands insulin secretion has followed the path of the identification of ion channels expressed in other tissues or organisms. Thus, as this work indicates, the complex electrophysiological behavior of the pancreatic islet may not be the result of the expression of a particular and conspicuous type of channel in the β-cell, but to the combined expression of a unique assortment of channels that allow the exquisite coupling of fuel metabolism to membrane potential modulation.

References

1. Dean PM, Matthews EK: Electrical activity in pancreatic islet cells. *Nature* 219:389,390, 1968.
2. Atwater I, Carroll PB, Li MX: Electrophysiology of the pancreatic B-cell. In *Molecular and Cellular Biology of Diabetes Mellitus,* Draznin B, Melmed S, LeRoith D, eds., Liss, New York, pp. 49–68, 1989.
3. Rosario LM, Atwater I, Scott AM: Pulsatile insulin release and electrical activity from single ob/ob mouse islets of Langerhans. *Adv Exp Med Biol* 211:413–425, 1986.
4. Santos RM, Rosario LM, Nadal A, Garcia-Sancho J, Soria B, Valdeolmillos M: Widespread synchronous [Ca^{2+}] oscillations due to bursting electrical activity in single pancreatic islets. *Pflugers Arch* 418:417–422, 1991.
5. Gilon P, Shepherd RM, Henquin JC: Oscillations of secretion driven by oscillations of cytoplasmic Ca^{2+} as evidenced in single pancreatic islets. *Biol Chem* 268:22,265–22,268, 1993.

5a. Rojas E, Santos RM, Atwater I: Role of membrane receptors in stimulus secretion coupling, in *Transduction in Biological Systems,* vol. 7, Plenum, New York, pp. 101–122.

6. Atwater I, Goncalves A, Herchuelz A, Lebrun P, Malaisse WJ, Rojas E, Scott A : Cooling dissociates glucose-induced insulin release from electrical activity and cation fluxes in rodent pancreatic islets. *J Physiol (Lond)* 348:615–627, 1984.
7. Henquin JC: D-glucose inhibits potassium efflux from pancreatic islet cells. *Nature* 271:271–273, 1978.

8. Atwater I, Ribalet B, Rojas E: Cyclic changes in potential and resistance of the beta-cell membrane induced by glucose in islets of Langerhans from mouse. *J Physiol (Lond)* 278:117–139, 1978.
9. Atwater I, Ribalet B, Rojas E: Mouse pancreatic beta-cells: tetraethylammonium blockage of the potassium permeability increase induced by depolarization. *J Physiol (Lond)* 288:561–574, 1979.
10. Ashcroft FM, Ashcroft SJH, Harrison DE: Properties of single potassium channels modulated by glucose in rat pancreatic B-cells. *J Physiol (Lond)* 400:501–527, 1988.
11. Cook DL, Hales CN: Intracellular ATP directly blocks K channels in pancreatic B-cells. *Nature* 211:269–271, 1984.
12. Carroll PB, Li MX, Rojas E, Atwater I: The ATP-sensitive potassium channels in pancreatic B-cells is inhibited in physiological bicarbonate buffer. *FEBS Lett* 234:208–212, 1988.
13. Dunne MJ, West-Jordan JA, Abraham RJ, Edwards RHT, Petersen OH: The gating of nucleotide-sensitive K^+ channels in insulin-secreting cells can be modulated by changes in the ratio ATP4-/ADP3- and by nonhydrolyzable derivatives of both ATP and ADP. *J Membrane Biol* 104:165–177, 1988.
14. Aguilar-Bryan L, Nichols C G, Rajan A S, Parker C, Bryan J: Co-expression of sulfonylurea receptors and KATP channels in hamster insulinoma tumor (HIT) cells. Evidence for direct association of the receptor with the channel. *J Biol Chem* 267:14,934–14,940, 1992.
15. Aguilar-Bryan L, Nelson DA, Vu QA, Humphrey MB, Boyd AE: Photoaffinity labeling and partial purification of the beta cell sulfonylurea receptor using a novel, biologically active glyburide analog. *J Biol Chem* 265:8218–8224, 1990.
16. Ho K, Nichols CG, Lederer WJ, Lytton J, Vassilev PM, Kanazirska MV, et al.: Cloning and expression of an inwardly rectifyng ATP-regulated potassium channel. *Nature* 362:31–38, 1993.
17. Sentenac H, Bonneaud N, Minet M, Lacroute F, Salmon J M, Gaymard F, Grignon C: Cloning and expression in yeast of a plant potassium ion transport system. *Science* 256:663–668, 1992.
18. Arispe N, Rojas E, Hartman J, Sorscher EJ, Pollard HB: Intrinsic anion channel activity of the recombinant first nucleotide binding fold domain of the cystic fibrosis transmembrane regulator protein. *Proc Natl Acad Sci USA* 89:1539–1543, 1992.
19. Sheppard DN, Welsh MJ: Effect of ATP-sensitive K^+ channel regulators on cystic fibrosis transmembrane conductance regulator chloride currents. *J Gen Physiol* 100:573–591, 1992.
20. Dawson CM, Atwater I, Rojas E: The response of pancreatic β-cell membrane potential to potassium-induced calcium influx in the presence of glucose. *Q J Exp Physiol* 69: 819–830, 1984.
21. Lebrun P, Atwater I, Claret M, Malaisse WJ, Herchuelz A: Resistance to apamin of the Ca^{2+}-activated K^+ permeability in pancreatic B-cells. *FEBS Lett* 161:41–44, 1983.

22. Cook DL, Ikeuchi M, Fujimoto WY: Lowering of pH_i inhibits Ca^{2+}-activated K^+ channels in pancreatic in pancreatic B-cells. *Nature* 311:269–271, 1984.
23. Eddlestone GT, Ribalet B, Ciani S: Comparative study of K channel behavior in β cell lines with different secretory responses to glucose. *J Membrane Biol* 109:123–134, 1989.
24. Kukuljan M, Goncalves AA, Atwater I: Charybdotoxin-sensitive K(Ca) channel is not involved in glucose-induced electrical activity in pancreatic B-cells. *J Membrane Biol* 119:187–195, 1991.
25. Ammala C, Larsson O, Berggren P O, Bokvist K, Juntti-Berggren L, Kindmark H, Rorsman P: Inositol trisphosphate-dependent periodic activation of a Ca^{2+}-activated K^+ conductance in glucose-stimulated pancreatic β-cells. *Nature* 353:849–852, 1991.
26. Stojilkovic SS, Kukuljan M, Iida T, Rojas E, Catt KJ: Integration of cytoplasmic calcium and membrane potential oscillations maintains calcium signaling in pituitary gonadotrophs. *Proc Natl Acad Sci USA* 89:4081–4085, 1992.
27. Butler A, Tsunoda S, McCobb DP, Wei A, Salkoff L: mSlo, a complex mouse gene encoding "maxi" calcium-activated potassium channels. *Science* 261:221–224, 1993.
28. Rorsman P, Trube G: Calcium and delayed potassium currents in mouse pancreatic β-cells under voltage-clamp conditions. *J Physiol (Lond)* 550:531–550, 1986.
29. Bokvist K, Rorsman P, Smith PA: Effects of external tetraethylamonium ions and quinine on delayed rectifying K^+ channels in mouse pancreatic β-cells. *J Physiol (Lond)* 423:311–325, 1990.
30. Betsholtz C, Baumann A, Kenna S, Ashcroft FM, Ashcroft SJH, Berggren PO, et al.: Expression of voltage-gated K^+ channels in insuling-producing cells. *FEBS Lett* 263:121–126, 1990.
31. Hoshi T, Zagotta WN: Recent advances in the understanding of potassium channel function. *Curr Opin Neurobiol* 3:283–290, 1993.
32. Mackinnon R: New insights into the structure and function of potassium channels. *Curr Opin Neurobiol* 1:14–19, 1991.
33. Rorsman P, Bokvist K, Ammala C, Arkhammar P, Berggren PO, Larsson O, et al.: Activation by adrenaline of a low-conductance G protein-dependent K^+ channel in mouse pancreatic β cells. *Nature* 349:77–79, 1991.
34. Santana de Sa S, Ferrer R, Rojas E, Atwater I: Effects of adrenaline and noradrenaline on glucose-induced electrical activity of mouse pancreatic beta cell. *Q J Exp Physiol* 68:247–258, 1983.
35. Atwater I, Dawson CM, Eddlestone GT, Rojas E: Voltage noise measurements across the pancreatic beta-cell membrane: calcium channel characteristics. *J Physiol (Lond)* 314:195–212, 1981.
36. Hiriart M, Matteson DR: Na channels and two types of Ca channels in rat pancreatic β cells identified with the reverse hemolytic plaque assay. *J Gen Physiol* 91:617–639, 1988.
37. Tsien RW, Tsien RY: Calcium channels, stores, and oscillations. *Annu Rev Cell Biol* 6:715–760, 1990.

38. Smith PA, Rorsman P, Ashcroft FM: Modulation of dihydropyridine-sensitive Ca^{2+} channels by glucose metabolism in mouse pancreatic B-cells. *Nature* 342:550–553, 1989.
39. Ammala C, Ashcroft FM, Rorsman P: Calcium-independent potentiation of insulin release by cyclic AMP in single β cells. *Nature* 363:356–358, 1993.
40. Satin LS, Cook DL: Calcium current inactivation in insulin-secreting cells is mediated by calcium influx and membrane depolarization. *Pflugers Arch* 414:1–10, 1989.
41. Seino S, Chen L, Seino M, Blondel O, Takeda J, Johnson J H, et al.: Cloning of the alpha 1 subunit of a voltage-dependent calcium channel expressed in pancreatic beta cells. *Proc Natl Acad Sci USA* 89:584–588, 1992.
42. Rojas E, Hidalgo J, Carroll PB, Atwater I: A new class of calcium channels activated by glucose in human pancreatic B-cells. *FEBS Lett* 261:265–270, 1990.
43. Pressel DM, Misler S: Sodium channels contribute to action potential generation in canine and human pancreatic islet β cells. *J Membrane Biol* 116:273–280, 1990.
44. Stühmer W, Parekh AB: The structure and function of Na^+ channels. *Curr Opin Neurobiol* 2:243–246, 1992.
45. Catterall WA: Structure and function of voltage-gated sodium and calcium channels. *Curr Opin Neurobiol* 1:5–13, 1991.
46. Smith PA, Ashcroft FM, Rorsman P: Simultaneous recordings of glucose dependent electrical activity and ATP-regulated K^+-currents in isolated mouse pancreatic beta-cells. *FEBS Lett* 261:187–190, 1990.
47. Sherman A, Rinzel J, Keizer J: Emergence of organized bursting in clusters of pancreatic beta-cells by channel sharing. *Biophys J* 54:411–425, 1988.
48. Orci L, Unger RH, Renold AE: Structural coupling between pancreatic islet cells. *Experientia* 29:1015–1018, 1973.
49. Beigelman PM, Thomas LJ, Slavin B, Shu MJ, Bessman SP: Insulin from individual isolated islets of Langerhans. I: response to glucose. *Biochem Med* 8:392–398, 1973.
50. Meda P, Atwater I, Goncalves A, Bangham A, Orci L, Rojas E: The topography of electricasl synchrony among B-cells in the mouse islet of Langerhans. *Quart J Exp Physiol* 69:831–839, 1984.
51. Pérez-Armendáriz E, Atwater I, Rojas E: Glucose induced oscillatory changes in the extracellular ionized potassium concentration in mouse islets of Langerhans. *Biophys J* 48:741–751, 1985.
52. Pérez-Armendáriz E, Atwater I: Glucose-evoked changes in K^+ and Ca^{2+} in the intracellular spaces of the mouse islet of Langerhans. *Adv Exptl Med. Biol* 211:31–51, 1986.
53. Meda P, Santos RM, Atwater I: Direct identification of electrophysiologically monitored cells within intact mouse islets of Langerhans. *Diabetes* 35:232–236, 1986.
54. Pérez-Armendáriz E, Roy C, Spray DC, Bennett MVL: Biophysical properties og gap junctions between freshly dispersed pairs of mouse pancreatic beta cells. *Biophys J* 59:76–90, 1991.

55. Eddlestone GT, Goncalves A, Bangham JA, Rojas E: Electical coupling between cells in islets of Langerhans from mouse. *J Membrane Biol* 77:1–12, 1984.
56. Stokes C, Rinzel J: Diffusion of extracellular K^+ can synchronize bursting oscillations in a model islet of Langerhans. *Biophys J* 65:597–607, 1993.
57. Rinzel J, Chay TR, Himmel D, Atwater I: Prediction of the glucose-induced changes in membrane permeability and cytosolic Ca^{2+} by mathematical modeling. In *Biophysics of the Pancreatic B-Cell*, Atwater I, Rojas E, Soria B, eds., Plenum, New York, pp. 247–263, 1987.
58. Atwater I, Rinzel J: The β-cell bursting pattern and intracellular calcium. In *Ionic Channels in Cells and Model Systems*, Latorre R, ed., Plenum, New York, pp. 304–316, 1986.
59. Sherman A., Carroll P, Santos RM, Atwater I: Glucose dose response curve of pancreatic β cells: experimental and theoretical results. In *Transduction in Biological Systems*, Hidalgo C, Bacigalupo J, Jaimovich E, Vergara J, eds., Plenum, New York, pp. 123–141, 1990.

Chapter 14

Molecular Biology of Gap Junction Proteins

Paolo Meda

Introduction

Virtually every animal cell type forms gap junctions, the specialized regions of the cell membrane where adjacent cells concentrate channels for direct cell-to-cell exchanges of cytoplasmic ions and small molecules *(1–4)*. Although the structure, tissue distribution and biophysical characteristics of gap junctions as well as the regulation of the intercellular communications they mediate have been the subject of numerous studies in the last three decades, an indepth analysis of the biochemistry of the proteins comprising gap junctions and of the molecular biology of the encoding genes has been possible only in the last few years *(2–4)*. These recent developments have not completely elucidated all the intriguing questions which are raised by the existence of direct exchanges of cytoplasmic constituents between nearby cells, particularly inasmuch as the physiological function and meaning of these exchanges is concerned. However, they have clearly identified gap junction proteins as the members of a multigene family of highly conserved molecules, which have rather unique characteristics and are essentially ubiquitous in multicellular, mesozoa, and metazoa organisms *(2–4)*.

From: *Molecular Biology of Diabetes, Part I*
Edited by: B. Draznin and D. LeRoith

In 1973, the Geneva group identified gap junctions between the endocrine cells of pancreatic islets *(5)*. Since, several groups have extended these studies, focusing almost exclusively on the insulin-producing B-cells. Collectively, this work has revealed that B-cell gap junctions and coupling show distinctive if not unique features, and, more importantly, that they are modulated in close association with insulin secretion *(6–7)*.

In this context, the purpose of this chapter is twofold. First, to review the most salient features of the cell and molecular biology of gap junction channels and of their constitutive connexin proteins. Second, to summarize our present knowledge about the gap junctions of pancreatic B-cells, with particular regard to their relationship to the biosynthesis, storage, and release of insulin.

Gap Junctions

Gap Junction Plaques

Gap junctions are surface structures made up by adjacent cells, at sites where two plasma membranes become closely apposed, reducing the interweening intercellular space, which is typically 100–250 nm wide, to a regular, narrow gap (which explains the name of the junctions) of about 2 nm *(8)*. In these regions, the two interacting membranes feature specialized microdomains characterized by the concentration of proteinaceous, tubular structures now called connexons *(9,10)*. Each connexon, which at the electron microscope level appears as a large and globular intramembrane particle (Figs. 1 and 2), spans the entire width of the phospholipid bilayer of one membrane. Thus, one end of each connexon extends in the cytoplasm, whereas the other end enters the intercellular space *(10)*. In the middle of such space, the connexons of one cell dock with the connexons made up by an adjacent cell (Fig. 1), hence establishing a continuous structure that bridges the intercellular space. The cell-to-cell docking of connexons appears quite strong since it is usually difficult to split apart the two halves of vertebrate gap junction plaques without using harsh treatments *(11)*.

Connexons

Each connexon is formed by the assembly of integral membrane proteins *(1–4,10–12)*, belonging to the connexin (Cx) family *(13,14)*, and that arrange as pentamers and/or hexamers around a central

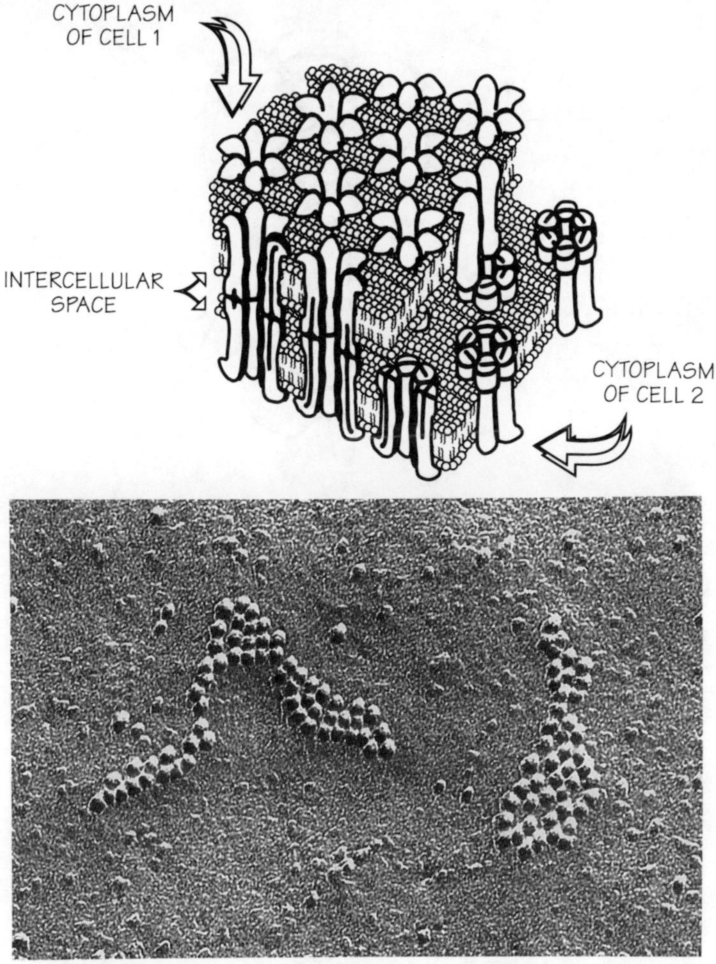

Fig. 1. A gap junction. Upper panel: The presently accepted model envisions this structure as an area where the membranes of two adjacent cells are closely apposed and are enriched in proteins of the connexin family. These proteins assemble in structures, called connexons, that span the phospholipid bilayer of each membrane, and extend across the intercellular space where they interact with the connexons made by another cell. The alignment of two opposed connexons is required to form the wall of a channel that directly links the cytoplasm of one cell to that of an adjacent cell. Lower panel: By freeze-fracture electron microscopy, gap junctions (here between two insulin-producing B-cells) are identified as intramembrane aggregates of uniformly large proteic particles, each of which represents a connexon.

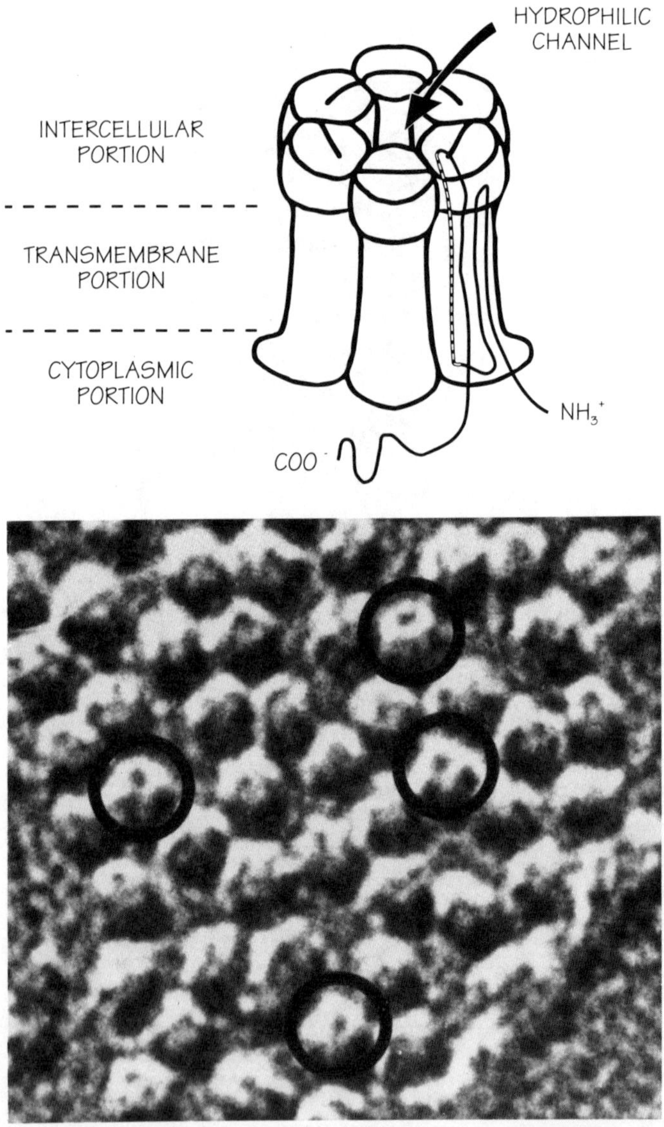

Fig. 2. A connexon. Upper panel: The half of each gap junction channel is envisioned as a tube made up of five or six connexin molecules, arranged around a central space. This space is a 2 nm wide hydrophilic channel that extends across the entire length of the connexon. Lower panel: At high magnification, freeze-fracture electron microscopy shows that connexons (some of which are circled) are formed by multiple subunits and feature a central dense spot that represents the intercellular opening of their hydrophilic channel.

hydrophilic space (Fig. 2). Thus, the wall of a complete gap junction channel comprises 10–12 connexin molecules *(10,12)*. Connexons and double membrane gap junctions can be generated by a single type of connexin *(15)*, and it is likely that different connexins produce channels with distinct unitary conductances and permeability *(2–4,13,14)*. Furthermore, expression of Cx43 in yeast, which does not have endogenous connexin genes, has led to the formation of double membrane structures resembling gap junctions, suggesting that no additional gap junction specific factor is required for the biosynthesis and assembly of a connexon *(3)*. However, the mere expression of a connexin will not necessarily result in a functional gap junction channel, since recent observations indicate that some connexins (e.g., Cx40), which can establish cell-to-cell communications when interacting with homologous molecules, cannot form functional gap junction channels after interaction with other types of connexins *(2,3,16)*. At least in some cases, hemichannels composed of one connexin (e.g., Cx32) may form junctions with hemichannels composed of a different connexin (e.g., Cx26), although the conductance and permeability of the presumptive heterotypic junctions may be smaller than that of homotypic junctions *(2,3,16,17)*. It is still a matter of debate whether different types of connexins may oligomerize within individual connexons.

The central hydrophilic space of each connexon, which is about 1.5 nm wide and 10 nm long, represents half of a gap junction channel *(10,17)*. Thus, a complete gap junction channel requires the precise end-to-end abutment of the central spaces of two connexons *(10)*, arranged in series (Fig. 1). Gap junction channels are relatively long because of this arrangement, and this length may explain why their unitary conductance (which may range from 40 to 150 pS) is comparable to that of other ionic channels, in spite of a much larger permeability to molecules *(1,2,17)*.

Connexins

Gap junctions are formed by a set of homologous integral membrane proteins, called connexins, which are encoded by a multigene family *(2–4,13,14)*. In mammals, twelve members of this family have been identified (Table 1). A few additional connexins, more or less analogous to the mammalian types, have been found in chickens and amphibians, and proteins related to connexins may also be

Table 1
Mammalian Gap Junction Connexins

Gene	Protein[a] size, kDa	mRNA size, kb	References	Pancreatic localization[b]
β_2	26.5	2.7	*J Cell Biol* 109:3391 (1989)	Acinar cells
β_5	30.3	3.2,1.8	*Eur J Cell Biol* 56:1 (1991)	ND[c]
β_3	31	2.3,1.7	*J Biol Chem* 266:6524 (1991)	ND
β_4	31.1	1.6	*Eur J Cell Biol* 56:1 (1991)	ND
β_1	32	1.6	*J Cell Biol* 103:123 1986) *J Cell Biol* 103:767 (1986)	Acinar cells
α_7	32.9	2.3	*J Biol Chem* 267:2057 (1992)	ND
α_4	37.6	1.7	*J Cell Biol* 114:1049 (1991)	Arterioles
α_5	40	3.5	*Eur J Cell Biol* 56:1 (1992) *J Biol Chem* 267:2057 (1992)	Arterioles
α_1	43	3.2	*J Cell Biol* 105:2621 (1987)	B-cells islet non-B-cells fibroblasts
α_6	45	2.3	*Eur J Cell Biol* 56:1 (1991)	ND
α_3	45	2.8	*J Biol Chem* 115:1077 (1991)	ND
α_8	50	3.8	*Mol Biol Cell* 3:711 (1992)	ND

[a]Predicted from cDNA analysis.
[b]*Exp Cell Res* 192:469–480 (1991); *Endocrinology* 133:2371–2378 (1993).
[c]ND = not determined.

expressed in higher plants. Virtually every type of connexin is expressed in more than one tissue, and a single cell type may express more than one connexin, either within the same gap junction or within different gap junction plaques *(2–4,13,14)*.

All connexins feature large analogies in membrane topology, as determined by sequencing their amino acids or fragments obtained by protease treatment of isolated gap junctions (these treatments are not expected to attack the portions of connexins exposed in the intercellular space and that are protected by the small size of the gap), as well as by immunolabeling of both intact and split open junctions with antibodies raised against selected epitopes. In combination, these approaches have indicated that connexins are ribbonlike molecules (Fig. 3) that have their N- and C-termini in the cytoplasm, four hydrophobic regions that presumably correspond to transmembrane domains and that are connected by a cytoplasmic loop and two extracellular loops *(2–4,10,11,13,14,18–22)*. The four hydrophobic regions cross the lipid bilayer probably as α-helices aligned in parallel and antiparallel directions. The corresponding connexin of the apposed cell membrane is thought to have the same orientation, so that each second membrane-spanning domain of one connexin would be aligned with the fourth membrane-spanning domain of the connexin facing it in the nearby cell. The third membrane-spanning region has polar, basic, and acidic groups that are conserved in all connexins. This region is thought to form an amphipathic helix, with the polar residue side lining the wall of the connexon channel *(2–4, 10,11,13,14,18–22)*.

All connexins also show large analogies in sequence *(2–4, 13,14)*. They all feature two highly conserved portions (>60% amino acid identity in the membrane-spanning regions and 50% in the N-terminus) and two unique regions that vary in both length and sequence in different connexins. Each of the two conserved portions (N-terminus + first membrane-spanning domain + first extracellular loop + second membrane-spanning domain and third membrane-spanning domain + second extracellular loop + fourth membrane-spanning domain) is about 100 amino acids long. Each of the two loops that extend across the intercellular space is about 40 amino acids long and contains a set of three cysteines that have conserved the same position and spacing in all connexins. These cysteines allow for intramolecular disulfide bonds that may be required to ensure a stable conformation of the extracellular loops *(2–4,23)*. This conformation, in turn, may be essential in permitting a proper docking between the connexins of adjacent cells. The variable regions of connexins are the cytoplasmic loop and the C-terminus. The latter region varies in length from 18 amino acids in Cx26 to 191 amino acids in Cx46, accounting for the different molecular weight of connexins, which ranges from 26–50 kDa (Table 1). The C-terminus also provides useful epitope sites for raising specific antibodies to selected connexins, which now permit the localization of these molecules at both light and electron microscope level (Fig. 3). The conserved regions are likely to be important for the proper functioning of gap junction channels, even though the significance of many of their portions is still uncertain, but most of the divergent regions are likely to be neutral. Some, however, may confer significantly distinct characteristics to different connexins, such as consen-

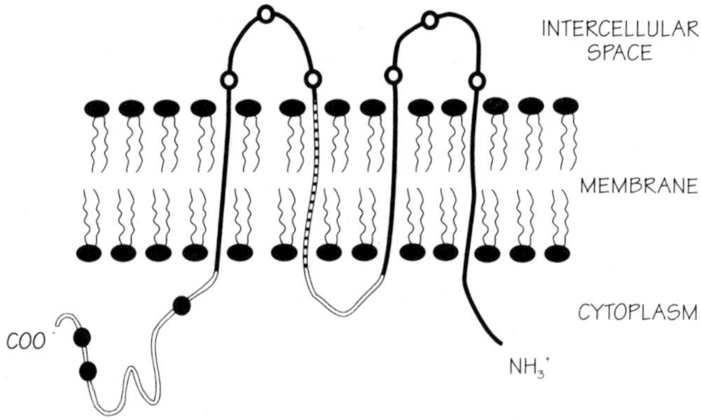

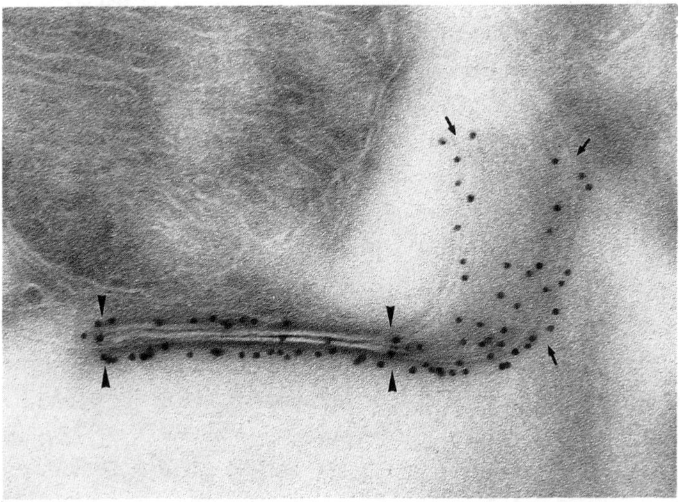

Fig. 3. A connexin. Upper panel: A gap junction protein is thought to be a ribbon-shaped molecule that crosses the phospholipid bilayer of the membrane four times, forms two loops in the intercellular space, and features both C- and N-termini in the cytoplasm. The third intramembranous portion of the molecule (dotted line) borders the central hydrophilic space of the connexon. All connexins feature three cysteine residues (open circles) in each of the two extracellular loops. Multiple serine and thyrosine residues (solid dots) that may be phosphorylated, are found along the C-terminus portion of some connexins. The aminoacid sequence of the four transmembrane domains and of the two extracellular loops (solid and dotted line portions) are highly conserved in all connexins. In contrast, the

sus sites for phosphorylation along the C-terminus, which are present in some (e.g., C32 and Cx43) but not all (e.g., Cx26) connexins *(2–4,24–27)*.

Phosphorylation is the only posttranslational modification detected in connexins and may take place at either serine (PKA- and PKC-induced) or thyrosine sites ($pp60_{sarc}$-induced) along the cytoplasmic C-terminus of the molecules *(24–27)*. At variance with numerous other membrane proteins, connexins have a rather short half life, typically less than 4–6 hours, and are not glycosylated *(2–4)*.

There is still some debate about how to name different connexins *(2–4)*. Throughout this text, the author has used the most widespread nomenclature that names these molecules according to their predicted molecular weight deduced from the corresponding cDNA (Table 1). Another nomenclature classes connexins in two groups, depending on the presence of some residues that are conserved in one group but not in the other, and on the length of the cytoplasmic loop, two differences that may or may not have physiological significance. In this second classification, connexins are referred to the α (short cytoplasmic loop) or β group (long cytoplasmic loop) and distinguished by a numerical subscript, according to the temporal sequence of identification (Table 1). Comparison of the available sequences suggests that the inferred gene duplication that permitted the divergence of the α and β groups must have occurred early in, or prior to, vertebrate evolution *(2,4)*.

---

cytoplasmic loop and the C-terminal (open line portions) show a rather variable sequence and length in different connexins. Lower panel: Immunostaining of a cryostat section of rat myocardium with an antibody directed against a 20 amino acid epitope of the C-terminus portion of Cx43, reveals a concentration of this protein at close membrane appositions typical of gap junctions. In en face views (arrows), the gold particles that were linked to a secondary antibody, reveal the two-dimensional, plaque arrangement of connexins. In sections perpendicular to the plane of the two interacting cell membranes (arrowheads), gold particles align along the two cytoplasmic faces of the gap junction, consistent with the cytoplasmic localization of the C-terminus epitope.

Connexin Genes

Screening of cDNA libraries with antibodies, synthetic oligonucleotides constructed on the basis of known connexin sequences and available connexin cDNAs, has shown that different connexins are encoded by single genes that hybridize as distinct mRNAs species *(2–4,16,19–22)*. The few connexin genes that have so far been characterized, show a conserved architecture characterized by two exons separated by one intron. The first exon is small and contains only a 5'-untranslated sequence. It is followed by an intron in the 5' nontranslated region, which has a variable length in different connexin genes and in all connexins features a possible splice acceptor site 16–33 bp upstream of the start translation codon. The intron is followed by the second exon, which is larger than the first exon and contains the entire coding sequence with an uninterrupted reading frame *(28,29)*. The absence of introns in the reading frame is at variance with what is observed for most other cell proteins that are usually encoded by mRNAs assembled from heterogeneous RNAs, which contain intron sequences dispersed among coding exon sequences. However, uninterrupted coding regions are also observed for other families of membrane channel proteins, such as those comprising K^+ channels.

Little is still known about the promoter/enhancer regions of connexin genes. So far, the analysis of consensus binding sites for transcription factors has revealed few common features in different connexin genes *(30)*, providing a possible molecular basis for a differential regulation of the expression of the cognate proteins. However, since the few putative regulatory elements that have been identified have not yet been functionally analyzed by protein binding assays and reporter gene constructs, it is still unclear whether and how the genomic organization of the connexin gene family reflects the pattern of expression of different gap junction proteins.

Most connexin genes are dispersed throughout human chromosomes (e.g., Cx32 on chromosome X, Cx43 on chromosome 6, a sequence that may represent a processed Cx43 pseudogene on chromosome 5), without evidence for large gene clusters *(14,28–31)*. However, some connexin genes have been found to be closely located on a same chromosome (e.g., Cx26 and Cx46 on chromosome

13, Cx37 and Cx40 on chromosome 1), suggesting that they may share common developmental and tissue regulatory gene sequences. Clearly, the relationship between chromosome clustering and connexin expression, if any, is not simple. For example, whereas Cx37 and Cx40 are usually expressed in the same tissues, Cx26 and Cx46 usually are not. Comparison with mice *(31)* show that a same connexin gene may be mapped to a different chromosome in different species. For example, whereas the Cx37 and the Cx40 genes are mapped to human chromosome 1, the corresponding mouse genes are located on chromosomes 3 and 4, respectively. Also, Cx26 and Cx46 genes are located on chromosome 13 in humans and on chromosome 14 in mice.

Gap Junctional Coupling

At gap junctions, the intercellular space is bridged by a continuous hydrophilic pathway, made up by the precise abutment of two connexons, and through which ions and small molecules may directly pass from the cytoplasm of one cell into the cytoplasm of an adjacent cell, without entering the intercellular fluid. This intercellular passage is also referred to as ionic and metabolic (cell-to-cell or junctional) coupling. Direct cell-to-cell exchange of ions may be demonstrated by the simultaneous recording of electrotonic potential changes, induced by current pulses, in both current-injected and nearby noninjected cells, by the direct measurement of junctional conductances at individual cell-to-cell interfaces, as well as by the synchronization of electrophysiological parameters across territories of coupled cells *(1,2)*. Direct cell-to-cell exchanges of several molecules, including nucleotides, amino acids, vitamin cofactors, and metabolites less than 900 Daltons, has been detected by autoradiography and microspectrofluorometry *(1,32,33)*. Experimentally, however, the direct intercellular exchange of molecules is most often tested using exogenous tracers. After microinjection into individual cells, the intercellular diffusion of these molecules, which cannot cross the cell membrane, can be directly visualized by fluorescence microscopy or immunohistochemical staining *(1,2,17,34,35)*. The intercellular passage of molecules through gap junctions is driven by diffusion and may be quite extensive. As much as 10^6 molecules of the size of cAMP may be exchanged per second between coupled cells, and such an exchange may take place over territories comprising up to one hundred cells *(32)*. On the other hand, organelles, proteins, nucleic acids, and molecules larger than 1 kDa may not cross gap junctions *(32)*.

Gap junction channels are unique in that they are obligatorily made up by two membranes, usually contributed by two different cells, do not show ion selectivity, and have a fairly large permeability. However, as other membrane channels, those forming gap junctions are modulated by second messengers, particularly H^+, Ca^{2+}, and arachidonic acid metabolites, and by both cAMP-dependent kinases and protein kinase C *(1–4)*. The effects of second messengers on gap junction channels vary widely depending on a number of parameters, including the type of cell, its state of activity, the type of connexin, and of the second messenger. Also, there might be fast (in the ms range) and slow changes (in the min-h range) of gap junctional communication. The fastest and reversible changes of junctional conductance are owing to open-close transitions of existing channels, presumably as a result of a conformational change of connexins. There is evidence that in closed channels, connexins are tilted along their axis, thereby reducing the central hydrophilic space of connexons *(2,3)*. The slower changes are owing to the formation or removal of channels, which may result from many different events, including insertion in the cell membrane of a premade connexin pool, changes in the transcription of connexin genes, in the levels and/or stability of the resulting mRNAs, in the translation of these transcripts, and in the degradation rate of connexins *(1–4)*.

Gap junctional coupling ensures the electrical synchronization of cells in excitable, neural, and muscular systems, and contributes to controlled cell growth and differentiation in several developing and tumoral tissues *(1–4,36)*. By contrast, the physiological functions of these structures are still largely unknown in a variety of adult tissues that function, under most physiological conditions, without changing the differentiation and growth status of their cells *(1–4,36)*. Most vertebrate glands fall into this category. Gap junctions and coupling appear to be obligatory attributes of virtually every endocrine and exocrine gland, including the pancreas *(37,38)*. It is in this organ that almost all the experimental evidence indicating a contribution of junctional coupling to the proper functioning of secretory cells has been gained *(6,7)*.

The Case of Insulin-Producing Cells

Gap Junctions and Coupling

Pancreatic B-cells are connected to each other and to other islet cell types by numerous and minute gap junctions *(5)* made exclusively of Cx43 *(38–40)*. In a resting B-cell, there are 800–2000 gap junction channels that, altogether, occupy less than 1 μm^2 of the plasma membrane *(40)*. These channels allow for the B-to-B-cell exchange of current-carrying ions, low molecular weight probes, nucleotides and glycolytic intermediates *(33,41–44)*. Ionic and metabolic coupling are not observed between all B-cells *(40)*, in agreement with the detection of gap junctions in only 30% of the B-to-B-cell interfaces, and at least metabolic coupling is spatially restricted to small groups of B-cells in both intact islets of Langerhans and monolayer cultures *(44)*. Hence, the 10–3000 B-cells that comprise a pancreatic islet may form a assemblies of multiple communication territories rather than a single syncytial unit.

Junctional Coupling and Insulin Secretion

Several lines of evidence indicate a contribution of B-cell coupling to the control of insulin secretion. First, single B-cells are either totally unresponsive to glucose and other stimuli or show a limited and perturbed secretion, as indicated by increased basal release of insulin, poor responsiveness to secretagogs, decreased protein biosynthesis, decreased basal expression of the insulin gene, and loss of its normal, cAMP-dependent control *(45–49)*. Restoration of B-to-B-cell contacts is paralleled by a rapid secretory improvement, as judged by a decrease in the basal release of insulin and an increased responsiveness to secretagogs, as well as by a larger protein biosynthesis and expression of the insulin gene *(45–49)*. The finding that a drug blocking gap junctions prevents the increase in insulin secretion that normally takes place as single B-cells interact to form pairs *(46,47)*, indicates that coupling may acutely control the recruitment of secreting B-cells as well as their individual level of activity.

Second, sustained stimulation of insulin release increases B-cell coupling in vivo as well as in vitro *(41,50)* owing, at least in some cases, to increased expression of gap junctions and Cx43 *(40,41)*. The almost immediate increase in coupling coefficient which is observed when islets are exposed to concentrations of glucose stimulating insulin release, further suggests that B-cell coupling may also be acutely regulated by changes in the conductance and/or permeability of existing gap junction channels *(42)*.

Third, conditions that inhibit insulin release decrease or abolish B-to-B-cell coupling in vitro *(50)* as well as in vivo *(51)*. In vivo, however, this effect may be overcome whenever inhibition of B-cell secretion results in hyperglycemia *(44,51)*, indicating that the level of circulating glucose and the ability of B-cells to properly recognize the sugar stimulus independently control junctional coupling.

Fourth, the acute pharmacological blockade of gap junction channels markedly alters B-cell function, as indicated by an increased basal insulin release and by a loss of stimulated insulin secretion from both isolated islets of Langerhans and intact pancreas *(49,52)*. These alterations appear specifically related to B-cell uncoupling since they could not be accounted for by consistent changes in the main second messengers that are known to control insulin secretion, they were rapidly and fully reversible after wash out of the uncoupling drugs, and they were not observed with single B-cells *(49,52)*.

Fifth, a number of tumoral and transformed insulin-producing cell lines (RIN, INS1, HIT, AtT20ins, CGT-5, CGT-6) that show abnormal or inexistant glucose sensitivity, do not express connexins and gap junctions and are essentially uncoupled *(39,53)*. This coupling deficiency cannot be simply explained by an in vitro down-regulation of gap junction channels, since primary B-cells in monolayer culture continue to express Cx43, gap junctions, and coupling *(39,53)*. It cannot be ascribed either solely to the proliferating ability of the cell lines, since the glucose-sensitive cells of a rat insulinoma, from which at least two of the communication-deficient clones (RIN and INS1) were derived, still express Cx43, gap junctions, and coupling in vivo *(53)*. Hence, coupling defects appear to be a shared attribute of cell lines showing abnormal sensitivity to glucose, whatever is their expression of several key factors (GLUT-2, glucokinase, hexokinase, and so on) that rate-limit the entry and early metabolic response to the sugar. Preliminary observations on INS cells that had been stably transfected with the gene coding for

Cx43, support this coupling–glucose responsiveness relationship. Indeed, as compared to wild type noncommunicating INS cells, a number of Cx43-transfected INS clones show a junctional coupling analogous to that of primary B-cells, and display a normal dose-response curve to glucose, and a marked increase in insulin content and in the expression of the insulin gene *(53)*.

Results of Junctional Coupling

The observations summarized above provide compelling evidence that the junctional communications and the secretory functioning of B-cells are tightly linked, and that this link is implicated in the moment-to-moment regulation of insulin release as well as in the more long-term control of the expression of the insulin gene. These observations also suggest that defective coupling may participate in the loss of B-cell responsiveness to secretagogs. However, the molecular mechanism underlying this link remains speculative, as is the reason why gap junctional communications are required, if not obligatory, for proper B-cell functioning.

As compared to other forms of cell-to-cell communications, the coupling mediated by gap junctions is unique in providing a direct mechanism to equilibrate ionic and molecular electrochemical gradients between nearby cells *(1)*. In such a system, the increase of cytoplasmic ions or molecules less than 900 Daltons into one cell is followed by its diffusion-driven passage into nearby cells. At steady state, this passage leads to the equilibration of electrochemical concentrations on the two sides of the channels. If the resulting concentration reaches a threshold level for activation of an effector mechanism, functioning will be modified not only in the one cell in which the ionic and molecular change first occurred, but also in all other cells coupled to it. In this way, junctional coupling may ensure the functional recruitment of cells that could not be directly activated *(1,53)*. Such a recruiting role of coupling has been experimentally verified in B-cell populations *(46,47)*. Furthermore, since the amounts of insulin secreted by individual B-cells are larger when these cells share gap junctions than when they are single *(46,47)*, the coupling-induced equilibration should also optimize the concentration of factors critical for insulin secretion. This view is consistent with the observation that the threshold level for activation of insulin secretion and biosynthesis is lowered under conditions promoting B-cell coupling *(54)*. Eventually, coupling would be expected to synchronize changes of factors exchanged through gap junctions. This expectation has also been verified for B-cells *(55,56)*.

This model implies that junctional coupling may be particularly advantageous in systems comprising functionally different cells *(53)*. Increasing evidence shows that individual B-cells indeed feature substantial heterogeneity in their ability to release secretory products, as revealed by the coexistence of actively secreting and nonsecreting B-cells, that are otherwise indistinguishable by their viability, their insulin content and their electrophysiological characteristics *(46,47,57)*. B-cells have also been shown to be heterogeneous in their ability to biosynthesize proteins, including insulin, and in their early metabolic response to glucose *(47,58,59)*. Conceivably, these disparities may result in the asynchronous function of individual cells. By equilibrating ionic and molecular gradients, junctional coupling could balance and coordinate these disparities and, thus, permit intrinsically different cells to function simultaneously and at the same rate.

The identification of an intrinsic heterogeneity of B-cells provides a first clue to conceptualize why and how junctional coupling could modulate insulin secretion. What is not determined is the molecular mechanism underlying this modulation. A first possibility is that coupling may enhance the secretagog-induced changes in free intracellular Ca^{2+}. The levels and oscillations of this cation, which plays a critical role in the control of insulin secretion, are differentially affected by the establishment of B-to-B-cell contacts *(55,56)*. Coupling may also regulate the electrophysiological characteristics of B-cells. It has been observed that resting membrane potentials and individual conductances become larger and more stable after establishment of cell-to-cell contacts, presumably because individual B-cells are equipped with so limited numbers of K^+ and Ca^{2+} channels that they cannot ensure stable ionic fluxes as channels fluctuate between the open and close state *(60)*. By mediating a non selective intercellular exchange of current-carrying ions, junctional coupling results in the functional sharing of ionic channels by several cells, thus ensuring that the number of opened channels be always sufficient *(60)*. This change may markedly promote the responsiveness of B-cells, since the activation of the distal, effector steps of their secretory machinery depends on proper control of membrane potentials and ionic fluxes. Third, coupling could ensure the spreading across large cell populations of signals controlling secretion. Secretagog-induced Ca^{2+} waves, indicating a temporally and spatially coordinated change in the levels of this ion across multiple cells, have been observed throughout intact islets of Langerhans *(55)*. These waves, which may result from the intercellular passage of Ca^{2+} or IP_3 via gap junctions, could mediate the rapid recruitment of secreting cells at distance from the site of signaling. In other systems, cells devoid of specific receptors have been shown to be nevertheless activated after establishment of junctional coupling with cells recognizing the cognate signal, probably as a result of a gap junction-mediated intercellular exchange of second messengers *(61)*. An analogous mechanism, resulting in the intercellular diffusion of Ca^{2+} *(55,56)* or cAMP *(43)*, may similarly ensure the rapid recruitment of "nonsecreting" B-cells *(46,47,57)*, some of which may be equipped with insufficient amounts of factors (GLUT-2, glucokinase, ATP-sensitive K^+ channels, and so on) that rate limit insulin secretion. By sharing gap junctions with nearby cells equipped with these essential molecules, the defective cells may be adequately activated to secrete, even though they may be unable to directly recognize stimuli.

Implications for Diabetes

The existence of direct communication between B-cells, and the major influences these communications may have on insulin secretion and biosynthesis, imply that alterations in gap junctional coupling may cause secretory defects that could play significant roles in the early pathogenesis of pancreatic diseases. This possibility is supported by the observation that the absence and blockade of B-cell gap junctions are associated with increased basal insulin release and loss of responsiveness to glucose *(45–49,52)*, two secretory defects which characterize type II diabetes. Also, several lines of insulin-producing cells that cannot be stimulated by glucose, do not express detectable connexins, gap junctions, and coupling *(39,53)*, and glibenclamide, a sulfonylurea which improves insulin secretion in diabetics, improves the expression of Cx43, gap junctions and coupling between B-cells *(40,41,44)*. It is therefore possible that B-cell connexins and coupling may be defective in type II diabetes and may contribute to the initial, and still obscure, derangements of intercellular signaling that start the process of this chronic disease.

Relevance of the B-Cell Data for Other Endocrine Cells

At variance with most other cell types that express multiple types of connexins, pancreatic B-cells, as well as the other endocrine islet cell types, express only Cx43 *(39)*, a protein that is not expressed by the nearby acinar cells of the exocrine pancreas *(38–40)*. Conversely, acinar cells express two connexins (Cx26 and Cx32) which are not found in pancreatic islets *(38–40)*. Conceivably, this distinct connexin pattern could account for the numerous differences in the electrical conductance, permeability to molecules, gating mechanisms and regulation by second messengers of B- and acinar cell gap junctions *(6,7)*. Still, the reason why B- and acinar cells have selected different types of gap junctions is unclear.

Screening of a variety of glands for connexins and their coding transcripts has revealed that endocrine cells always express Cx43 and usually no Cx32, as insulin-producing B-cells, whereas exocrine cells always express Cx32 and usually no Cx43, as pancreatic acinar cells *(38)*. This alternative connexin distribution was observed in glands derived from the three germ layers, and irrespective both of the spatial arrangement and the metabolic differentiation of their secretory cells, suggesting that the expression of gap junction proteins may be differentially regulated depending on whether a secretory cell becomes part of an endocrine or of an exocrine gland *(38)*. In this perspective, it is intriguing that the segregation of endocrine and exocrine cells into distinct glands occurred in the early vertebrates, at about the same time that a gene duplication permitted the divergence of Cx43, and other connexins of group β, from Cx26 and Cx32, and other connexins of group α *(2–4)*.

Perspectives

We are now entering the third decade since the first identification of gap junctions and the discovery that adjacent cells that share these structures directly exchange current-carrying ions and small cytoplasmic molecules. In this time period, a lot has been learned about the structure of gap junctions, their membrane topography, their tissue distribution, the characteristics of their constitutive connexin proteins, the biophysical characteristics of their channels and their regulation in a variety of systems, and the molecular characterization of the encoding genes has begun. It is now clear that gap junctions, and the direct cell-to-cell communications they mediate, are obligatory features of virtually every cell type, throughout the phylogenetic scale. Furthermore, we have begun to appreciate the numerous variations in gap junction composition, structure, and regulation that have developed with evolution, cell differentiation, and tissue morphogenesis. Analysis of genomic sequences and of relevant transcription factors now provides a lead for further investigation of this unexpected diversity and of the mechanisms that ensure the control of the differential expression of distinct connexins. In parallel, further biochemical and biophysical studies on gap junction channels should contribute to a better understanding of the reasons for the multiplicity of connexins and of their evolution changes. Comparison of different connexins should also guide the preparation of mutant gap junction proteins that will be essential tools to explore structure–function relationships and to clarify how molecules pass through gap junctions, how these structures are formed, and how they are gated.

As yet, a major unresolved question in the field is, what is (are) the physiological function(s) of gap junctions. It is now accepted that gap junctional communications play a regulatory role in the electrical and mechanical coupling of different types of muscle cells, in the control of cell growth and differentiation in developing systems and in the regulation of adult gland secretion *(1–4,36)*. However, even in these cases, a definitive demonstration that such roles are specifically and obligatorily fulfilled by gap junctions has not yet been provided, particularly under conditions of physiological relevance, i.e., within intact tissues and organs in vivo. Also, quite limited evidence is presently available to understand why gap junctional communications are required for such functions. The study of secretory cells, and in particular of pancreatic B-cells, has been instructive in this respect, and, we believe, still offers a number of unique advantages for addressing these central questions.

Insulin secretion from pancreatic islets is the result of the activity of multiple and functionally heterogeneous B-cells, whose integration obligatorily depends on proper intercommunications. As the mechanisms for such communications are unraveled, it becomes evident that full control of B-cell function cannot be ascribed to a sole regulatory mechanism at the expense or exclusion of the others, but rather to the interaction between multiple mechanisms that involve cell-to-cell signaling by nutrients, intrinsic and extrinsic neural inputs, local and circulating hormones, and direct interactions between adjacent cells. In this context, our work has revealed that gap junctional communications play a significant role under conditions abolishing other forms of cell-to-cell communications, indicating a fundamental, hitherto disregarded, implication of cell-to-cell coupling. In view of the functional heterogeneity of B-cells, it is probable that this mechanism has become an obligatory feature in the evolution of pancreas, and of other glands, since it provides the most direct way to compensate intrinsic metabolic and effector differences of secretory cells. At this time, however, the molecular mechanism underlying the relationship between the control of B-cell coupling and of insulin secretion remains to be unraveled, and our understanding of whether such a relationship is causal remains, at best, quite limited. Would future experiments ascertain a direct involvement of B-cell coupling in the control of insulin secretion, it would also be necessary to assess whether and how coupling defects participate in the early, and still obscure, pathogenesis of pancreatic dysfunctions of major relevance to human medicine, and in particular in type II diabetes.

Direct experimental testing of some of these crucial questions is now conceivable, because of the recent availability of novel cell and molecular biology methodologies and systems that should permit us to specifically interfere with the building and functioning of gap junction channels as well as with selected steps of secretory machineries, in vitro as well as in vivo.

Acknowledgments

This chapter was supported by grants from the Swiss National Science Foundation (32-34090.92), the Sir Jules Thorn Charitable Overseas Trust, the Juvenile Diabetes Foundation International (192467), and the commission of the European communities (SC1*-CT92-0833).

References

1. Loewenstein WR: Junctional intercellular communication. The cell-to-cell membrane channel. *Physiol Rev* 61:829–913, 1981.
2. Bennett MVL, Barrio LC, Bargiello TA, Spray DC, Hertzberg E, Saez JC: Gap junctions: New tools, new answers, new questions. *Neuron* 6:305–320, 1991.
3. Kumar NM, Gilula NB: Molecular biology and genetics of gap junction channels. *Sem Cell Biol* 3:3–16, 1992.
4. Beyer EC: Gap junctions. *Int Rev Cytol* 137C:1–37, 1993.
5. Orci L, Unger RH, Renold AE: Structural coupling between pancreatic islet cells. *Experientia* 29:1015–1018, 1973.
6. Meda P, Bosco D, Giordano E, Chanson M: Junctional coupling modulation by secretagogues in two-cell pancreatic systems. In *Biophysics of Gap Junction Channels*, Peracchia C, ed. CRC, Boca Raton, FL, pp. 191–208, 1991.
7. Meda P: Gap junctional coupling and secretion in endocrine and exocrine pancreas. In *Cell Interactions and Gap Junctions*, Sperelakis N, Cole WC, eds. CRC, Boca Raton, FL, pp. 59–83, 1989.
8. Revel J-P, Karnovsky MJ: Hexagonal array of subunits in intercellular junctions of the mouse heart and liver. *J Cell Biol* 33:C7–C12, 1967.
9. Bullivant S: Freeze-fracturing of biological materials. *Micron* 1:46–51, 1969.
10. Makowski L, Caspar DL, Phillips WC, Goodenough DA: Gap junction structures. II. Analysis of the x-ray diffraction data. *J Cell Biol* 74:629–645, 1977.
11. Goodenough DA, Paul DL, Jesaitis L: Topological distribution of two connexin32 antigenic sites in intact and split rodent hepatocyte gap junctions. *J Cell Biol* 107:1817–1824, 1988.
12. Unwin PNT, Ennis PD: Two configurations of a channel-forming membrane protein. *Nature (London)* 307:609–613, 1984.
13. Beyer EC, Paul DL, Goodenough DA: Connexin family of gap junction proteins. *J Membr Biol* 116:187–194, 1990.
14. Willecke K, Hennemann H, Dahl E, Jungbluth S, Heynkes R: The diversity of connexin genes encoding gap junctional proteins. *Eur J Cell Biol* 56:1–7, 1991.
15. Werner R, Miller T, Azarnia R, Dahl G: Translation and functional expression of cell-cell channel mRNA in *Xenopus* oocytes. *J Membr Biol* 87:253–268, 1985.
16. Bruzzone R, Haefliger J-A, Gimlich RL, Paul DL: Connexin40, a component of gap junctions in vascular endothelium, is restricted in its ability to interact with other connexins. *Mol Biol Cell* 4:7–20, 1993.
17. Schwarzmann G, Wiegandt H, Rose B, Zimmerman A, Ben Haim D, Loewenstein WR: Diameter of the cell-to-cell junctional membrane channels as probed with neutral molecules. *Science* 213:551–553, 1981.
18. Zimmer DB, Green CR, Evans WH, Gilula NB: Topological analysis of the major protein in isolated intact rat liver gap junctions and gap junction-derived single-membrane structures. *J Biol Chem* 262:7751–7763, 1987.

19. Kumar NM, Gilula NB: Cloning and characterization of human and rat liver cDNAs coding for a gap junction protein. *J Cell Biol* 103:767–776, 1986.
20. Paul D: Molecular cloning of cDNA for rat liver gap junction protein. *J Cell Biol* 103:123–134, 1986.
21. Beyer EC, Paul DL, Goodenough DA: Connexin 43: A protein from rat heart homologous to a gap junction protein from liver. *J Cell Biol* 105:2621–2629, 1987.
22. Zhang J-T, Nicholson BJ: Sequence and tissue distribution of a second protein of hepatic gap junctions, Cx 26, as deduced from its cDNA. *J Cell Biol* 109:3391–3401, 1989.
23. Dupont E, El Aoumari A, Briand JP, Fromaget C, Gros D: Cross linking of cardiac gap junction connexons by thiol/disulfide exchanges. *J Membr Biol* 108:247–252, 1989.
24. Sáez JC, Spray DC, Nairn AC, Hertzberg EL, Greengard P, Bennett MVL: cAMP increases junctional conductance and stimulates phosphorylation of the 27-kDa principal gap junction polypeptide. *Proc Natl Acad Sci USA* 83:2473–2477, 1986.
25. Musil LS, Beyer EC, Goodenough DA: Expression of the gap junction protein connexin 43 in embryonic chick lens: molecular cloning, ultrastructural localization, and post-translational phosphorylation. *J Membr Biol* 116:163–175, 1990.
26. Gimlich RL, Kumar NM, Gilula NB: Sequence and developmental expression of mRNA coding for a gap junction protein in *Xenopus*. *J Cell Biol* 107:1065–1073, 1988.
27. Crow DS, Beyer EC, Paul DL, Kobe SS, Lau AF: Phosphorylation of connexin43 gap junction protein in uninfected and Rous sarcoma virus-transformed mammalian fibroblasts. *Mol Cell Biol* 10:1754–1763, 1990.
28. Miller T, Dahl G, Werner R: Structure of a gap junction gene: rat connexin 32. *Biosci Rep* 8:455–464, 1988.
29. Fishman GI, Eddy RL, Shows TB, Rosenthal L, Leinwand LA: The human connexin gene family of gap junction proteins: distinct chromosomal locations but similar structure. *Genomics* 10:250–256, 1991.
30. Hennemann H, Kozjek G, Dahl E, Nicholson B, Willecke K: Molecular cloning of mouse connexins26 and -32: similar genomic organization but distinct promoter sequences of two gap junction genes. *Eur J Cell Biol* 58:81–89, 1992.
31. Hsieh C-L, Kumar NM, Gilula NB, Francke U: Distribution of genes for gap junction membrane channel proteins on human and mouse chromosomes. *Somatic Cell Mol Genet* 17:191–200, 1991.
32. Hooper ML, Subak-Sharpe JH: Metabolic co-operation between cells. *Int Rev Cytol* 69:46–104, 1981.
33. Kohen E, Kohen C, Thorell B, Mintz DH, Rabinovitch A: Intercellular communication in pancreatic islet monolayer cultures: a microfluorometric study. *Science* 204:862–865, 1979.
34. Stewart WW: Functional connections between cells as revealed by dye-coupling with a highly fluorescent naphthalimide tracer. *Cell* 14:741–759, 1978.

35. Vaney DI: Many diverse types of retinal neurons show tracer coupling when injected with biocytin or Neurobiotin. *Neurosc Let* 125:187–190, 1991.
36. Meda P, Spray DC: Gap junction function. In *Adv Mol Cell Biol*, in press.
37. Meda P, Perrelet A, Orci L: Gap junctions and cell-to-cell coupling in endocrine glands. *Mod Cell Biol* 3:131–196, 1984.
38. Meda P, Pepper M, Traub O, Willecke K, Gros D, Beyer E, Nicholson B, Paul D, Orci L: Differential expression of gap junction connexins in endocrine and exocrine glands. *Endocrinology* 133:2371–2378, 1993.
39. Ullrich S, Vozzi C, Meda P: Connexins of insulin-secreting cells: Quantification of mRNA by polymerase chain reaction. *Diabetologia* 36(Suppl 1):A5, 1993.
40. Meda P, Chanson M, Pepper M, Giordano E, Bosco D, Traub O, Willecke K, El Aoumari A, Gros D, Beyer E, Orci L, Spray DC: In vivo modulation of connexin 43 gene expression and junctional coupling of pancreatic B-cells. *Exp Cell Res* 192:469–480, 1991.
41. Meda P, Perrelet A, Orci L: Increase of gap junctions between pancreatic B-cells during stimulation of insulin secretion. *J Cell Biol* 82:441–448, 1979.
42. Eddlestone GT, Gonçalves A, Bangham JA, Rojas E: Electrical coupling between cells in islets of Langerhans from mouse. *J Membr Biol* 77:1–14, 1984.
43. Meda P, Amherdt M, Perrelet A, Orci L: Metabolic coupling between cultured pancreatic B-cells. *Exp Cell Res* 133:421–430, 1981.
44. Meda P, Michaels RL, Halban PA, Orci L, Sheridan JD: In vivo modulation of gap junctions and dye coupling between B-cells of the intact pancreatic islet. *Diabetes* 32:858–868, 1983.
45. Lernmark A: The preparation of, and studies on, free cell suspensions from mouse pancreatic islets. *Diabetologia* 10:431–438, 1974.
46. Salomon D, Meda P: Heterogeneity and contact-dependent regulation of hormone secretion by individual B cells. *Exp Cell Res* 162:507–520, 1986.
47. Bosco D, Meda P; Actively synthetizing B-cells secrete preferentially during glucose stimulation. *Endocrinology* 129:3157–3166, 1992.
48. Philippe J, Giordano E, Gjinovci A, Meda P: cAMP prevents the glucocorticoid-mediated inhibition of insulin gene expression in rodent islet cells. *J Clin Invest* 90:2228–2233, 1992.
49. Meda P, Bosco D, Chanson M, Giordano E, Vallar L, Wollheim C, Orci L: Rapid and reversible secretion changes during uncoupling of rat insulin-producing cells. *J Clin Invest* 86:759–768, 1990.
50. Kohen E, Kohen C, Rabinovitch A: Cell-to-cell communication in rat pancreatic islet monolayer cultures is modulated by agents affecting islet cell secretory activity. *Diabetes* 32:95–98, 1983.
51. Appel MC, O'Neill, JJ, Meda P: Effects of glucose on islet gap junctional communication. *Diabetes* 37(suppl 1)47A, 1988.
52. Bruzzone R, Meda P: The gap junction: a channel for multiple functions? *Eur J Clin Invest* 18:444–453, 1988.

53. Vozzi C, Ullrich S, Bosco D, Dupont E, Meda P: Glucose-unresponsive insulin-producing cells show defects in gap junction coupling and improved secretion after Cx43 transfection. *Acta Anat*, in press.
54. Sorenson RL, Parsons JA: Insulin secretion in mammosomatotropic tumor-bearing and pregnant rats. A role for lactogens. *Diabetes* 34:338–341, 1985.
55. Santos RM, Rosario LM, Ndala A, Garcia-Sancho J, Soria B, Valdeomillos M: Widespread synchronous $[Ca^{2+}]_i$ oscillations due to bursting electrical activity in single pancreatic islets. *Pflugers Arch* 418:417–422, 1991.
56. Gylfe E, Grapengiesser E, Hellman B: Propagation of cytoplasmic Ca^{2+} oscillations in clusters of pancreatic β-cells exposed to glucose. *Cell Calcium* 12:229–240, 1991.
57. Soria B, Chanson M, Giordano E, Bosco D, Meda P: Ion channels of glucose-responsive and -unresponsive B-cells. *Diabetes* 40:1069–1078, 1991
58. Schuit FC, In't Veld PA, Pipeleers DG: Glucose stimulates proinsulin biosynthesis by a dose-dependent recruitment of pancreatic beta cells. *Proc Natl Acad Sci USA* 85:3865–3869, 1988.
59. Kiekens R, In't Veld P, Mahler T, Schuit F, Van De Winkel M, Pipeleers D: Differences in glucose recognition by individual rat pancreatic B cells are associated with intercellular differencesin glucose-induced biosynthetic activity. *J Clin Invest* 89:117–125, 1992.
60. Atwater I, Rosario L, Rojas E: Properties of the Ca-activated K^+ channel in pancreatic B-cells. *Cell calcium* 4:451–461, 1983.
61. Lawrence TS, Beers WH, Gilula NB: Transmission of hormonal stimulation by cell-to-cell communication. *Nature* 272:501–506, 1978.

Chapter 15

The Gluco-Incretin Hormone Glucagon-Like Peptide-1 and Its β-Cell Receptor

Bernard Thorens

Introduction

Glucose-induced insulin secretion can be stimulated or inhibited by a number of hormones or neurotransmitters. In particular, gut hormones have been suggested to have profound effects on the β-cells secretory activity. Indeed, it has been known for a long time that oral glucose ingestion induced a considerably greater elevation in plasma insulin levels compared to an intravenous glucose injection producing the same glycemia *(1–3)* and the existence of an "entero-insular axis," which refers to the action of these putative intestinal hormones on the the endocrine pancreas, has been suggested *(3)*. A number of peptides have been purified from intestinal extracts such as secretin, cholecystokinin (CCK), gastrin, gastrin releasing peptide, vasoactive intestinal polypeptide (VIP), or enteroglucagon *(1–3)*, which were able to stimulate insulin secretion in the presence of normal or slightly elevated glucose concentrations. The "insulinotropic" or "gluco-incretin" activity of these peptides was, however, weak even at high pharmacological concentrations. Today, two principal gluco-incretins have been characterized: Gastric inhibitory

From: *Molecular Biology of Diabetes, Part I*
Edited by: B. Draznin and D. LeRoith

peptide (GIP), also referred to as glucose-dependent insulinotropic polypeptide, and truncated forms of glucagon-like peptide 1, GLP-1(7-37) or GLP-1(7-36)amide.

GIP is a 42 amino acid long peptide produced by K-cells from the duodenum and the upper jejunum and is secreted both in response to oral absorption of glucose or fatty acids *(2,4)*. It has an insulinotropic action at physiological concentrations and its effect on insulin secretion requires the presence of glucose at concentrations slightly above the normal value of about 5 m*M*. GIP apparently also stimulates glucagon secretion. Experiments by Creutzfeld and his collaborators have demonstrated that immunodepletion of GIP from gut extracts removed only about 50% of the gluco-incretin potency of these extracts. This strongly suggested the presence of additional incretin hormone(s) in the gut *(5)*. The recent characterization of GLP-1, a product of the preproglucagon gene secreted by intestinal endocrine cells, together with the demonstration of its strong potentiation effect on insulin secretion has established this peptide as a major new gluco-incretin.

Glucagon-Like Peptide-1

The structure of the preproglucagon molecule was established by molecular cloning of its cDNA from a hamster islet cDNA library *(6)* and the structure of the glucagon gene *(7)* was determined from analysis of human genomic DNA clones. Analysis of the preproglucagon molecule (Fig. 1) revealed, in addition to glucagon itself, the presence of peptides of related sequence, referred to as glucagon-like peptides. Preproglucagon is 180 amino acids long. The first 20 amino acids form the leader sequence. The glucagon sequence is present at position 33-61 of proglucagon. The two glucagon-like peptides (GLP-1 and GLP-2) are located at position 72-108 and 126-158. These internal peptides are separated by dibasic amino acid residues that are potential sites for cleavage by proteolytic enzymes involved in the maturation of peptidic hormones *(8)*.

Analysis of the proglucagon-derived products in the pancreas and the intestine revealed a strikingly different pattern of proteolytic processing. In pancreatic α-cells, the major preproglucagon-derived products are glucagon (corresponding to preproglucagon 33-61), glicentin related pancreatic polypeptide (GRPP, proglucagon 1-69),

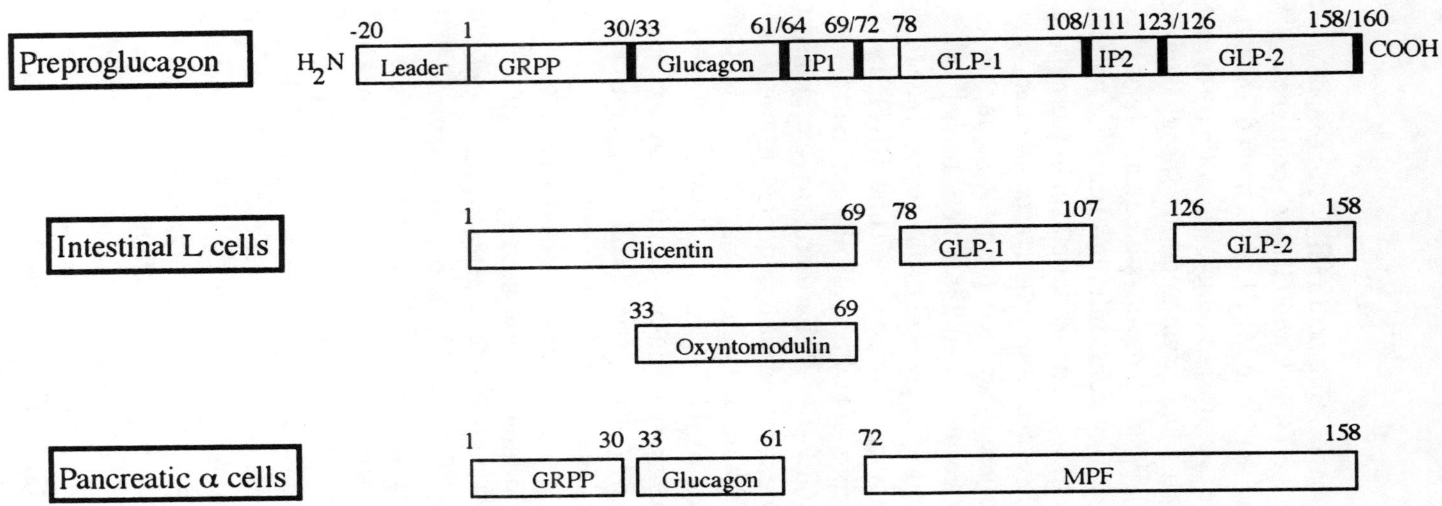

Fig. 1. Schematic representation of the preproglucagon molecule and of its major proteolytic fragments produced in intestinal L-cells and in pancreatic α-cells. Sequence from position 1 to 160: proglucagon. Heavy vertical bars: site of dibasic amino acid residues where proteolytic processing of proglucagon takes place. At position 77, a single arginine residue is the recognition signal for proteolytic cleavage of GLP-1 in the active form GLP-1(7-36)amide. GRPP: glicentin related polypeptide, IP1 and IP2: intervening peptide 1 and 2, GLP-1 and GLP-2: glucagon-like peptide 1 and 2, MPF: major proglucagon fragment. Reprinted from ref. *81* with permission from ADA.

and the major proglucagon fragment (MPF, proglucagon 72-158), which contains both the GLP-1 and GLP-2 sequences *(9,10)*. No physiological role for GRPP and MPF has yet been demonstrated. In intestine, major peptides corresponding to glicentin (proglucagon 1-69, or "enteroglucagon") and oxyntomodulin (proglucagon 33-69) were detected *(10,11)*. Whereas the physiological role of glicentin is not clearly established, oxyntomodulin has been shown to have an inhibitory effect on acid secretion by parietal cells from the stomach *(12)* and also to stimulate insulin secretion by pancreatic β-cells *(13)*. These effects are observed at elevated, probably supraphysiological, concentrations of this hormone and it is not clear whether a specific oxyntomodulin receptor is expressed in any tissue. Indeed, binding of oxyntomodulin to a somatostatinoma cell line (RINT3) was shown to be to the GLP-1 receptor but with an affinity constant one hundred-fold higher than for GLP-1 *(14)*. Furthermore, the cloned GLP-1 receptor *(see below)* expressed in transfected fibroblasts, bound oxyntomodulin with pharmacological characteristics identical to binding of this peptide to RINT3 cells. Therefore, the previously ascribed effects of oxyntomodulin on insulin secretion and hydrochloric acid secretion by gastric parietal cells may have been owing to binding of this peptide to the GLP-1 receptor.

Two additional peptides characterized as products of proglucagon processing in intestine, but not in pancreas, were GLP-1 and GLP-2 *(9)* (Fig. 1). GLP-1 was detected in several different molecular forms. GLP-1(72-108) and two truncated forms of this last peptide: GLP-1(79-108) and GLP-1(78-107)amide. These truncated forms of GLP-1 are produced by proteolytic cleavage of GLP-1(72-108) at a single arginine present at position 77. The presence of a glycine residue (position 108) followed by an arginine (position 109) is often used as an amidation signal. Indeed, purification of truncated GLP-1 from pig and human intestine and structural analysis revealed that the amidated form of the peptide represented 66% of the naturally occurring peptides, whereas the nonamidated form accounted for 33% of the truncated GLP-1 *(15,16)*. The only biologically active forms of the glucagon-like peptides are the truncated forms of GLP-1, GLP-1(78-108) or GLP-1(78-107)amide. These forms are very often referred to in the literature as GLP-1(7-37) or GLP-1(7-36)amide, using a numbering relative to the GLP-1 molecule. For the sake of simplicity we will use in the rest of the text the term GLP-1 to refer to GLP-1(7-36), amide which is the predominant active form of the peptide.

Morphological analysis of GLP-1-containing cells in the gastrointestinal tract showed that immunoreactivity was present in endocrine cells present in the distal jejunum, the colon, and the rectum of human, pig, and rat *(17)*, and that the same cells were positive for glicentin, GLP-1, and GLP-2 *(9)*.

Biological Actions of GLP-1

Pancreatic Actions

The stimulatory action of GLP-1 on glucose-induced insulin secretion was first demonstrated in the perfused rat pancreas system *(18,19)*. In these experiments, GLP-1(7-37) or GLP-1(7-36)amide were shown to have identical effects on the β-cell secretory response. The stimulation of insulin secretion was detected at concentrations of peptide as low as 1–10 p*M* *(20)*. The stimulatory effect of these peptides was shown to be glucose-dependent. No insulin secretion could be elicited by GLP-1 with 2.8 m*M* glucose in the perfusate. However, with 6.6 m*M* glucose in the perfusate, a strong potentiation of insulin secretion was induced by GLP-1. A similar glucose dependency has also been described for GIP action *(1,2)*. A further characteristic of the action of these hormones is their priming effect on β-cell response to glucose, as shown in studies by Fehman et al. *(21)*. These authors first perfused pancreas with GLP-1 (or GIP) at concentrations within the normal physiological range (10–1000 p*M*) and in the presence of substimulatory glucose concentrations (2.8 m*M*). Following a 10-min washout period they could show that the response to a high glucose challenge was markedly stimulated by the preexposure to the gluco-incretins. Interestingly, the first phase of secretion was much more sensitive to the priming effect than the second phase.

A gluco-incretin effect of GLP-1 in humans has also been demonstrated. Increase in circulating insulin levels and inhibition of glucagon secretion have been observed in the fasted state as a result of GLP-1 infusion. The insulin secretory effect was further enhanced following an intravenous glucose infusion *(22)*. In the same set of experiments, the efficiency of GIP as an incretin was shown to be less than that of GLP-1. In humans, as in rat, the amidated and nonamidated forms of GLP-1 have indistiguishable effects on stimulation of insulin secretion, decrease in glucagon release, and on lowering of blood glucose concentrations *(23)*.

In addition to the stimulatory effect on glucose-induced insulin secretion, GLP-1 also stimulates insulin gene transcription. This has been shown to result in the accumulation of insulin in secretory granules, at least as measured on insulinoma cell lines *(24,25)*. Since the GLP-1 receptor is coupled to activation of adenylyl cyclase, transcriptional regulation of the insulin gene may be mediated by cAMP and a cAMP-responsive element binding protein (CREB) *(26)*. These additional effects of GLP-1 provide a means to stimulate the replenishment of insulin stores and prevent exhaustion of the β-cells.

Extrapancreatic Actions

A number of extrapancreatic effects of GLP-1 have been reported. Probably the most clearly established effect is on hydrochloric acid secretion by gastric parietal cells. In in vivo experiments, GLP-1 induces inhibition of acid secretion and a decreased rate of gastric emptying *(27,28)*. It is not yet clear whether the effect on acid secretion is a direct or indirect one. Indeed, in rat isolated parietal cells, GLP-1 has been reported to rather stimulate acid secretion *(29)*. Therefore, the inhibitory effect observed in vivo may result from the stimulation by GLP-1 of somatostatin release from stomach D-cells that, in turn, inhibits the secretory activity of parietal cells *(14)*. Binding sites for GLP-1 have been described on somatostatinoma cell lines *(14)*.

An extrapancreatic effect of GLP-1 on the control of blood glucose levels has been suggested *(30)*. Although the exact mechanism that could account for this blood-lowering effect is not known, GLP-1 binding sites have been characterized in adipocytes *(31)* and the addition of GLP-1 or GIP to explants of rat adipose tissue has been reported to stimulate fatty acid synthesis *(32)*. GLP-1 has also been reported to decrease circulating levels of free fatty acid *(23)*. The molecular nature of this putative adipocytes GLP-1 receptor is not known, nor whether it is related to the cloned β-cell GLP-1 receptor *(see below)*.

GLP-1 binding sites have been detected in lung membranes *(33,34)* and mRNA species for the GLP-1 receptor identical to those present in β-cell have indeed been detected in lung RNA preparations *(35)*. The role of GLP-1 in lung physiology is not yet clearly established. The presence of GLP-1 binding sites in different regions of the brain has also been reported *(36,37)*. The role of this peptide in the brain is not known.

The Glucagon-Like Peptide-1 Receptor

Structure of a β-Cell Receptor

A rat pancreatic islet cDNA clone for the GLP-1 receptor was recently isolated by an expression cloning strategy *(35)*. This technology involves the construction of a cDNA library in a plasmid vector that, when transfected in Cos cells, permits high expression of the cloned receptor at the cell surface *(38)*. Identification of receptor-expressing cells is then performed by binding and crosslinking of the radioiodinated ligand to the receptor. This is followed by exposure of the cells to a photographic emulsion and subsequent screening under the microscope: Cells expressing the receptor are covered by reduced silver grains that appear bright in the darkfield and are easily identified. The initial cloning of a rat receptor allowed the isolation of a cDNA clone for the human pancreatic islet GLP-1 receptor by standard nucleic acid hybridization screening of a human islet cDNA library *(39)*. Characterization of rat and human GLP-1 receptors in transfected Cos cells (35) or Chinese hamster lung fibroblasts *(14,39)* showed that the receptor had a high affinity for GLP-1 (kDa = 0.2–0.6 n*M*), whereas peptides of related structure such as GIP, VIP, or secretin did not bind to the receptor, even at concentrations up to 1μ*M*. Oxyntomodulin and glucagon bound to the receptor but with affinities 100 and >1000 times lower than GLP-1, respectively. Interestingly, two peptides isolated from the venom of the lizard *Heloderma suspectum,* exendin-4 and exendin-(9-39) *(40,41)* bind to the cloned GLP-1 receptor with affinities identical to GLP-1 binding *(39)*. Out of the eight first amino-terminal amino acids of exendin-4 and GLP-1, seven are identical. On the remainder or the peptides, only 9 out of 22 amino acids are identical. The truncated form of exendin, exendin (9-39) therefore lacks the region of high identity with GLP-1. However, it binds to the receptor with the same affinity as GLP-1 but, in contrast to GLP-1 and exendin-4, it is not able to induce cAMP formation. In contrast, it can completely inhibit GLP-

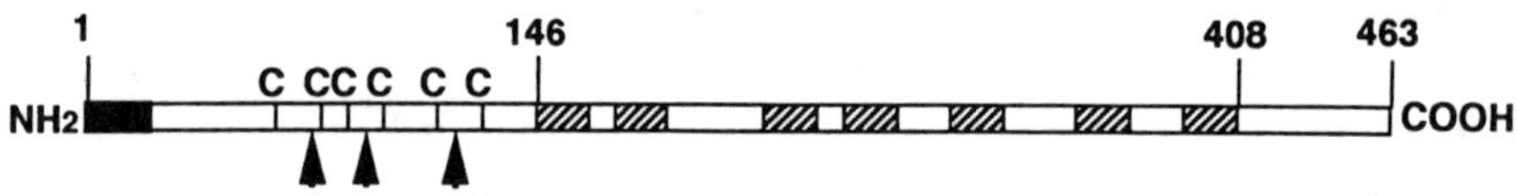

Fig. 2. Schematic representation of the structure of the GLP-1 receptor. The primary amino acid sequence contains eight hydrophobic domains. The amino terminal one (black box) is a leader sequence and the seven other hydrophobic segments (stippled boxes) represent transmembrane domains. C: cysteines residues of the amino-terminal extracellular domain that are conserved in number and location between the members of this new subfamily of G-coupled receptors (*see text* and Fig. 3). Arrowheads indicate *N*-glycosylation sites. Numbers refer to the position in the amino acid sequence.

1-induced cAMP formation. Therefore, although exendin-4 is an agonist, exendin-(9-39) is a perfect antagonist of the receptor *(39)*.

Analysis of the nucleotide sequence of the cloned receptor cDNAs and of the deduced amino acid sequences revealed several important features. Hydropathy analysis indicated that the receptor contained eight hydrophobic segments. The amino-terminal one is most probably a leader sequence, whereas the seven other are putative transmembrane domains (Fig. 2). This receptor thus belongs to the superfamily of receptors coupled to activation of heterotrimeric G-proteins. Interestingly, however, the GLP-1 receptor showed significant sequence similarity only to the receptors for glucagon *(42)* secretin *(43)*, VIP (44), PTH *(45)*, calcitonin *(46)*, and GRF *(47)*, which form a newly described subfamily of G-coupled receptors. Sequence identitiy between these receptor range is from 27 to 49% (Table 1). Interestingly, the receptors most closely related in sequence (Fig. 3), like the receptors for glucagon, GLP-1, secretin, and VIP, bind peptides which are also the most closely related in sequence. From these observations one can predict that receptors for GIP and PACAP (pituitary adenylate cyclase activating peptide) will also be of the same subfamily. The receptors from this newly characterized subfamily share less than 10% sequence identity with the other G-coupled receptors such as the adrenergic, tachikinin, or olfactory receptors. One particular structural feature of these receptors is the

Table 1
Amino Acid Sequence Identity Between the Members of the GLP-1/Glucagon Receptor Family

	rGLUCR	rVIPR	rSECR	rPTHR	rGRFR	pCTR
rGLP1R	49	41	40	32	36	28
rGLUCR		38	39	34	32	31
rVIPR			49	38	43	28
rSECR				42	40	30
rPTHR					36	32
rGRFR						25

presence of a relatively long (~120 amino acids) amino terminal extracellular domain (Fig. 2). The amino acid sequence of this domain is poorly conserved between the different receptors except for six cysteines distributed at identical positions. These cysteines may form intrachain disulfide bonds important for the proper three-dimensional structure of this region.

Signaling by the Receptor

Understanding which intracellular second messengers are activated by GLP-1 binding to its receptor on β-cells is of critical importance for the comprehension of the crosstalk between the GLP-1 and glucose signaling pathways. Studies with insulinoma or somatostatinoma cells expressing the endogenous GLP-1 receptor have shown that the receptor was coupled to activation of adenylate cyclase and production of cAMP *(14,24,48)*. Signal transduction by the cloned GLP-1 receptor has been studied after transient expression in Cos cells or in stably transfected Chinese hamster lung fibroblasts. Binding of GLP-1 induced a dose-dependent accumulation of intracellular cAMP with EC50 of about 0.1–1 n*M*, a value close to the Kd of GLP-1 binding to the receptor *(14,39,48a)*. In insulinomas, transfected fibroblasts and Cos cells no coupling to inositol phosphate production nor mobilization of calcium from intracellular stores could be recorded *(48a)*. However, a recent publication described an increased production of inositol phosphate and a raise in intracellular Ca^{2+} following exposure to GLP-1 of Cos cells transiently transfected with the receptor *(49)*. The reasons for the different observations in receptor-transfected Cos cells is not clear but may represent a cell-

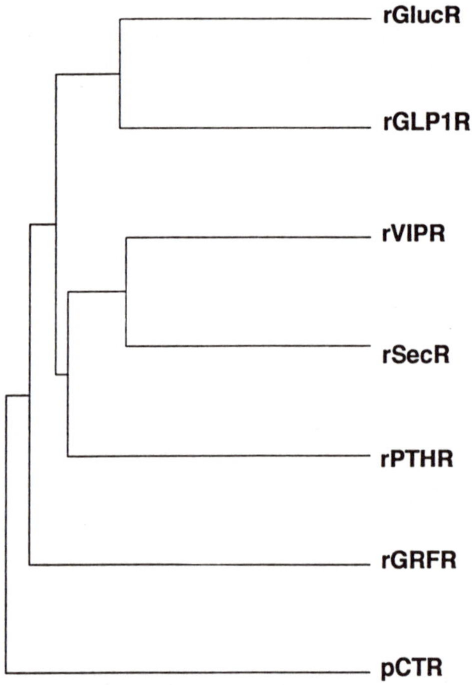

Fig. 3. Dendogram displaying the relative sequence identity between members of this subfamily of G-coupled receptors. rGlucR: rat glucagon receptor, rGLP1R, rat GLP-1 receptor, rVIPR: rat vasointestinal polypeptide receptor, rSecR: rat secretin receptor, rPTHR: rat parathyroid hormone receptor, rGRFR: rat growth hormone releasing factor receptor, pCTR: pig calcitonin receptor. For the extent of identity between receptors, *see* Table 1.

specific coupling of the receptor. However, in insulinomas or β-cells coupling to inositol phosphate production has never been observed in response to GLP-1. Different authors have also suggested that production of cAMP by gluco-incretins was also glucose-dependent. A possible explanation for this observation is that the β-cell adenylate cyclase may be regulated by calcium and calmodulin *(50)*. Increase in intracellular Ca^{2+} concentration consequent to glucose stimulation of β-cells may provide a link between glucose signaling and increased cAMP production. Together, the present evidences indicate that the β-cell GLP-1 receptor is probably only coupled to activation of adenylate cyclase and production of cAMP. The gluco-incretin effect of GLP-1 should therefore be mediated by activation of cAMP-dependent protein kinase (protein kinase A) and the phosphorylation of different proteins involved in glucose-induced insulin secretion.

Intracellular Events Controlled by cAMP

Intracellular events mediated by cAMP may be separated in two main categories:

1. Acute effects, probably mediated by phosphorylation of effector proteins such as those participating in glucose signaling; and
2. Long-term effects, mediated by transcriptional activation of genes such as the insulin gene.

The acute effects can be further classified in two groups: those responsible for the gluco-incretin effect (the stimulation of the secretory response to glucose), and those required to maintain β-cells in a glucose-competent state. Whether these two groups of effects represent different phenomena or merely a gradation in the phosphorylation state of elements of the glucose signaling pathway is not yet known and will require an understanding of the molecular details of the phosphorylation reactions controlled by protein kinase A. Here we are not going to address the transcriptional control of the cAMP-responsive genes, except to mention that stimulation of insulin gene transcription by GLP-1 and cAMP is probably an important action of this hormone, which helps replenish insulin stores. We will now first discuss the glucose competence concept and then the possible sites of interaction between GLP-1 and glucose signaling.

Glucose Competence

The concept of cAMP as a competence factor was first derived from studies on isolated β-cells performed by Pipeleers et al. *(51,52)*. These authors observed that isolated β-cells were poorly responsive to glucose and that this correlated with a low intracellular level of cAMP as compared to cells in intact islets. Elevation of intracellular cAMP by addition either of isobutylmethyl xanthine (IBMX, an inhibitor of phosphodiesterase), glucagon or by reaggregating β-cells with α-cells, enhanced considerably the glucose-dependent secretory response. This strongly supported the hypothesis that cAMP was necessary to allow β-cells to respond to glucose stimulation.

They further suggested that glucagon, secreted within the islet, was responsible for maintaining an adequate cAMP level in β-cells.

The importance of cAMP for the glucose competence state of single beta cells has also been assessed by recording the depolarization of the plasma membrane potential following exposure to glucose and/or GLP-1 *(53)* or by microfluorimetry recordings of intracellular Ca^{2+} in isolated β-cells exposed to 20 m*M* glucose *(54)*. In the work of Holz et al. *(53)*, single β-cells were divided into three subgroups:

1. One composed of cells that could never be made responsive to glucose;
2. A second group in which cells responded well to 10 m*M* glucose; and
3. A group of cells that did not respond to 10 m*M* glucose but could be made responsive by GLP-1.

Since analogs of cAMP could also render this last subgroup of cells responsive to glucose, the effect of GLP-1 was probably through activation of cAMP production. This experiment clearly indicated that a basal level of cAMP and consequently a basal level of phosphorylation was required to allow the cells to respond to glucose. Moreover, in these experiments, GLP-1 could prime the cells to respond to subsequent exposure to glucose, provided that the time interval between the application of the two components was not too long. Inversely, glucose preexposure to glucose rendered β-cells responsive to subsequent exposure to GLP-1. Measurements of intracellular Ca^{2+} in single β-cells following exposure to 20 m*M* glucose also revealed a marked heterogeneity among β-cells *(54)*. As in the previous case, a subpopulation of β-cells were not responsive to glucose but were induced to respond following increase in intracellular cAMP induced by theophylline or glucagon. Together these informations strongly suggest that a basal level of cAMP is important for the glucose-competence state of the β-cells.

In in vivo situtations, which hormone control β-cells cAMP level? Glucagon secretion within the islets may possibly affect β-cells in direct contact to α-cells. However, since the blood flow first reaches β-cells then α-cells and finally δ-cells *(55)* most β-cells are probably not directly influenced by paracrine glucagon secretion *(56)*. Instead, they are probably exposed only to circulating levels of this hormone, whose concentration varies between 10–50 p*M*. At these concentrations, glucagon displays only a very small stimulatory effect on insulin secretion *(20)* and a small or undetectable effect on intracellular cAMP in purified β-cells or intact islets *(52)*. In contrast, circulating levels of GLP-1 or GIP, which may vary between 10–100 p*M* *(57,58)*, are sufficient to markedly stimulate cAMP production and glucose-induced insulin secretion *(20,21,24)*. These hormones may therefore be of crucial importance to maintain the glucose competence of β-cells in the basal state. Why some isolated β-cells are not glucose-responsive while others respond well to this stimulus is not known. A possible reason might be that gluco-incretin receptor expression in β-cells is heterogenous. This could lead to differential production of cAMP and consequently to different transcriptional activation of certain genes required for glucose-sensitivity of individual β-cells.

Crosstalk Between GLP-1 and Glucose Signaling Pathways

The potentiation effect of GLP-1 on glucose-induced insulin secretion implies that production of cAMP and activation of protein kinase A will interfere with the glucose signaling pathway most probably as a result of phosphorylation of proteins involved in the control of insulin secretion. Figure 4 schematically depicts the steps involved in glucose-induced insulin secretion and the possible sites of interaction between the two signaling pathways. Glucose signaling involves the following steps:

1. Glucose uptake into β-cells by the facilitated diffusion glucose transporter GLUT2;
2. Phosphorylation of glucose by glucokinase, glucose catabolism, and production of ATP;
3. Closure of an ATP-dependent K^+ channel, probably as a consequence of a change in the intracellular ATP/ADP ratio; this closure induces depolarization of the plasma membrane;
4. Opening of a voltage-dependent Ca^{2+} channel; and
5. Increase in intracellular Ca^{2+} concentration which leads to exocytosis of insulin granules *(59-61)*.

Direct evidence for the phosphorylation of elements of the glucose signaling pathway are still missing. Indirect evidence has been gathered that shows that increase in cAMP and consequently activation of protein kinase A may regulate the activity of different steps in glucose signaling.

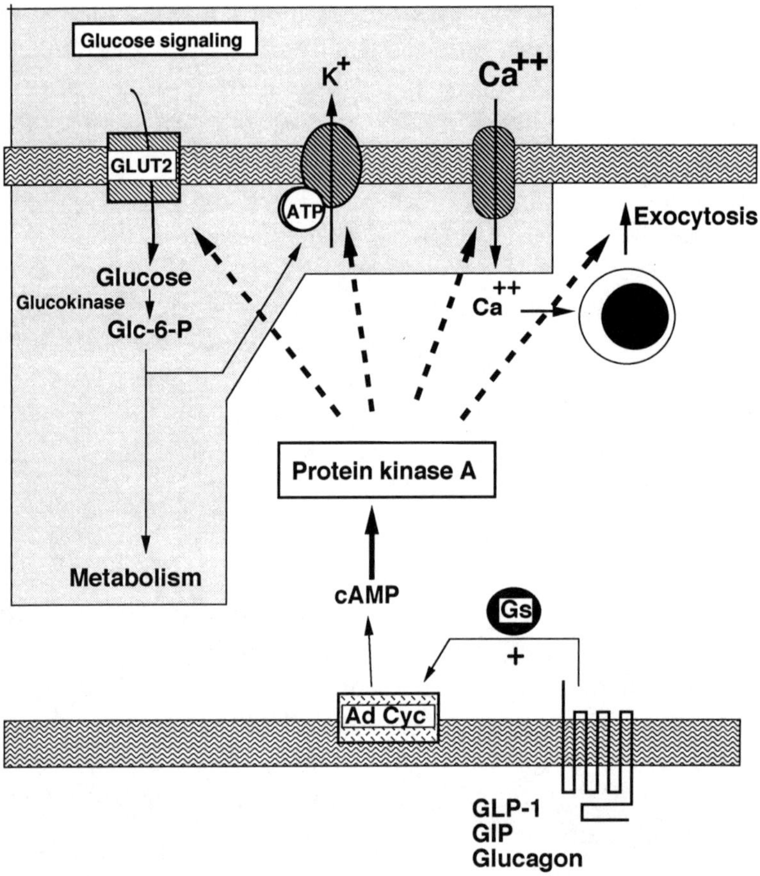

Fig 4. Schematic representation of the possible interactions between glucose and gluco-incretin hormones signaling. Glucose uptake by GLUT2 is followed by its catalytic phosphorylation by glucokinase. ATP or a change in the ATP/ADP ratio consequent to glucose catabolism induces the closure of ATP-dependent K^+ channels. The consequent depolarization of the plasma membrane induces the opening of dihydropyridine-sensitive Ca^{2+} channels. The increase in intracellular Ca^{2+} concentration initiates a cascade of events resulting in insulin secretion. Gluco-incretins binding to their receptors stimulate the production of intracellular cAMP probably by stimulating adenylate cyclase via activation of the α subunit of the heterotrimeric GTP-binding protein Gs. The consequent activation of cAMP-dependent protein kinase (protein kinase A) can modulate by phosphorylation a number of elements of the glucose signaling pathway, as indicated by the broken arrows and discussed in detail in the text. Reprinted from ref. *81* with permission from ADA.

Electrophysiological measurements in the cell-attached patch configuration have demonstrated that closure of the ATP-dependent K^+ channel could be induced by GLP-1 in the subgroup of cells that were responsive to glucose after priming with the gluco-incretin *(53)*. In addition, depolarization in the presence of 10 m*M* glucose but in the absence of GLP-1 could be induced by Sp-cAMPS, an agonist of cAMP. Conversely, the effects on depolarization induced by glucose and GLP-1 were blocked by Rp-cAMPS, an antagonist of cAMP. Thus, GLP-1 priming effect on beta cells may, at least in part, be mediated by a sensitization of the K^+_{ATP} channel resulting from activation of protein kinase A. It is not clear, however, whether the channel itself can be phosphorylated or whether the observed effect on channel activity is indirect. A previous electrophysiological study *(62)* on RINm5F insulinoma cells indeed failed to detect any modulation of this channel activity by increased intracellular cAMP levels or by exposure to the catalytic subunit of protein kinase A in the presence of ATP.

GLP-1, GIP or cAMP analogue have been shown to elevate cytosolic Ca^{2+} in the HIT hamster insulinoma cell line, as measured by the fluorescent indicator Fura-2 *(63–65)*. The elevation in intracellular Ca^{2+} was, however, dependent on the presence of glucose at stimulatory levels and was blocked by depletion of extracellular calcium with EGTA or by the L-type calcium channel blockers nimodipine, verapamil, and nifedipine. In a study already mentioned *(54)*, the calcium response to 20 m*M* glucose of single β-cells was either dependent on prior elevation in cAMP levels by glucagon or theophylline, or if the cells were already responsive to glucose, the response could be further stimulated by these agents. This report did not determine whether Ca^{2+} was coming from intracellular stores or from uptake of extracellular calcium. Together these data suggest that phosphorylation of the Ca^{2+} channel may be a way to control its function and indeed, in mouse β-cells, analogs of cAMP induced a threefold increase in Ca^{2+} channel activity *(66)*. Similarly, in heart, the L-type Ca^{2+} channel has been shown to be modulated by phosphorylation *(67)*.

The importance of cAMP in the control of the exocytic process has been reported by several groups. In digitonin-permeabilized islet cells *(68)* or RINm5F cells *(69)* insulin secretion stimulated by fixed concentrations of Ca^{2+} could be further increased by addition of cAMP. In isolated β-cells exposed to 5 m*M* glucose, potentiation of insulin secretion by cAMP was observed to result mostly from an effect on the exocytic machinery itself rather than on Ca^{2+} uptake by the L-type channels *(62)*. Therefore, activation by GLP-1 or GIP of protein kinase A may stimulate exocytosis of secretory granules. Other potential targets of protein kinase A that could modulate glucose-induced insulin secretion could be the glucose transporter GLUT2 or glucokinase that catalyze the first two steps in glucose signaling: glucose uptake and phosphorylation.

From the results described above it is clear that activation of protein kinase A is mediating the gluco-incretin effect. However, very little is yet known in molecular details about which proteins are phosphorylated, which phosphorylation events are necessary to maintain the glucose competence state of the β-cells, and which are inducing the potentiation effect of GLP-1.

GLP-1 in Noninsulin-Dependent Diabetes Mellitus

The increase in plasma insulin and C-peptide concentrations following oral glucose is considerably greater than the increase following intravenous infusion of glucose producing the same glycemia. This differential effect of oral glucose absorption on insulin secretion, which is due to gluco-incretin secretion from intestine endocrine cells, is markedly reduced in type II diabetic patients *(1,70–72)*. This indicates that beside the well-characterized glucose-unresponsiveness of β-cells *(73–76)*, the gluco-incretin effect is also reduced in diabetic patients. The molecular basis of this reduced effect is not completely understood. However available data indicate that there is no correlation between the reduced gluco-incretin effect and basal or stimulated levels of immunoreactive GIP *(71,72)* or GLP-1 *(57)*. A similar impaired sensitivity of pancreatic β-cells to GIP and GLP-1 has also been demonstrated in an animal model of type II diabetes, the neonatal streptozocin rat *(77)*. This decreased sensitivity to gluco-incretins was not improved by previous insulin treatment.

Altogether these studies suggest that the diminished incretin effect observed in diabetes does not result from impaired GLP-1 or GIP secretion. This implies that signaling by these hormones at the β-cell level may be altered. This could be either because of a decreased expression of their β-cell receptors or because of an inefficient coupling of the receptors to intracellular second messengers. Whether a decreased gluco-incretin effect precedes or follows development of diabetes is not known. It is, however, conceivable that impaired signaling by GIP or GLP-1 receptors may lead to a loss of β-cell glucose competence and/or a diminished potentiation effect that could cause the reduced insulin secretory capability of β-cells from diabetic individuals.

In spite of the reduced insulinotropic effect of GLP-1 in diabetes, infusion of this peptide at pharmacological concentrations, but not of GIP, is able to stimulate postprandial insulin secretion, decrease glucagon release, and increase glucose disposal *(30,78,79)*. These studies therefore led to two conclusions: first, even if the total incretin effect in diabetic patients is reduced, pharmacological doses of GLP-1 can still display an incretin effect. Second, GIP receptor signaling in β-cells from diabetic patients is probably impaired to a greater extent than signaling through GLP-1 receptors. Also, since the effect of GLP-1 is glucose-dependent, it has been suggested that agonists of its receptor may be used as therapeutic agents in NIDDM. Such compounds would indeed not risk inducing hypoglycemia, a complication frequently associated with the currently used sulfonylureas *(80)*.

Conclusions

GLP-1 is a recently described gastrointestinal hormone. Considerable interest in this peptide has arisen mostly because of its very strong potentiation effect on glucose-induced insulin secretion. More recently, the cloning of its β-cell receptor has opened new ways to understand the physiology of this peptide. In particular, coupling of the receptor to activation of adenylate cyclase and production of cAMP could be ascertained by expressing the cloned receptor in different cell lines. The cDNA for this receptor should allow to address a number of questions: whether the receptor is regulated in different conditions of imbalanced glucose homeostasis, in particular in the development of type II diabetes; whether the receptor is heterogenously expressed in different subpopulations of β-cells; how the receptor is desensitized following exposure to GLP-1; and, finally, how GLP-1 signaling interacts with glucose-induced insulin secretion.

Also important, since pharmacological doses of GLP-1 can ameliorate postprandial glucose disposal in diabetic patients, the availability of a human pancreatic islet GLP-1 receptor cDNA will contribute to the characterization of agonists of the receptor that could be used in the treatment of diabetes.

Acknowledgments

This work has been supported by Grants No. 31-30313.90 from the Swiss National Science Foundation and Grant No. 192038 from Juvenile Diabetes Foundation International. BT is the recipient of a Career Development Award from the Swiss National Science Foundation.

References

1. Ebert R, Creutzfeld W: Gastrointestinal peptides and insulin secretion. *Diab Met Rev* 3:1–16, 1987.
2. Dupre J: Influences of the gut on the endocrine pancreas An overview of established and potential physiological mechanisms. In *The Endocrine Pancreas,* Samols E, ed. Raven, New York, pp. 253–281, 1991.
3. Unger RH, Eisentraut AM: Entero-insular axis. *Arch Intern Med* 123:261–266, 1969.
4. Krarup T: Immunoreactive gastric inhibitory polypeptide. *Endocrine Rev* 9:122–134, 1988.
5. Ebert R, Unger H, Creutzfeld W: Preservation of incretin activity after removal of gastric inhibitory polypeptide (GIP) from rat gut extracts by immunoadsorption. *Diabetologia* 24:449–454, 1983.
6. Bell GI, Santerre RF, Mullenbach GT: Hamster preproglucagon contains the sequence of glucagon and two related peptides *Nature* 302:716–718, 1983.
7. Bell GI, Sanchez-Pescador R, Laybourn PJ, Najarian RC: Exon duplication and divergence in the human preproglucagon gene. *Nature* 304:368–371, 1983.
8. Steiner DF, Smeekens SP, Ohagi S, Chan SJ: The new enzymology of precursor processing endoproteases. *J Biol Chem* 267:23,435–23,438, 1992.
9. Mojsov S, Heinrich G, Wilson IB, Ravazzola M, Orci L: Preproglucagon gene expression in pancreas and intestine diversifies at the level of post-translational processing. *J Biol Chem* 261:11,880–11,889, 1986.
10. Ørskov C: Glucagon-like peptide-1 a new hormone of the entero-insular axis *Diabetologia* 35:701–711, 1992.
11. Habener JF, Drucker DJ, Mojsov S, Knepel W, Philippe J: Biosynthesis of glucagon. In *The Endocrine Pancreas,* Samols E, ed. Raven, New York, pp. 53–71, 1991.
12. Jarousse C, Niel H, Audousset-Puech M-P, Martinez J, Bataille D: Oxyntomodulin and its C-terminal octapeptide inhibit liquid meal-stimulated acid secretion. *Peptides* 7:253–256, 1986.

13. Jarousse C, Bataille D, Jeanrenaud B: A pure enteroglucagon oxyntomodulin (glucagon 37) stimulates insulin release in perfused rat pancreas. *Endocrinol* 115:102–105, 1984.
14. Gros L, Thorens B, Bataille D, Kervran A: Glucagon-like peptide-1(7-36)amide oxyntomodulin and glucagon interact with a common receptor in a somatostatin-secreting cell line. *Endocrinology* 133:631–638, 1993.
15. Ørskov C, Bersani M, Johnsen AH, Hojrup P, Holst JJ: Complete sequences of glucagon-like peptide-1 from human and pig small intestine. *J Biol Chem* 264:12,826–12,829,1989.
16. Mojsov S, Kopzynski MG, Habener JF: Both amidated and nonamidated forms of glucagon-like peptide-1 are synthesized in the rat intestine and the pancreas. *J Biol Chem* 265:8001–8008, 1990.
17. Eissele R, Göke R, Harthus H-P, Vermeer H, Arnold R, Göke B: Glucagon-like peptide-1 cells in the gastrointestinal tract of pancreas of rat pig and man. *Eur J Clin Invest* 22:283–291, 1992.
18. Holst JJ, Ørskov C, Vagn Nielsen O, Schwartz TW: Truncated glucagon-like peptide 1 an insulin-releasing hormone from the distal gut. *FEBS Lett* 211:169–174, 1987.
19. Mojsov S, Weir GC, Habener JF: Insulinotropin: glucagon-like peptide 1(7-37) co-encoded in the glucagon gene is a potent stimulator of insulin release in the perfused rat pancreas. *J Clin Invest* 79:616–619, 1987.
20. Weir GC, Mojsov S, Hendrick GK, Habener JF: Glucagon-like peptide 1 (7-37) actions on endocrine pancreas. *Diabetes* 38:338–342, 1989.
21. Fehmann H-C, Göke R, Göke B, Bächle R, Wagner B, Arnold R: Priming effect of glucagon-like peptide-1 (7-36)amide glucose-dependent insulinotropic polypeptide and cholecystokinine-8 at the isolated perfused rat pancreas. *Biochem Biophys Acta* 1091:356–363, 1991.
22. Kreymann B, GhateiMA, William G, Bloom SR: Glucagon-like peptide-1 7-36: a physiological incretin in man. *Lancet* II:1300–1304, 1987.
23. Ørskov C, Wettergren A, Holst JJ: Biological effects and metabolic rates of glucagon-like peptide-1 7-36 amide and glucagonlike peptide-1 7-37 in healthy subjects are indistinguishable. *Diabetes* 42:658–661, 1993.
24. Drucker DJ, Philippe J, Mojsov S, Chick WL, Habener JF: Glucagon-like peptide I stimulates insulin gene expression and increases cyclic AMP levels in rat islet cell line. *Proc Natl Acad Sci USA* 84:3434–3438,1987.
25. Fehmann H-C, Habener JF: Insulinotropic hormone glucagon-like peptide-I(7-37) stimulation of proinsulin gene expression and proinsulin biosynthesis in insulinom a βTC-1 cells. *Endocrinology* 130:159–166, 1992.
26. Philippe J, Missotten M: Functional characterization of a cAMP-responsive element of the rat insulin I gene. *J Biol Chem* 265:1465–1469, 1990.
27. Schjoldager BTG, Mortensen PE, Christiansen J, Ørskov C, Holst JJ: GLP-1 (glucagon-like peptide 1) and truncated GLP-1 fragments of human proglucagon inhibit gastric acid secretion in humans. *Dig Dis Sci* 34:703–708, 1989.
28. Wettergren A, Schjoldager B, Mortensen PE, Myhre J, Christiansen J, Holst JJ: Truncated GLP-1 (proglucagon 78-107-amide) inhibits gastric and pancreaic functions in man. *Dig Dis Sci* 38:665–673, 1993.

29. Schmidtler J, Schepp W, Janczewska I, Weigert N, Fürlinger C, Schusdziarra V, et al.: GLP-1-(7-36)amide -(1-37) and -(1-36)amide: potent cAMP-dependent stimuli of rat parietal cell function. *Am J Physiol* 260:G940–G950, 1991.
30. Gutniak M, Ørskov C, Holst JJ, Ahrén B, Efendic S: Antidiabetogenic effect of glucagon-like peptide-1 (7-36)amide in normal subjects and patients with diabetes mellitus. *N Engl J Med* 326:1316–1322, 1992.
31. Valverde I, Merida E, Trapote MA, Villanueva-Penacarrillo ML: Presence and characterization of glucagon-like peptide-1(7-36)amide receptors in solubilized membranes of rat adipose tissue. *Endocrinology* 132:75–79, 1993.
32. Oben J, Morgan L, Fletcher J, Marks V: Effect of entero-pancreatic hormones gastric inhibitory polypeptide and glucagon-like polypeptide-1(7-36)amide on fatty acid synthesis in explants of rat adipose tissue. *J Endocrin* 130:267–272, 1991.
33. Richter G, Göke R, Höke B, Arnold R: Characterization of receptors for glucagon-like peptide-1 (7-36)amide on rat lung membranes. *FEBS Lett* 267:78–80, 1990.
34. Göke R, Kolligs F, Richter G, Lankat-Buttgereit B, Göke B: Solubilization of active receptors for glucagon-like peptide-1(7-36)amide from rat lung membranes. *Am J Physiol* 264:L146–L152, 1993.
35. Thorens B: Expression cloning of the pancreatic beta cell receptor for the gluco-incretin hormone glucagon-like peptide I. *Proc Natl Acad Sci USA* 89:8641–8645, 1992.
36. Uttenthal LO, Toledano A, Blazquez E: Autoradiographic localization of receptors for glucagon-like peptide-1(7-36)amide in the rat brain. *Neuropeptide* 21:143–146, 1992.
37. Shimizu I, Hirota M, Ohboshi C, Shima K: Identification and localization of glucagon-like peptide-1 and its receptor in rat brain. *Endocrinology* 121:1076–1082, 1987.
38. Aruffo A, Seed B: Molecular cloning of a CD28 cDNA by a high-efficiency COS cell expression system. *Proc Natl Acad Sci USA* 84:8573–8577, 1987.
39. Thorens B, Porret A, Bühler L, Deng S-P, Morel P, Widmann C: Cloning and functional expression of the human islet GLP-1 receptor: demonstration that exendin-4 is an agonist and exendin-(9-39) an antagonist of the receptor. *Diabetes* 42:1678–1682, 1993.
40. Eng J, Kleinman WA, Singh L, Singh G, Raufman J-P: Isolation and characterization of exendin-4 an exendin-3 analogue from heloderma suspectum venom Further evidence for an exendin receptor on dispersed acini from guinea pig pancreas. *J Biol Chem* 267:7402–7405,1992.
41. Raufman JP, Singh L, Singh G, Eng J: Truncated glucagon-like peptide-1 interacts with exendin receptors on dispersed acini from guinea pig pancreas. *J Biol Chem* 267:21,432–21,437, 1992.
42. Jelinek LJ, Lok S, Rosenberg GB, Smith RA, Grant FJ, Biggs S, et al.: Expression cloning and signaling properties of the rat glucagon receptor. *Science* 259:1614–1616, 1993.

43. Ishihara T, Nakamura S, Kaziro Y, Takahashi T, Takahashi K, Nagata S: Molecular cloning and expression of a cDNA encoding the secretin receptor. *EMBO J* 10:1635–1641, 1991.
44. Ishihara T, Shigemoto R, Mori K, Takahashi K, Nagata S: Functional expression and tissue distribution of a novel receptor for vasoactive intestinal polypeptide. *Neuron* 8:811–819, 1992.
45. Abou-Samra A-B, Jüppner H, Force T, Freeman MW, Kong X-F, Schipani E, et al.: Expression cloning of a common receptor for parathyroid hormone and parathyroid hormone-related peptide from rat osteoblast-like cells: a single receptor stimulates intracellular accumulation of both cAMP and inositol triphosphates and increases intracellular free calcium. *Proc Natl Acad Sci USA* 89:2732–2736, 1992.
46. Lin HY, Harris TL, Flannery MS, Aruffo A, Kaji EH, Gorn A, et al.: Expression cloning of an adenylate cyclase-coupled calcitonin receptor. *Science* 254:1022–1024, 1991.
47. Lin C, Lin S-C, Chang C-P, Rosenfeld MG: Pit-1-dependent expression of the receptor for growth hormone releasing factor mediates pituitary cell growth. *Nature* 360:765–768, 1992.
48. Göke R, Trautmann ME, Haus E, Richter G, Fehmann H-C, Arnold R, et al.: Signal transmission after GLP-1(7-36)amide binding in RINm5F cells. *Am J Physiol* 257:G397–G401, 1989.
48a. Widmann C, Bürki E, Dolci W, Thorens B: Signal transduction by the cloned glucagon-like peptide-1 receptor: comparison with signaling by the endogenous receptors of B-cell lines. *Mol Pharmacol,* in press, 1994.
49. Wheeler MB, Lu M, Dillon JS, Leng XH, Chen C, Boyd III AE: Functional expression of the rat glucagon-like peptide-1 receptor evidence for coupling to both adenylyl cyclase and phospholipase C. *Endocrinology* 133:57–62, 1993.
50. Valverde I, Vandermeers A, Anjaneyulu R, Malaisse WJ: Calmodulin activation of adenylate cyclase in pancreatic islets. *Science* 206:225–227, 1979.
51. Pipeleers DG, Schuit FC, In't Veld PA, Maes E, Hooghe-Peters EL, Van De Winkel M, et al.: Interplay of nutrients and hormones in the regulation of insulin release. *Endocrinology* 117:824–833, 1985.
52. Schuit FC, Pipeleers DG: Regulation of 3'5'-monophosphate levels in the pancreatic B-cell. *Endocrinology* 117:834–840, 1985.
53. Holz IV GG, Kühtreiber WM, Habener JF: Pancreatic beta-cells are rendered glucose-competent by the insulinotropic hormone glucagon-like peptide-1 (7-37). *Nature* 361:362–365, 1993.
54. Wang JL, Corbett JA, Marshall CA, McDaniel ML: Glucose-induced insulin secretion from purified beta-cells A role for modulation of Ca^{2+} influx by cAMP- and protein kinase C-dependent signal transduction pathways. *J Biol Chem* 268:7785–7791, 1993.
55. Bonner-Weir S, Orci L: New perpective on the microvasculature of the islets of Langerhans in the rat. *Diabetes* 31:883–889, 1982.
56. Asfari M, Janjic D, Meda P, Li G, Halban PA, Wollheim CB: Establishment of 2-mercaptoethanol-dependent differentiated insulin-secretin cell lines. *Endocrinology* 130:167–178, 1992.

57. Ørskov C, Jeppesen J, Madsbad S, Holst JJ: Proglucagon products in plasma of noninsulin-dependent diabetics and nondiabetic controls in the fasting state and after oral glucose and intravenous arginine. *J Clin Invest* 87:415–423, 1991.
58. Alam MJ, Kerr JI, Cormican K, Buchanan KD: Gastric inhibitory polypeptide (GIP) response in diabetes using a highly specific antiserum. *Diab Med* 9:542–545, 1992.
59. Henquin JC, Debuyser A, Drews G, Plant TD: Regulation of K+ permeability and membrane potential in insulin-secreting cells. In *Nutrient Regulation of Insulin Secretion.* FlattPR, ed. Portland Press, London, pp. 173–191, 1992.
60. Ashcroft FM, Williams B, Smith PA, Fewtrell CMS: Ion channels involved in the regulation of nutrient-stimulated insulin secretion. In *Nutrient Regulation of Insulin Secretion.* Flatt PR, ed. Portland Press, London, pp. 193–212, 1992.
61. Hellman B, Gylfe E, Grapengiesser E, Lund P-E, Marcström A: Cytoplasmic calcium and insulin secretion. In *Nutrient Regulation of Insulin Secretion.* Flatt PR, ed. Portland Press, London, pp. 213–246, 1992.
62. de Weille JR, Schmid-Antomarchi H, Fosset M, Lazdunski M: Regulation of ATP-sensitive K+ channels in insulinoma cells: activation by somatostatin and protein kinase C and the role of cAMP. *Proc Natl Acad Sci USA* 86:2971–2975, 1989.
63. Prentki M, Glennon MC, Geschwing J-F, Matschinski FM, Corkey BE: Cyclic AMP raises cytosolic Ca^{2+} and promotes Ca^{2+} influx in a clonal pancreatic b-cell line (HIT T-15). *FEBS Lett* 220:103–107, 1987.
64. Rajan AS, Hill RS, Boyd AE III: Effect of rise in cAMP levels on Ca^{2+} influx through voltage-dependent Ca^{2+} channels in HIT cells Seond-messenger synarchy in b-cells. *Diabetes* 38:874–880, 1989.
65. Lu M M, Wheeler B, Leng X-H, Boyd AE III: The role of the free cytosolic calcium level in b-cell signal transduction by gastric inhibitory polypeptide and glucagon-like peptide I(7-37). *Endocrinology* 132:94–100, 1993.
66. Smith PA, Fewtrell CMS, Ashcroft FM: Cyclic AMP potentiates L-type Ca-channel activity in murine pancreatic β cells. *Diabetologia* 33:A104, 1990.
67. Catterall WA, Epstein PN: Ion channels. *Diabetologia* 35 (suppl. 2):S23–S33, 1992.
68. Tamagawa T, Niki H, Niki A: Insulin release independentof a rise in cytosolic free Ca^{2+} by forskolin and phorbol ester. *FEBS l* 183:430–432, 1985.
69. Vallar L,Biden TJ , Wollheim CB: Guanine nucleotide induce Ca^{2+}-independent insulin secretion from permeabilized RINm5F cells. *J Biol Chem* 262:5049–5056, 1987.
70. Perley MJ, Kipnis DM: Plasma insulin responses to oral and intravenous glucose: studies in normal and diabetic subjects. *J Clin Invest* 46:1954–1962, 1967.
71. Creutzfeld W, Ebert W, Nauck M, Stöckmann F: Disturbances of the entero-insular axis. *Scand J Gastroenterol*(suppl.)83:111–119, 1983.
72. Nauck M, Stöckmann F, Ebert R, Creutzfeld W: Reduced incretin effect in type 2 (non-insulin-dependent) diabetes. *Diabetologia* 29:46–52, 1986.

73. Decker T, Lauridsen UB, Madsen SN, Mogesen P: Insulin response to glucose tolbutamide secretin and isoprenaline in maturity-onset diabetes mellitus. *Dan Med Bull* 19:222–226, 1972.
74. Cerasi E, Luft R, Efendic S: Decreased sensitivity of the pancreatic β cells to glucose in prediabetic and diabetic subjects *Diabetes* 21:224–234, 1971.
75. Robertson RP, Porte D Jr: The glucose receptor: a defective mechanism in diabetes mellitus distinct from the beta adrenergic receptor *J Clin Invest* 52:870–876, 1973.
76. Aronoff SL, Bennett PH, Rushforth NB, Miller M, Unger RH: Normal glucagon response to arginine infusion in "prediabetic" Pima Indians. *J Clin End Metab* 43:279–286, 1976.
77. Suzuki S, Kawai K, Ohashi S, Mukai H, Murayama Y, Yamashita K: Reduced insulinotropic effects of glucagonlike peptide I-(7-36)-amide and gastric inhibitory polypeptide in isolated perfused diabetic rat pancreas. *Diabetes* 39:1320–1325, 1990.
78. Nathan DM Schreiber E, Fogel H, Mojsov S, Habener JF: Insulinotropic action of glucagonlike peptide-1-(7-37) in diabetic and nondiabetic subjects. *Diabetes Care* 15:270–276, 1992.
79. Nauck MA, Heimesaat MM, Ørskov C, Holst JJ, Ebert R, Creutzfeld W: Preserved incretin activity of glucagon-like peptide 1 (7-36)amide but not of synthetic human gastric inhibitory polypeptide in patients with type-2 diabetes mellitus. *J Clin Invest* 91:301–307, 1993.
80. Kahn CR, Shechter Y: Insulin oral hypoglycemic agents and the pharmacology of the endocrine pancreas. In *The Pharmacological Basis of Therapeutics.* Gilman AG, Rall TW, Nies AS, Taylor P, ed. Pergamon, New York, pp. 1463–1494, 1990.
81. Waeber G. and Thorens B.: Glucagon-like peptide-1 and the control of insulin secretion in the normal state and in NIDDM. *Diabetes* 42:1219–1225, 1993.

Chapter 16

Islet Amyloid Polypeptide (IAPP) and Insulin Secretion

Peter C. Butler, Norman L. Eberhardt, and Timothy D. O'Brien

Introduction

Although it has been known for almost a century that there are marked abnormalities in the morphology of islets in patients with non-insulin-dependent diabetes mellitus (i.e., islet amyloid and loss of β-cell volume), interest in the cause of these abnormalities and their potential mechanistic significance in the pathogenesis of NIDDM has been subject to renewed interest recently. This interest has transpired from an increasing emphasis of the role of impaired insulin secretion vs insulin resistance in the pathogenesis of NIDDM, and the recent identification of a constitutive peptide present in islet amyloid, islet amyloid polypeptide (IAPP). In this chapter, we briefly review the epidemiology and the islet morphology in NIDDM before focusing on the molecular properties of amyloid in general and IAPP in particular. Finally, we focus on potential mechanisms of islet amyloidosis and propose a hypothetical model that invokes a central role for IAPP induced amyloidosis in pathogenesis in NIDDM.

From: *Molecular Biology of Diabetes, Part I*
Edited by: B. Draznin and D. LeRoith

Pathogenesis of NIDDM: Insulin Secretion or Action?

It is clear that both genetic and environmental factors contribute to the pathogenesis of NIDDM, which is characterized by both insulin resistance *(1)* and a progressive defect in insulin secretion *(2)*. The cause of insulin resistance is most likely multifactorial. Each of the recognized risk factors for development of NIDDM (obesity *[3]*, multiparity *[4]*, and corticosteroid *[5]*, or growth hormone excess *[6]*) cause insulin resistance. It is therefore possible that insulin resistance represents the common pathway through which these risk factors induce expression of NIDDM in subjects genetically predisposed. However, unlike insulin-dependent diabetes mellitus (IDDM), in which an autoimmune β-cell destructive process is well recognized *(7)*, no clearcut pancreatic cause for NIDDM has been found, although the coexistence of islet amyloid and partial β-cell loss has long been described *(8)*. Furthermore, unlike IDDM in which insulin secretion is negligible, plasma insulin concentrations in patients with NIDDM have been reported to be comparable or even greater than those present in nondiabetic subjects *(9)*.

However, it has been known since the classical studies of Yalow and Berson that the insulin response to glucose is impaired in NIDDM *(10)*, a defect that is even more apparent when the plasma glucose concentration is matched in diabetic and nondiabetic subjects *(11)*. In fact, a progressive defect in insulin secretion is characteristic of the development of NIDDM (Fig. 1). It has been argued that since insulin resistance has been identified prior to impaired insulin secretion in patients at risk of development of NIDDM, the former must be the primary and therefore presumably the genetic defect *(12)*. However, these studies have not allowed for the fact that more sophisticated techniques were employed to assess insulin action than insulin secretion, so that early defects in insulin secretion may not have been detected. If insulin resistance was truly the primary determinant of NIDDM, it would be anticipated that all subjects with prolonged insulin resistance would develop NIDDM. In fact, the majority of patients with longstanding insulin resistance do not develop NIDDM. Thus, ~20% of patients with massive obesity *(13)*, acromegaly *(14)* or Cushing's syndrome *(15)* (all characterized by insulin resistance) develop NIDDM, whereas notably ~80% of these patients compensate adequately with islet hyperplasia and increased insulin secre-

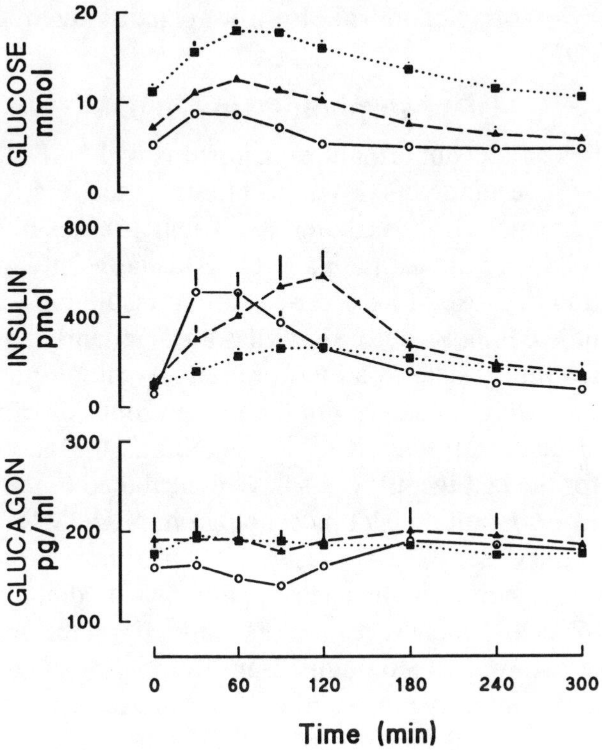

Fig. 1. Glucose, insulin, and glucagon concentrations before and after meal ingestion in nondiabetic (○), glucose-intolerant (▲), and patients with non-insulin-dependent diabetes mellitus (■). Note the progressive decrease in rate and magnitude of insulin response to meal ingestion, and the associated failure of suppression of glucagon. Reprinted with permission from ref. *11a*.

tion. Furthermore, there is considerable overlap in insulin sensitivity between patients with NIDDM and nondiabetic subjects, implying that factors other than insulin sensitivity determine predisposition to NIDDM. It would therefore appear that, although insulin resistance is undoubtedly important in NIDDM, an underlying defect in insulin secretion is necessary for development of the disease.

Taken together, these observations have recently focused attention on the role of impaired insulin secretion in the pathogenesis of NIDDM. In turn, the latter has resulted in a renewed interest in abnormalities of islet morphology long recognized in patients with NIDDM.

Islet Morphology in NIDDM

Studies of islet abnormalities in humans with NIDDM are confounded by several factors. First, islet tissue is scattered throughout the exocrine pancreas and is therefore difficult to assess morphologically. Second, in humans the pancreas is usually only available at autopsy; and because of autolysis, is often unsuitable for morphological studies. Finally, autopsy studies are frequently hampered by inadequate clinical data to allow for clinical–pathological correlation. These factors together with the major emphasis of the role of insulin resistance vs impaired insulin secretion in the pathogenesis of NIDDM for the last twenty years have contributed to the slow evolution of information on islet morphology in NIDDM.

Opie first described the presence of "hyalinosis" (nonspecific extracellular material) in the islets of patients with diabetes mellitus in 1901 *(16)*. Subsequent investigators reported that this material was amyloid in nature and, although absent from islets of patients with IDDM, was commonly present in islets from patients with NIDDM *(17)*. Similar amyloid deposits are present in the islets of other mammals affected with NIDDM (e.g., monkeys *[18]*, cats *[19]*), and also in insulinoma tissue *(20)*. In patients with NIDDM, up to 80% of the β-cell volume may be destroyed and yet the mean islet area remains comparable to that in nondiabetic patients *(21)*. This observation suggests that the area of the islet occupied by amyloid corresponds to the area formerly occupied by β-cells. The concept that islet amyloid replaces the area occupied by destroyed β-cells is supported by the only available prospective study that reports the progression of islet morphological abnormalities during the pathogenesis of NIDDM in monkeys *(22)*. Howard, in this remarkable 18-yr prospective study, performed sequential pancreatic biopsies and intravenous glucose tolerance tests in monkeys (Macaca Nigra) as they developed NIDDM *(22)*. The mean area of islet occupied by amyloid progressed from 1% in the nondiabetic state to 31% with development of glucose intolerance and 63% with establishment of NIDDM; the area occupied by β-cells declined concurrently. These findings were supported by a more recent cross-sectional study demonstrating an inverse relationship between the volume of islet amyloid and β-cell volume with a progressive decline in β-cell volume in obese monkeys *(23)*. In humans with NIDDM, the abundance of amyloid in islets shows regional variation in the pancreas that mirrors the regional variation of the abundance of β-cells, i.e., most frequent in the tail and least frequent in the polypeptide rich lobule of the head *(24)*. However, even within a particular region, the extent of amyloid is highly variable from islet to islet. The reported prevalence of islet amyloid in humans with NIDDM varies from 40–100% *(25,26)*. Small amounts of islet amyloid are reported in a proportion of nondiabetic patients with a prevalence that increases with age *(27)*. Thus, although studies to date indicate that islet amyloid is associated with the development of NIDDM, the question posed in 1952 by Warren and LeCompte, "Is hyalinization of the islands the result of, or the cause of diabetes?" remains to be answered *(28)*. Fortunately, since 1952 the advent of electron microscopy, immunohistochemistry molecular biology, and, most recently, Fourier Transform Infrared Spectroscopy (FTIR) have provided important new insights into the nature of amyloid.

Amyloid

Amyloid was originally defined as an insoluble protein aggregate with the following three criteria:

1. Birefringent staining with Congo red;
2. An unbranched fibrillar morphology composed of rigid nonbranching fibrils of 75–100 A in diameter *(29)*, as determined by electron microscopy; and
3. A specific X-ray diffraction pattern *(30)*.

Lansbury recently reviewed these criteria and pointed out that considerable uncertainty remains as to the molecular basis of amyloid *(31)*. However, generally it is assumed that these fibrils are proteins consisting of multiple repeated units of a single constitutive peptide, in a β-pleated sheet crosslinked configuration *(30)*. Employing FTIR IAPP fibrils have been shown to have a cross β-fibril structure *(31)*.

Recently the constitutive peptide of most amyloids have been determined. Amyloidogenic potential may be anticipated from the amino acid sequence when secondary structural predictions are performed *(32)*. The latter calculations may be confirmed by demonstrating fibril formation in vitro in a solution of the free peptide. The latter experiments indicate that fibril formation is concentration dependent, i.e., occurs after a critical concentration is reached *(33)*. In vitro studies have also shown that fibril formation is enhanced by seeding (i.e., by the presence of a nidus of amyloid) *(34)*.

In some of the hereditary amyloidosis, a genetic mutation has been identified that confers the constitutive peptide with amyloidogenic properties *(35)* through a single amino acid substitution. In other amyloids, the normal peptide is amyloidogenic; for example, immunoglobulin light chains in myeloma *(36)*, and therefore amyloidosis in these diseases presumably reflects aggregation of a normal protein into amyloid because of an abnormality in the processing, trafficking, or local environment of the protein. Thus, if the amyloidogenic properties of the constitutive peptide are not caused by changes in the primary structure (i.e., mutations), then the possibility that amyloidosis reflects:

1. A local high concentration of the peptide;
2. Deficiency of protective elements that generally prevent amyloidosis;
3. Seeding of amyloidogenesis protein on nidi of amyloid; and
4. An abnormal local environment (e.g., pH) warrant investigation.

The recent isolation and identification of the constitutive peptide present in islet amyloid has resulted in new opportunities to investigate both the cause and significance of this abnormality.

IAPP: Identification and Location

As long ago as 1928, Opie predicted that source of islet amyloid was secreted locally in the islet *(37)*. However, identification of the precursor molecule of islet amyloid was not accomplished until 1989 following the purification and sequencing of amyloid proteins derived from cats and humans *(38,39)*. The resulting peptide, IAPP, was found to have a previously undescribed amino acid sequence of 37 amino acids and a theoretical molecular mass of 3,850 daltons *(38)*. IAPP derived from human insulinoma tissue *(38)* is identical to that present in islet amyloid from patients with NIDDM (40) (and IAPP in healthy humans from cDNA predictions) *(41,42)*. Immunohistochemical studies in several species (human, cat, dog, celebese macaque, mouse, rat, guinea pig, hamster, and degu) show that IAPP immunoreactivity is almost exclusively located in the pancreatic β-cells *(17,38,43,44)*. Furthermore, *in situ* hybridization studies in the rat confirm that IAPP mRNA is predominantly located in β-cells *(45)*. Ultrastructurally, IAPP immunoreactivity (in humans and cats) is predominantly in β-cell secretory granules *(43,44,46)*. The colocalization of IAPP and insulin in β-cell secretory granules predicted the subsequent observation that these peptides are cosecreted following appropriate stimuli *(47–49)*. It is of note that regulation of synthesis of insulin and IAPP is also closely linked *(50)*.

IAPP: Amyloidogenic Properties

IAPP structure shows close sequence homology between all species in both the amino-terminal (residues 1–19) and carboxy-terminal (residues 30–37) regions *(51,52)*. Less homology is present in the portion of the molecule spanning residues 20–29, especially between rodents and other mammalian species (Fig. 2). Secondary structural predictions of this region of the human IAPP molecule indicate a propensity to form amyloid fibrils *(51)*. These predictions have been confirmed in vitro with synthetic peptides corresponding to the amino acid sequence of human and cat IAPP in the 20–29 region that, under conditions of high concentration, form amyloid fibrils *(52)* with cross β-sheet structure *(31)*. In contrast, under similar circumstances the corresponding synthetic peptides in the rat, guinea pig, and mouse do not form amyloid fibrils *(52)*. The 25–28 region of human, monkey, and cat IAPP is identical in structure (i.e., Ala-Ile-Leu-Ser [AILS]) and appears to be the most important amyloidogenic sequence (Fig. 2). Thus, substitutions of single amino acids in the 25–28 region of synthetic human IAPP 20–29 significantly reduces or eliminates the amyloidogenicity of these peptides *(52)*. In conclusion, IAPP in healthy humans (and cats) has the necessary properties to form cross β-sheets and hence amyloid. This tendency depends upon a specific amino acid sequence, AILS, in the midportion of the molecule. The sequence of IAPP in humans (and cats) with or without NIDDM is identical. Thus, although the potential for IAPP to form amyloid is clear, the questions remain, Why (and where) does IAPP precipitate in amyloid fibrils in patients with

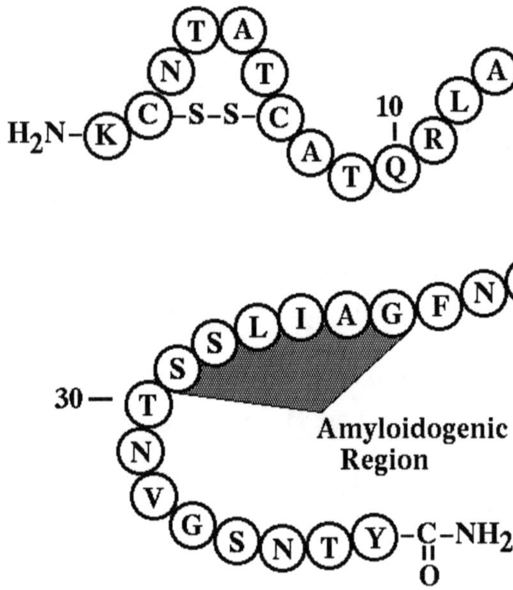

Fig. 2. Amino acid sequence of human IAPP showing the amyloidogenic central region.

NIDDM, and Is islet amyloid of mechanistic significance in the pathogenesis of NIDDM or merely a secondary marker of the underlying disease process?

Where and Why Does IAPP Amyloid Form in NIDDM?

Several lines of evidence suggest that islet amyloid forms intracellularly. First, we *(52)* and others *(54)* have shown that IAPP-derived amyloid forms intracellularly in human insulinoma tissue. Intracellular formation of IAPP-derived amyloid has also been demonstrated in β-cells of cats with early NIDDM (Fig. 3) *(55)*; although owing to the unavailability of tissue appropriate for EM studies, this has not been shown in humans to date. It is noteworthy that several other related endocrine amyloid deposits (e.g., growth hormone in growth hormone secreting pituitary tumors) have also recently been shown to be formed intracellularly *(56)*. Since human IAPP forms amyloid fibrils in vitro concentrations of approx 10^{-9} molar and the concentration of IAPP in the endoplasm reticulum, Golgi, and secre-

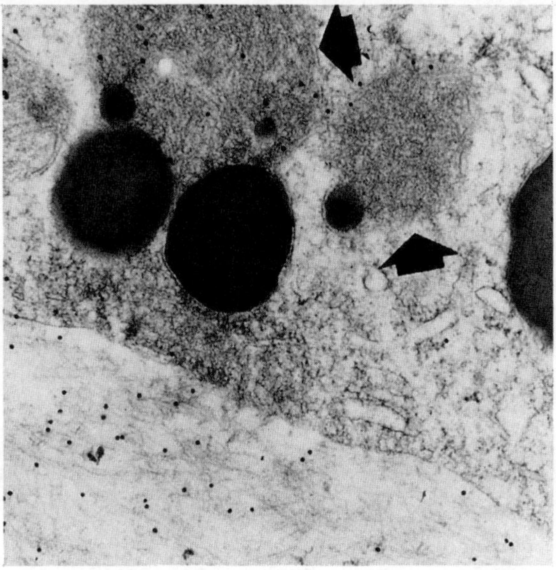

Fig. 3. EM intra- (arrows) and extracellular amyloid labels with IAPP immunogold in cat with early NIDDM. Reprinted with permission from ref. *43*.

tory granules of health human β-cells must far exceed this concentration, it is reasonable to pose the question, Why does human IAPP *not* form amyloid fibrils in the endoplasm reticulum, Golgi, and secretory granules of all β-cells? It would thus appear that a mechanism must be present in normal β-cells that prevents the aggregation of IAPP in fibrils.

Recent interest has focused on the role of heat shock (chaperon) proteins in the folding and trafficking of proteins within the cell as well as their role in preventing inappropriate aggregation of normal proteins *(57)*. Knowledge about chaperon proteins is developing rapidly in a recently emerged field *(58,59)*. Studies to date suggest that there exists a series of distinct chaperons that transiently associate with many cellular proteins at distinct points in the protein trafficking pathway in eucaryotic cells. These chaperon proteins appear to be essential in the prevention of abnormal aggregates of normally expressed proteins intracellularly. The latter is particularly likely if the protein contains a strong hydrophobic sequence such as that

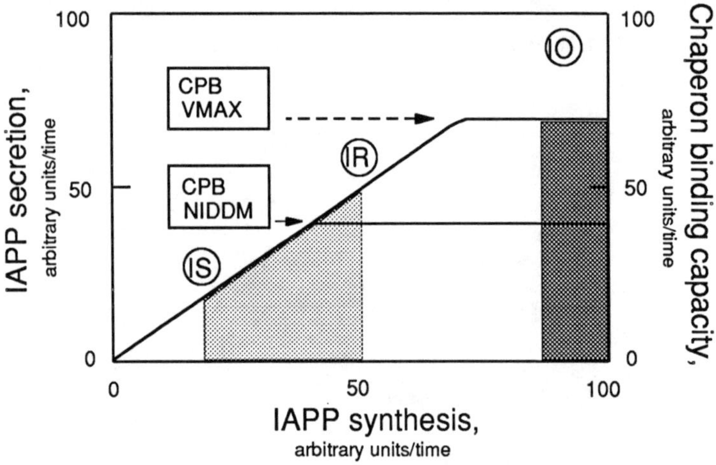

Fig. 4. Theoretical model to account for intracellular IAPP-amyloidosis in insulinoma (IO) and NIDDM. The figure shows the theoretical relationship between the rate of IAPP synthesis and secretion, in arbitrary units, over 24 h by a single β-cell. In an insulin resistant (IR) individual the rate of synthesis and secretion in a representative β-cell exceed those of a β-cell of an insulin sensitive (IS) individual. If the successful trafficking of IAPP requires chaperon proteins, the maximal available chaperon binding capacity (CPBVmax) may be exceeded in β-cells of an insulinoma (resulting in free IAPP and IAPP-amyloidosis). This model proposes that one or several genetic defects that result in a decrease in chaperon binding (CPB-NIDDM) may, in the setting of insulin resistance, result in intracellular IAPP-amyloid and β-cell death.

present in human IAPP. One potential mechanism for the formation of intracellular IAPP amyloid may therefore be that there is either inadequate availability of one or more chaperon proteins within the protein trafficking pathway for IAPP. Thus, under conditions of supraphysiological rates of IAPP synthesis (as may occur in insulinoma) chaperon protein availability could be overcome, and the resulting free IAPP form intracellular fibrils. In patients with NIDDM, it is plausible that there is a genetic defect that results in a decreased availability of one or more chaperon proteins, and that under conditions of chronic insulin resistance (i.e., recognized risk factors for NIDDM) accumulation of free IAPP within β-cells that, in turn, results in intracellular islet amyloid. This hypothetical model to account for the formation of islet amyloid in NIDDM is illustrated in Fig. 4.

Other potential causes of IAPP-amyloid exist. Thus, the pH or other environmental properties of the secretory vesicles, endoplasmic reticulum, and so on, may be abnormal as a consequence of metabolic perturbations in the β-cell that are primary or secondary to diabetes mellitus. Such environmental changes potentially could favor IAPP aggregation, resulting in a nidus of amyloid that could, in turn, promote additional amyloidogenesis *(34)*. Whatever the mechanism of intracellular IAPP amyloidogensis, it is plausible that intracellular amyloid is cytotoxic since large aggregations of intracellular hydrophobic protein would most likely be deleterious to normal cellular function (particularly properties of membranes). Cytotoxicity of intracellular amyloid may provide the link between loss of β-cell volume and accumulation of an equivalent volume of islet amyloid.

As is clear from the above discussion, it is not clear at present whether IAPP-derived amyloid is primary or secondary to the underlying defects in β-cell function in NIDDM. However, there is sufficient evidence available to create a compelling argument that IAPP-amyloid at least contributes to β-cell destruction, and that further studies are needed to address these questions.

Role of IAPP in Insulin Secretion and Insulin Action

Since IAPP is secreted with insulin following β-cell stimulation, it has been suggested that IAPP may function as a hormone. Earlier observations employing $10^{-9}M$ IAPP extracted from human pancreas tissue demonstrated that IAPP causes impaired insulin action in skeletal muscle *(60)*. However, numerous studies have now been reported showing that the concentration of IAPP circulating in plasma under physiological conditions is in the range of 1–20 pmol/L *(47,61,62,63)* (Fig. 5). No studies have yet shown that IAPP perturbs insulin action within this concentration range in humans *(64)* or other mammals (65). Furthermore, recent studies with transgenic mice with high concentrations of circulating IAPP have not demonstrated any evidence of insulin resistance or diabetes *(66)*. Since IAPP has approx 50% sequence homology with calcitonin gene related peptide (CGRP), high concentrations of IAPP most likely interact with the CGRP receptor *(67)*. Some *(68)* but not all *(69)* evidence to date suggests that the effects of supraphysiological con-

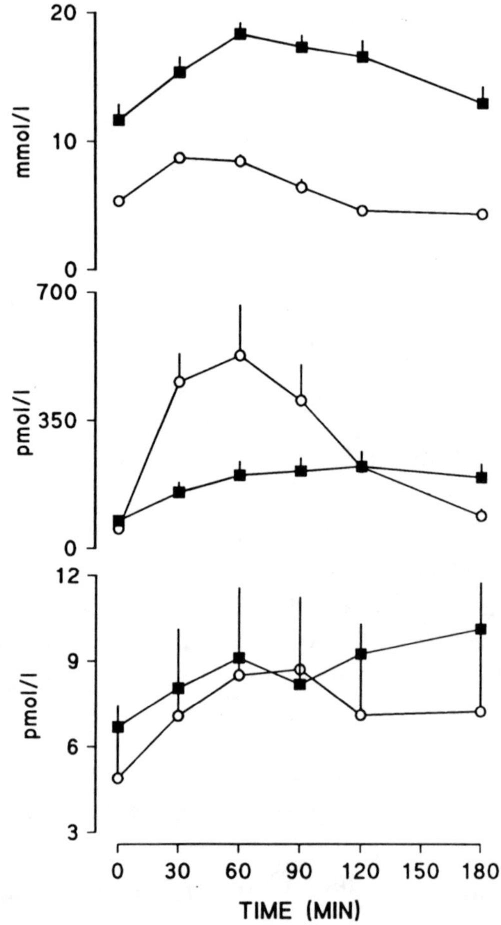

Fig. 5. Glucose (top panel), insulin (middle panel), and IAPP (bottom panel) concentrations in patients with NIDDM vs age, weight, sex matched following nondiabetic subjects following an overnight fast (0 min) and following a mixed meal. Reprinted with permission from ref. *47*.

centrations of IAPP are mediated through the CGRP receptor (possibly reflecting receptor spillover).

The potential effects of IAPP on insulin secretion are also controversial. Several *(70,71,72)*, but not all *(72,73)*, studies published to date have suggested that IAPP inhibits insulin secretion. However, since β-cells may be exposed to very high local concentrations of IAPP (i.e., a paracrine effect), a search for potential effects of IAPP on insulin secretion should not be limited to the concentration present in the circulation.

Conclusions

Islet IAPP amyloid is clearly associated with NIDDM. However, it remains uncertain what, if any, mechanistic significance IAPP-amyloid has in the pathogenesis of β-cell loss and NIDDM. Recent studies suggest IAPP-amyloid forms intracellularly where it may be cytotoxic. If the latter is true, it is important to establish why IAPP forms intracellular amyloid deposits in NIDDM but not in health. A better understanding of the molecular mechanism of IAPP-amyloidosis may then provide therapeutic options for the prevention and treatment of NIDDM.

Acknowledgment

Peter C. Butler is supported by PHS grants DK-44341, RR-00585, Pfizer Pharmaceutical, and Mayo Foundation.

References

1. DeFronzo R, Deibart D. Hendler R, Felig P, Soman V: Insulin sensitivity and insulin binding to monocytes in maturity-onset diabetes. *J Clin Invest* 63:939–946, 1979.
2. Robertson RP, Porte D: The glucose receptor. A defective mechanism in diabetes mellitus distinct from the beta adrenergic receptor. *J Clin Invest* 52:870–976, 1973.
3. Saad MF, Knowler WC, Pettitt DJ, Nelson RG, Mott DM, Bennett PH: The natural history of impaired glucose tolerance in the Pina Indians. *N Engl J Med* 319:1500–1506, 1988.
4. Fitzgerald MG, Malins JM, O'Sullivan DJ, Wall M: Effect of sex and parity on the incidence of diabetes mellitus. *Quart J Med* 30:57–70, 1961.
5. Conn J, Fajans S: Symposium on diabetes: Influence of adrenal cortisol steroids on carbohydrate metabolism in man. *Metabolism* 5:114–120, 1956.
6. Butler PC, Kryshak EJ, Rizza RA: Mechanism of growth hormone-induced postprandial carbohydrate intolerance in humans. *Am J Physiol* 260 (*Endocrinol Metab* 23):E513–E520, 1991.
7. Eisenbarth GS: Type 1 diabetes mellitus: A chronic autoimmune disease. *N Engl J Med* 314:1360–1368, 1986.
8. Ehrlich JC, Ratner JM: Amyloidosis of the islets of Langerhans: a restudy of islet hyalin in diabetic and nondiabetic individuals. *Am J Pathol* 38:49–59, 1961.
9. Niskanen LK, Uusitupa MI, Sarlund H, Siitonen O, Pyorala K: Five-year follow-up study on plasma insulin levels in newly diagnosed NIDDM patients and nondiabetic subjects. *Diabetes Care* 13:41–48, 1990.

10. Yalow RS, Berson SA: Plasma insulin concentrations in nondiabetic and early diabetic subjects. Determination by a new sensitive immuno-assay technic. *Diabetes* 9:254–260, 1960.
11. Perley M, Kipnis DM: Plasma insulin responses to glucose and tolbutamide of normal weight and obese diabetic and nondiabetic subjects. *Diabetes* 15:867–874, 1966.
11a. Butler PC, Rizza RA: Contribution to postprandial hyperglucemia and effect on initial glucose clearance of hepatic glucose cycling in glucose-intolerant or NIDDM patients. *Diabetes* 40:1:73–81.
12. Eriksson J, Franssila-Kallunki A, Ekstrand A, Saloranta C, Widen E, Schalin C, Groop L: Early metabolic defects in persons at increased risk for Non-insulin-dependent diabetic mellitus. *N Engl J Med* 321:337–343, 1989.
13. Felber JP, Golay A, Jéquier E, Curchod B, Temler E, DeFronzo RA, et al.: The metabolic consequences of long-term human obesity. *Int J Obes* 12:377–389, 1988.
14. Wright AD, Hill DM, Lowry C, Fraser TR: Mortality in acromegaly. *Q J Med* 39:1–13, 1970.
15. Wajchenberg BL, Leme CE, Lerario AC, Toledo T, Souza IT, Rodbard HW, Rodbard D: Insulin resistance in Cushing's syndrome. Evaluation by studies of insulin binding to erythrocytes. *Diabetes* 33:455–459, 1984.
16. Opie EL: On the relation of chronic interstitial pancreatitis to the islands of Langerhans and to diabetes mellitus. *J Exp Med* 5:397, 1901.
17. Westermark P, Wilander E, Westermark GT, Johnson KH: Islet amyloid polypeptide-like immunoreactivity in the islet B cells of type 2 (non-insulin-dependent) diabetic and non-diabetic individuals. *Diabetologia* 30: 887, 1987.
18. Howard CF Jr: Insular amyloidosis and diabetes in Macaca nigra. *Diabetes* 27:357, 1978.
19. Johnson KH, Stevens JB: Light and electron microscopic studies of islet amyloid in diabetic cats. *Diabetes* 22:81, 1973.
20. O'Brien TD, Hayden DW, O'Leary TP, Caywood DD, Johnson KH: Canine pancreatic endocrine tumors: immunohistochemical analysis of the hormone content and amyloid. *Vet Pathol* 24:308–314, 1987.
21. Westermark P, Wilander E: The influence of amyloid deposits on the islet volume in maturity onset diabetes mellitus. *Diabetologia* 15:417, 1978.
22. Howard CF: Longitudinal studies on the development of diabetes in individual Macaca nigra. *Diabetologia* 29:301–306, 1986.
23. de Koning EJP, Bodkin NL, Hansen BC, Clark A: Diabetes mellitus in Macaca mulatta monkeys is characterised by islet amyloidosis and reduction in beta-cell population. *Diabetologia* 36:378–384, 1993.
24. Clark A, Holman RR, Matthews DR, Holkaday TDR, Turner RC: Non-uniform distribution of islet amyloid in the pancreas of maturity onset diabetic patients. Diabetologia 27:527,528, 1984.
25. Melato M, Antonutto G, Ferronato E: Amyloidosis of the islets of Langerhans in relation to diabetes mellitus and aging. *Beitr Pathol* 160:73–81, 1977.

26. Narita R, Toshimori H, Nakazato M, Kuribayashi T, Toshimori T, Kawabata K, et al.: Islet amyloid polypeptide (IAPP) and pancreatic islet amyloid deposition in diabetic and non-diabetic patients. *Diabetes Res Clin Pract* 15:3–14, 1992.
27. Maloy AL, Longnecker DS, Greenberg ER: The relation of islet amyloid to the clinical type of diabetes. *Hum Pathol* 12:917–922, 1981.
28. Warren S, LeCompte PM: The pancreas in diabetes mellitus. In *The Pathology of Diabetes Mellitus,* Lea and Febiger, Philadelphia, 1952, pp. 31–75.
29. Cohen AS, Calkins E: Electron microscopic observations on a fibrous component in amyloid of diverse origins. *Nature* 183:1202,1203, 1959.
30. Eanes ED, Glenner GG: X-ray diffraction studies of amyloid filaments. *J Histochem Cytochem* 16:673–677, 1986.
31. Lansbury PT: In pursuit of the molecular structure of amyloid plaque: new technology provides unexpected and critical information. *Biochemistry* 31:6865–6870, 1992.
32. Glenner GG, Eanes ED, Wiley CA: Amyloid fibrils formed from a segment of the pancreatic islet amyloid protein. *Biochem Biophys Res Comm* 155:608–614, 1988.
33. Betsholtz C, Christmanson L, Engström U, Rorsman F, Jordan K, O'Brien TD, et al.: Structure of cat islet amyloid polypeptide and identification of amino acid residues of potential significance for islet amyloid formation. *Diabetes* 39:118–122, 1990.
34. Jarrett JT, Lansbury PT: Seeding "one-dimensional crystallization" of amyloid: a pathogenic mechanism in Alzheimer's disease and scrapie? *Cell* 73:1055–1058, 1993.
35. Levy E, Carmen MD, Fernandez-Madrid IJ, Power MD, Lieberburg I, Van Duinen SG, Bots GT, Luyendijk W, Frangione B: Mutation of the Alzheimer's disease amyloid gene in hereditary cerebral hemorrhage, Dutch type. *Science* 248:1124–1126, 1990.
36. Drurie BGM, Perskey B, Soehnlen BJ, Grogan TM, Salmon SE: Amyloid production in human myeloma stem-cell culture, with morphological evidence of amyloid secretion by associated macrophages. *N Engl J Med* 307:1689–1692, 1982.
37. Opie L: Cytology of the pancreas. In *The Form and Function of the Cell in Health and Disease.* Cowdrey EV, ed. Hoeber, New York, pp. 239–272, 1928.
38. Westermark P, Wernstedt C, Wilander E, Hayden DW, O'Brien TD, Johnson KH: Amyloid fibrils in human insulinoma and islets of Langerhans of the diabetic cat are derived from a neuropeptide-like protein also present in normal islet cells. *Proc Natl Acad Sci USA* 84:3881, 1987.
39. Westermark P, Wernstedt C, Wilander E, Sletten K: A novel peptide in the calcitonin gene related family as an amyloid fibril protein in the endocrine pancreas. *Biochem Biophys Res Commun* 140:827, 1986.
40. Cooper GJS, Willis AC, Clark A, Turner RC, Sim RB, Reid KBM: Purification and characterization of a peptide from amyloid-rich pancreases of type 2 diabetic patients. *Proc Natl Acad Sci USA* 84:8628, 1987.

41. Nakazato M, Asai J, Miyazato M, Mitsukura S, Kangawa K, Matsuo H: Isolation and identification of islet amyloid polypeptide in normal human pancreas. *Regul Pept* 31:179, 1990.
42. Nishi M, Bell GI, Steiner DF: Islet amyloid polypeptide (amylin): no evidence of an abnormal precursor sequence in 25 type 2 (non-insulin-dependent) diabetic patients. *Diabetologia* 33:628–630, 1990.
43. Johnson KH, O'Brien TD, Hayden DW, Jordan K, Ghobrial HKG, Mahoney WC, et al.: Immunolocalization of islet amyloid polypeptide (IAPP) in pancreatic beta cells by means of peroxidase-antiperoxidase (PAP) and protein A-gold techniques. *Am J Pathol* 130:1–8, 1988.
44. Lukinius A, Wilander E, Westermark GT, Engstrom U, Westermark P: Co-localization of islet amyloid polypeptide and insulin in the B cell secretory granules of the human pancreatic islets. *Diabetologia* 32:240, 1989.
45. Leffert JD, Newgard CB, Okamoto H, Milburn JL, Luskey KL: Rat amylin: cloning and tissue specific expression in pancreatic islets. *Proc Natl Acad Sci USA* 86:3127, 1989.
46. Clark A, Edwards CA, Ostle LR, Stutton R, Rothbard JB: Localization of islet amyloid peptide in lipofuscin bodies and secretory granules of human B-cells and in islets of type 2 diabetic subjects. *Cell Tissue Res* 257:179, 1989.
47. Butler PC, Chou J, Carter WB, Wang Y-N, Bu B-H, et al.: Effects of meal ingestion on plasma amylin concentrations in NIDDM and nondiabetic humans. *Diabetes* 39:752–756, 1990.
48. Hartter E, Svoboda T, Ludvik, B, Schuller M, Lell B, Kuenburg E: Basal and stimulated plasma levels of pancreatic amylin indicate its co-secretion with insulin in humans. *Diabetologia* 34:52–54, 1991.
49. Mitsukawa T, Takemura J, Asai J, Nakazato M, Kangawa K, Matsuo H, et al.: Islet amyloid polypeptide response to glucose, insulin, and somatostatin analogue administration. *Diabetes* 39:639, 1990.
50. Bretherton-Watt D, Ghetei MH, Bloom SR, Jamal H, Ferrier GJM, Girgis SI, et al.: Altered islet amyloid polypeptide (amylin) gene expression is rat models of diabetes. *Diabetologia* 32:881, 1989.
51. Betsholz C, Svensson V, Rorsman F, Engstrom U, Westermark GT, Wilander E: Islet amyloid polypeptide (IAPP): cDNA cloning and identification of an amyloidogenic region associated with the species-specific occurrence of age-related diabetes mellitus. *Exp Cell Res* 183:484–493, 1989.
52. Westermark P, Engström U, Johnson KH, Westermark GT, Betsholtz C: Islet amyloid polypeptide: pinpointing amino acid residues linked to amyloid fibril formation. *Proc Natl Acad Sci USA* 87:5036–5040, 1990.
53. O'Brien TD, Butler AE, Johnson KH, Roche PC, Butler PC: Islet amyloid polypeptide (IAPP) in human insulinomas: evidence for intracellular amyloidogenesis. *Diabetes* 43:329–336, 1993.
54. Toshimori H, Narita R, Nakazato M, Asai J, Mitsukawa T, Kangawa K, et al.: Islet amyloid polypeptide in insulinoma and in the islet of the pancreas of non-diabetic and diabetic subjects. *Virchows Archiv A Pathol Anat* 418:411–417, 1991.

55. Yano BL, Hayden DW, Johnson KH: Feline insular amyloid: ultrastructural evidence for intracellular formation by nonendocrine cells. *Lab Invest* 45:149–156, 1981.
56. Mori H, Mori S, Saitoh Y, Moriwaki K, Iida S, Matsumoto K: Growth hormone-producing pituitary adenoma with crystal-like amyloid immunohistochemically positive for growth hormone. *Cancer* 55:96–102, 1985.
57. Rothman JE: Polypeptide chain binding proteins: catalysts of protein folding and related processes in cells. *Cell* 59:591–601, 1989.
58. Hightower LE: Heat shock, stress proteins, chaperones, and proteotoxicity. *Cell Press* 66:191–197, 1991.
59. Ellis RJ: The molecular chaperone concept. *Cell Biology* 1:1–9, 1990.
60. Leighton B, Cooper GJS: Pancreatic amylin and calcitonin gene-related peptide cause resistance to insulin in skeletal muscle in vitro. *Nature* 335:632–635, 1988.
61. Eriksson J, Nakazato M, Miyazato M, Shiomi K, Matsukura S, Groop L: Islet amyloid polypeptide plasma concentrations in individuals at increased risk of developing Type 2 (non-insulin-dependent) diabetes mellitus. *Diabetologia* 35:291–293, 1992.
62. Enoki S, Mitsukawa T, Takemura J, Nakazato M, Aburaya J, Toshimori H, et al.: Plasma islet amyloid polypeptide levels in obesity, impaired glucose tolerance and non-insulin-dependent diabetes mellitus. *Diabetes Res Clin Pract* 15:97–102, 1992.
63. Ludvik B, Clodi M, Kautzky-Willer A, Capek M, Hartter E, Pacini G, Prager R: Effect of dexamethasone on insulin sensitivity, islet amyloid polypeptide and insulin secretion in humans. *Diabetologia* 36:84–87, 1993.
64. Bretherton-Watt D, Gilbey SG, Ghatei MA, Beacham J, Bloom SR: Failure to establish islet amyloid polypeptide (amylin) as a circulating beta cell inhibiting hormone in man. *Diabetologia* 33:115–117, 1990.
65. Kassir AA, Upadhyay AK, Lim TJ, Moossa AR, Olefsky JM: Lack of effect of islet amyloid polypeptide in causing insulin resistance in conscious dogs during euglycemic clamp studies. *Diabetes* 40:998–1004, 1991.
66. Fox N, Schrementi J, Nishi M, Ohagi S, Chan SJ, Heisserman JA, et al.: Human islet amyloid polypeptide transgenic mice as a model of non-insulin-dependent diabetes mellitus (NIDDM). *FEBS* 323:40–44, 1993.
67. Galeazza MT, O'Brien TD, Johnson KH, Seybold VS: Islet amyloid polypeptide (IAPP) competes for two binding sites of CGRP. *Peptides* 12:585–591, 1991.
68. Morishita T, Yamaguchi A, Fujita T, Chiba T: Activation of adenylate cyclase by islet amyloid polypeptide with COOH-terminal amide via calcitonin gene-related peptide receptors on rat liver plasma membranes. *Diabetes* 39:875–877, 1990.
69. Kreutter D, Orena SJ, Torchia AJ, Contillo LG, Andrews GC, Stevenson RW: Amylin and CGRP induce insulin resistance via a receptor distinct from cAMP-coupled CGRP receptor. *Am J Physiol* 264:E606–E613, 1993.

70. Ohsawa H, Kanatsuka A, Yamaguchi T, Makino H, Yoshida S: Islet amyloid polypeptide inhibits glucose-stimulated insulin secretion from isolated rat pancreatic islets. *Biochem Biophys Res Commun* 160:961–967, 1989.
71. Silvestre RA, Pieró E, Dégano P, Miralles P, Marco J: Inhibitory effect of rat amylin on the insulin responses to glucose and arginine in the perfused rat pancreas. *Regul Pept* 31:23–31, 1990.
72. Wang Z-L, Bennet WM, Ghatei MA, Byfield PGH, Smith DM, Bloom SR: Influence of islet amyloid polypeptide and the 8-37 fragment of islet amyloid polypeptide on insulin release from perifused rat islets. *Diabetes* 42:330–335, 1993.
73. Nagamatsu S, Carroll RJ, Grodsky GM, Steiner DF: Lack of islet amyloid polypeptide regulation of insulin biosynthesis or secretion in normal rat islets. *Diabetes* 39:871–874, 1990.
74. Broderick CL, Brooke GS, DiMarchi RD, Gold G: Human and rat amylin have no effects on insulin secretion in isolated rat pancreatic islets. *Biochem Biophys Res Commun* 117:932–938, 1991.

Index